ECHOCARDIOGRAPHY – NEW TECHNIQUES

Edited by **Gani Bajraktari**

Echocardiography – New Techniques
Edited by Gani Bajraktari

Published by InTech
Janeza Trdine 9, 51000 Rijeka, Croatia

Publishing Process Manager Gorana Scerbe

Technical Editor Teodora Smiljanic

Cover Designer InTech Design Team

Additional hard copies can be obtained from orders@intechopen.com

Echocardiography – New Techniques, Edited by Gani Bajraktari
p. cm.
ISBN 978-953-307-762-8

For EU product safety concerns:
IN TECH d.o.o., Prolaz Marije Krucifikse Kozulić 3, 51000 Rijeka, Croatia,
info@intechopen.com or visit our website at intechopen.com.

Meet the editor

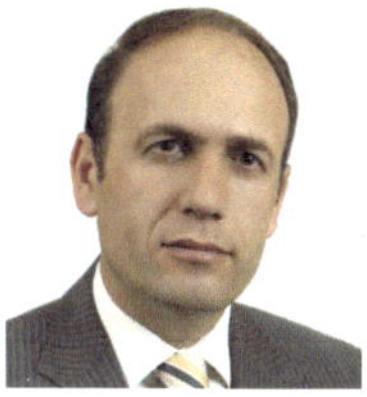

Dr. Gani Bajraktari graduated in Medicine at the University of Prishtina (Kosovo) in 1990 and completed his specialization in cardiology at the Second Clinic of Cardiology, University Clinical Center "Mother Teresa", Tirana (Albania), in 1997. He finished his postgraduate studies, defending the Master's thesis at Medical Faculty of Zagreb (Croatia) in 2000, in the field of stress-echocardiography, whereas he defended his doctoral thesis in 2002, at Medical Faculty of the University of Prishtina. He finished his PhD studies at Semelweis University in Budapest (Hungary), defending the Ph.D. thesis in 2007. In two mandates (2001-2003 and 2007-2009) he was the director of Internal Medicine Clinic, University Clinical Centre of Kosova, Prishtina. He was elected as Professor of Internal Medicine - Cardiology at Medical Faculty in 2006, whereas in 2009, he was elected as Dean of Medical Faculty, University of Prishtina.His clinical and research interests include echocardiography, diastology, diabetes and heart failure. He published 30 articles in these fields. He is the author of three books. Dr. Bajraktari is a Fellow of European Society of Cardiology and a Fellow of American College of Cardiology.

Contents

Preface

Echocardiography, as an integral part of clinical cardiology, is playing an increasingly important role in routine examinations of all cardiac patients. Echocardiography targets not only the diagnosis of cardiovascular diseases, but also clinical decision making, follow-up, and predicting cardiac events in patients. Despite the development of other competitive imaging techniques in the past few decades, echocardiography remains the gold standard for clinical examinations in cardiology.

The book *Echocardiography – New Techniques* brings worldwide contributions from highly acclaimed clinical and imaging science investigators, and representatives from academic medical centers. Each chapter is designed and written to be accessible to those with a basic knowledge of echocardiography. Additionally, the chapters are meant to be stimulating and educational to the experts and investigators in the field of echocardiography. This book is aimed primarily at cardiology fellows on their basic echocardiography rotation, fellows in general internal medicine, radiology and emergency medicine, and experts in the arena of echocardiography.

Over the last few decades, the rate of technological advancements has developed dramatically, resulting in new techniques and improved echocardiographic imaging. The authors of this book focused on presenting the most advanced techniques useful in today's research and in daily clinical practice. The advanced techniques are utilized in the detection of different cardiac pathologies in patients, in contributing to their clinical decision, as well as follow-up and outcome predictions. In addition to the advanced techniques covered, this book expounds upon several special pathologies with respect to the functions of echocardiography.

Finally, it is our hope that future decades will bring even greater advances in this field, and that this book will motivate other scientists toward future developments. We hope scientists will make use of these echo modalities for implementation in their daily practice, for the development of new future techniques, and for the better assessment of heart structure and its function. Collectively, we hope that this book will contribute to the improved treatment of patients.

I would like to thank all of the authors for their valuable contributions. I would also like to thank the staff at InTech, particularly Gorana Scerbe, who answered all of my questions and kept me on track during the entire process.

Prof.Asoc. Gani Bajraktari, MD, MSc, PhD, FESC, FACC
Service of Cardiology, Internal Medicine Clinic,
University Clinical Centre of Kosova, Prishtina
Republic of Kosovo

Part 1

Spackle Tracking Echocardiography

1

Assessment of Regional Longitudinal Stain by Using Speckle Tracking Echocardiography – A Validation Study

Vitek Nili[1], Bachner-Hinenzon Noa[1], Lempel Meytal[1], Friedman Zvi[2], Reisner Shimon[3], Beyar Rafael[1] and Adam Dan[1]
[1]*The Faculty of Biomedical Engineering, Technion-Israel Institute of Technology, Haifa,*
[2]*General Electric Healthcare,*
[3]*Department of Cardiology, Rambam Medical Center, Faculty of Medicine, Technion-Israel Institute of Technology, Haifa*
Israel

1. Introduction

Recently, there is an increasing body of evidence supporting the clinical importance of assessment of regional myocardial function as an essential tool for the evaluation of heart disease (Helm et al. 2005; Voigt et al. 2004, Liel-Cohen et al. 2010). In particular, numerous reports support the notion that diagnosis and management of coronary heart disease require the ability to adequately assess regional changes in myocardial function (Zwanenburg et al. 2005). Typical examples are the detection of ischemia or post acute myocardial infarction (AMI) during a stress test, even for nonocclusive coronary stenosis (Yip et al. 2004); Voigt and Flachskampf 2004), the differentiation of non-transmural vs. transmural infarct infarction, or of a reversible from non-reversible ischemic functional impairment.

One of the techniques currently in use for functional assessment of the cardiac muscle is Doppler based analysis of motion and deformation (Desco et al. 2002; Herbots et al. 2004; Voigt and Flachskampf 2004; Yip et al. 2003). The Doppler based techniques suffer from a number of critical limitations, the most significant one is that they are one dimensional and angle-dependent, leading to motion underestimation when the motion is not in the same orientation as the ultrasound beam at the point of measurement. Also, due to the cardiac movement during contraction, the segment being measured by the stable, but one dimensional beam, may be different at each moment. This limitation is significant since cardiac motion is very complex - at each location it consists of components that may either be independent from each other, such as heart translation, rotation and the active myocardial contraction, or that are physiologically related such as shortening along the myocardial fiber axis while thickening perpendicular to the fiber axis. These disadvantages limit the measurement to some sections of the heart, e.g. the septum and the free wall.

Ultrasound speckle tracking has been suggested for tissue strain and motion measurements (Bertrand et al., 1989; O'Donnell et al., 1991; O'Donnell et al., 1994). Recently, a different approach was suggested (Rappaport et al. 2006), also based on tracking of speckles (reflectors) in B-mode grayscale image sequences, which was reliable and efficient enough to be implemented in commercial systems. It suggested using an Acoustic Tagging method, which defines specific points that are being tracked over the time and finally the velocity in each Tracking Point (TP) is calculated (Behar et al. 2004). Acoustic Tagging is mimicking the idea used in tagged MRI, and the application of tagging for strain measurements. The implementation (AFI, GE Healthcare, Inc.) in the clinical setting allows computing motion and contraction information within the whole myocardial cross-section, directly from echocardiographic B-mode sequences. It provided in numerous clinical studies efficient diagnosis of myocardial dysfunction (De Boeck et al. 2006; Leitman et al. 2004; Reisner et al. 2004; Suffoletto et al. 2006; Yip et al. 2004; Zwanenburg et al. 2005).

The AFI tool is based on automatic initial selection (within the myocardial wall) of predominant features according to their brightness, size and persistence, and tracking them from one frame to the next. The changes in a feature position allow determining its velocity. The velocity field of these features is very noisy, thus at the center of each image section, e.g. of 50x50 pixels, a 'TP' is defined, with velocity value of the average movement of that section. The TP's are aligned within a grid along the myocardium, to finally form 4 lines of points. The velocities of these points are filtered again, to allow calculation of the longitudinal Strain Rate (SR) by the derivative of longitudinal velocity component along the line of points, and the transverse SR by the derivative of transverse velocity component perpendicular to the line of points. Strain is calculated by time-integration of the SR. The 'AFI' averages the velocity field of the 4 lines of TP's into one line of 'knots' along the longitudinal orientation of the wall, thus variations between myocardial layers cannot be detected. It also employs robust smoothing, thus the spatial resolution is relatively low.

The present study was designed to replace the exceedingly smoothing method (performed on the results of the tracking) used by the 'AFI', by a more elaborate smoothing scheme that would reveal motion information of the different myocardial layers. This would allow obtaining 2D Strain and SR tensors at multiple points along and across the myocardial wall, allowing analysis and observation of local deformations (orientations and magnitudes).

The smoothing scheme used here is based on the wavelet shrinkage method, which is efficient in noise rejection by cancelling certain components, as a result of thresholding in the wavelet domain (Donoho 1995; Donoho and Johnstone 1994; Mallat 1998; Unser 1996). The threshold must be selected so that noisy and unrealistic movements/velocities are cancelled, while changes of the Strain and SR over time, along and across the myocardial wall, could be analyzed. The wavelet shrinkage denoising algorithm used here follows a method suggested to suppress Gaussian noise (Donoho and Johnstone 1994), which selects the thresholds depending on the variance of the noise components of the signal. The efficiency of this denoising algorithm relies on the choice of the wavelet basis, the estimation of noise level, the method of threshold selection and parameters specific to the application.

2. Methods

The raw data for this study comprised of the regional velocities, estimated from the B-mode cine loops by the speckle tracking algorithm, before application of any smoothing or filtration. The raw data may be viewed as a velocity function, sampled at 4 transmural locations across ("transverse" - T) the myocardial wall, and at 50-58 locations along ("longitudinal" - L) the LV cross-section, from base to apex and back to the other base along the myocardium (TP's), and along one cardiac cycle. The ultrasound imaging system performs at frame rates of 60-90 fps, thus the number of samples along time is 60 to 90 accordingly.

The L and T components of the velocity are smoothed separately, by using a transformation from the Cartesian coordinate system to an (L,T) coordinate system, as follows: For each transversal line of four points - the inward direction is defined as the T axis, and the orthogonal direction is defined as the L axis.

2.1 De-noising using wavelet functions

The wavelet shrinkage method was applied to the myocardial velocities as described by Bachner-Hinenzon et al. (2010). At first, low tracking quality data points are replaced by a weighted average of their neighboring data points. Thereafter, an interpolation along the transmural orientation is performed. Subsequently, 3D wavelet de-noising is applied to the interpolated data. Following the wavelet decomposition, the Detail coefficients are thresholded by hard and soft threshold. For the first level, the Detail coefficients are removed completely (hard threshold) and for the second and third levels a soft universal threshold was used (Bachner-Hinenzon et al. 2010). Finally, to obtain the smoothed signal, the inverse of 3D discrete wavelet transform is computed using reconstruction filters in an iterated process.

The effectiveness of the wavelet shrinkage method was compared with a second smoothing method - a polynomial curve fitting method, which for the 3D case required 22 coefficients that were empirically chosen to estimate a polynomial of order 2 in space and of order 4 in time.

2.2 Strain and SR calculation

The tracking algorithm causes artifacts when the image quality is low, and even after the wavelet shrinkage smoothing operation, additional smoothing operation must be performed before regional Strain and SR are calculated. Strain is calculated at the center of each segment containing 12 TP's - 6 points along the L orientation, and 2 along the T orientation (2 adjacent layers across the LV wall). First, the center of such segment is calculated as a weighted moving average. Then, the location of each center in the next frame is found from the weighted average of the point's velocity.

Let Rn be the distance between two adjacent segment centers on the longitudinal axis at the n'th frame, and Rn+1 be the distance between the same two centers at the next frame. The relative shortening of the segment occurring between these two frames is:

$$dSL(n) = \frac{R_{n+1} - R_n}{R_n}$$

The accumulative strain of the segment at the n'th frame, relative to its initial length is:

$$SL(n) = SL(n-1) + dSL(n)(1 + SL(n-1))$$

The SR is calculated as the time derivative of the Strain.

2.3 Evaluation of the methods using simulated data

Sequences of velocity data have been generated by a software program, which modeled different movements, in order to accurately analyze the influence of different parameters of the algorithm and to allow quantification of the accuracy of measurement of smoothed motions. The simulated data also allowed accurate and reliable comparison between the wavelet shrinkage method and a second smoothing method - polynomial curve fitting method.

2.3.1 Simulation of normal cardiac motion

The complex myocardial motion was modeled by construction of a simplified heart motion model. A set of data points, taken from a clinical data set at end-diastole, served as the initial conditions (location of points) for the simulated contraction (Fig. 1(a)). To this set of data points, an analytic motion model was applied, as described in Fig. 1(b). The model describes the displacement of each point in the transmural and longitudinal direction, between 2 frames (i.e. 2 time samples), with delays among the 4 layers. It also includes a time dependant component common to all points, which describes the contraction and relaxations phases. By differentiating the displacement curves, the synthetic velocities in each layer are produced. The derived velocities (in each layer) are obtained in the transmural and longitudinal directions (see below). In order to test the algorithm under more realistic conditions, a random Gaussian noise was added (Noise ~ $N(0,\sigma)$, σ=10% of maximal velocity in each direction) to the velocities values. The quality of the results of each smoothing method were quantified in terms of the sum of square errors (SSE) between the denoised velocities (i.e. after applying the smoothing algorithm) and the original simulated velocities (before adding noise).

2.3.2 Simulation of an infarcted myocardium

Since the purpose of the method presented here is to enable measuring Strain and SR at myocardial layers across the LV wall, the locality of the Strain calculations was tested by modifying the above model to simulate a condition of an infarct. At one segment, the longitudinal velocity gradient was set to zero for two layers (out of 4), as if that part of the muscle does not actively contract, but only dragged by other segments. Random Gaussian noise was added to the velocities (Noise ~ $N(0,\sigma)$, σ=10% of maximal velocity in each direction.).

2.4 Application to clinical data

The method was applied in two clinical studies, to test its capability to quantitatively analyze the LV regional function. In the first study, the results of the analysis were compared with diagnosis made by an expert echocardiographer, and in the second with angiographic findings. The two studies included patients who were admitted to St. Vinzenz-Hospital for acute myocardial infarction (AMI), defined according to the Guidelines of the European Society of Cardiology. The studies were performed according to the regulations of the local ethical committee, which approved each study design. All patients gave informed consent for further evaluation of the anonymous results of their echocardiographic and heart catheterization examinations.

1(a)

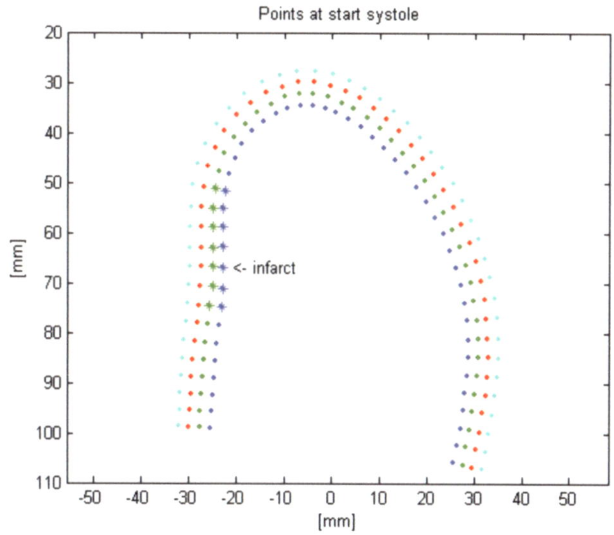

1(b)

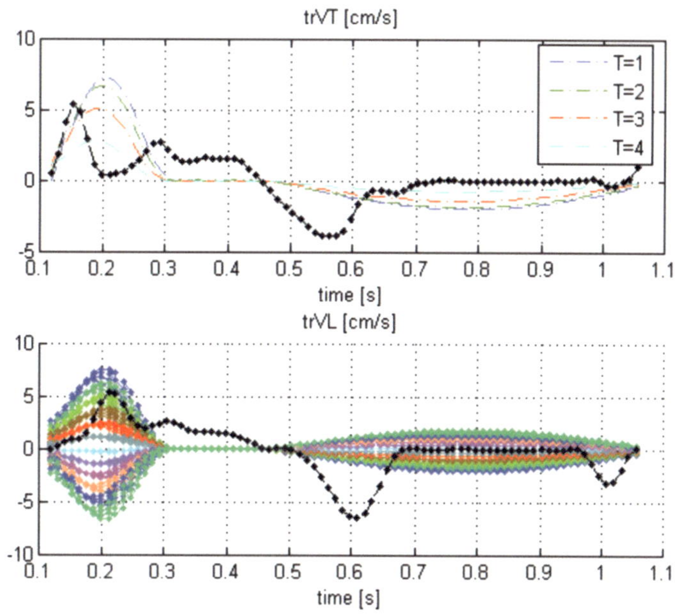

Fig. 1. (a): A model used for simulation of a non-transmural, regional infarct. A set of TP's (marked by '*'), located at the inner 2 layers of the second segment, does not actively contract. The results of the analysis of the data generated by this model are displayed in Fig. 2. Fig. 1(b): Simulated velocities [cm/sec] of the TP's of Fig. 1(a) plotted as a function of time. Upper subplot – transmural velocities at the 4 lines of points (layers) from the endocardium (T=1) to the epicardium (T=4). Bottom subplot -56 colored curves (colors used just to differentiate among the curves) depicting longitudinal velocities, as the function of time, at 56 TP's along the LV long axis (from the basal-septal region, to the apex and then to the basal-freewall). The dotted black lines denote example of genuine myocardial velocities. To these velocities, random Gaussian noise was added. Noise ~ N(0,σ) , σ= 10% of maximal velocity in each direction.

2.4.1 Comparison with an expert echocardiographer

Echocardiographic examination usually includes qualitative assessment of wall motion, by inspection of the changes of length and thickening of each myocardial segment, where each segment comprises the whole width of the myocardial wall (Cerqueira et al., 2002). This process is usually denoted as 'regional analysis' and is applied by sectioning the LV myocardium to 18 myocardial segments, as proposed by the American Society of Echocardiography (Cerqueira, et al., 2002).

The patient group consisted of 9 patients (mean age 63 ± 14 years), who had symptoms occur within twelve hours of admission, and all were immediately transferred to the catheterization laboratory for coronary angiography and percutaneous coronary intervention. Based on the results of coronary angiography, 1 was diagnosed as having no coronary obstruction, and 8 diagnosed as suffering from stenosis in one of their main coronary arteries. Standard echocardiographic examinations were performed within 48 hours of admission, following the in-hospital routine patient management. For each subject - 3 apical views were acquired (2 Chamber, 4 Chamber and Apical long-axis (Aplax) views), yielding a total of 162 segments. For each view and each myocardial segment, a score was given by an expert Echocardiographer studying the B-mode grey scale cine-loops. The score given: 1 - segment with normal kinematics; 2 - hypo-kinetic segment; 3 - a-kinetic segment; 4 - diskinetic segment.

The study focused on the systolic function, using two common measures - peak systolic Strain and peak systolic SR. These measures were compared to the score given by the expert. Longitudinal and transmural Strain and SR were calculated for each TP as explained above, and for each segment by averaging for all TP's of this segment. Peak systolic strain values were determined for each segment by finding during systole the minimal strain value in the longitudinal direction (contraction), and maximal strain values in the transmural direction (thickening).

2.4.2 Statistical analysis

The analysis of the results for all (n=9) subjects above included calculation of the significance of the separation of the (162) segments into the four kinetic groups, according to the two motion parameters. Analysis of variance (ANOVA) was used to estimate the difference between the four groups. When the ANOVA test resulted in positive significance, post hoc tests (Scheffe) were used. The analysis was performed for the results of the smoothing performed by the wavelets method and by the polynomial fitting method.

2.4.3 Comparison with angiographic results – Qualitative study

A different patient group consisted of 21 patients (mean age 64 ± 12 years), selected following emergency admission for AMI. They had symptoms occur within twelve hours of admission, and all were immediately transferred to the catheterization laboratory for coronary angiography and percutaneous coronary intervention. Based on the results of coronary angiography, 5 were diagnosed as having no coronary obstruction and 16 diagnosed as patients who suffer from stenosis in one of their main coronary arteries. Standard echocardiographic examinations were performed within 48 hours of admission, following the in-hospital routine patient management.

For each subject, three apical views were acquired (2ch, 4ch and Aplax) as well as short axis views at the basal-papillary level. The B-mode cine-loops were processed as described above, the data velocity data was smoothed as above, and the Strain and SR parameters were derived as described above. The evaluation was done by producing M-mode maps that help visualize each parameter as a function of time and the longitudinal location along the septal base - the apex – the lateral base. Such maps were produced for each of the above parameters, for each of the three myocardial layers. The M-mode maps, especially the Strain and SR maps, allow straightforward recognition of regions of reduced contractibility. These regions were visually compared with the areas of perfusion of the corresponding narrowed coronary artery, where the areas of perfusion of the main coronary arteries were divided according to the standard division of LV into 16 segments (Cerqueira et al., 2002). These results were also compared with the 'AFI' method, which performs over-smoothing of the data and does not provide resolution across the LV wall.

3. Results

3.1 Simulated data - A normal myocardium

The results obtained when using the polynomial curve fitting method yielded errors calculated to be SSE= 549.6, while the wavelet shrinkage (with the best choice of parameters) method yielded an error 2/3 smaller (383.2 in terms of SSE).

3.2 Simulated data - An infarcted myocardium

Fig. 2 shows the longitudinal velocities after de-noising/smoothing, as performed by either the wavelet shrinkage method or the polynomial curve fitting method. Each subplot in the figure depicts the longitudinal velocities at one of the four myocardial layers (left – endocardium, the 2 at the center – midwall, right- epicardium), as the function of time during the cardiac cycle. In each subplot, the vertical axis depicts the location along the anatomical M-mode line, starting from the septal base, through the apex and ending at the lateral base. The first row of four subplots presents the results of the wavelet denoising method, the middle row presents the results of the polynomial curve fitting method and the bottom row presents the original simulated velocities before the addition of noise. The arrows in the subplots of the 2nd column, point at the segment of infarction at the subendocardial-midwall layers, while the arrows in the subplots of the 3rd column point at the adjacent normal segment at the midwall-epicardial layers. The original simulated velocities (bottom row) display the difference between the normal and infarcted layers: the normal segment has a smooth longitudinal gradient of velocities, which does not exist in the infarcted layers. As can be seen from this figure, the difference of the velocities distribution between the two inner layers and the two outer layers is still apparent after the smoothing operation performed by either the wavelet method or the polynomial curve fitting method.

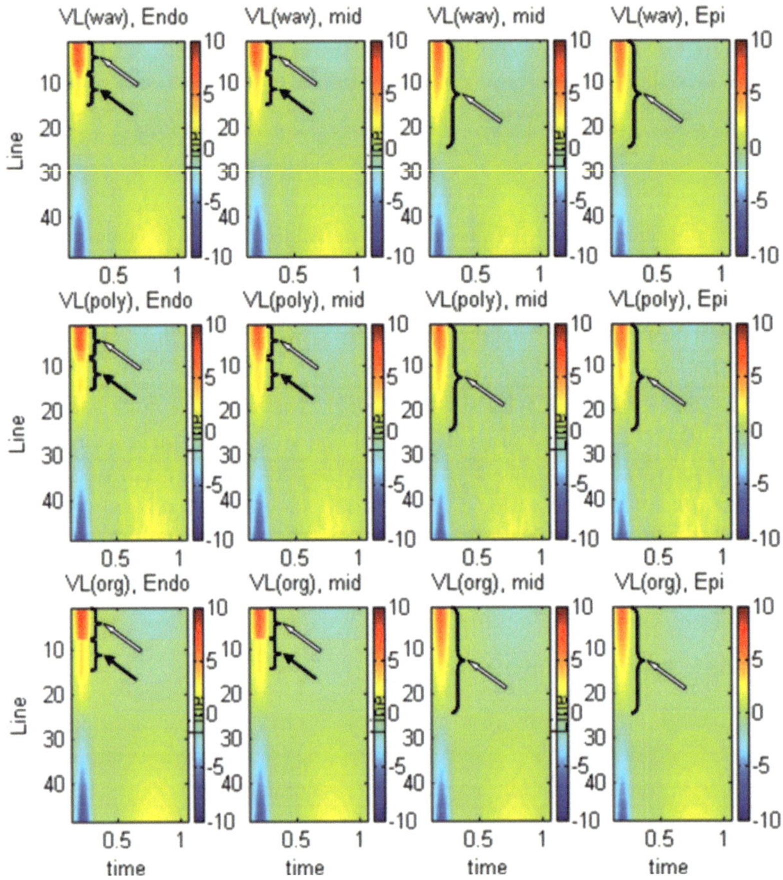

Fig. 2. Comparison of the de-noised longitudinal velocities, as performed by the wavelet vs. the polynomial fitting methods. Lower row - the original velocity distribution; Middle row - de-noising by polynomial fitting; Upper row - de-noising by wavelets. Each subplot is an M-mode plot of longitudinal velocities of the TP's (i.e. the ordinate depicts their longitudinal location) along the cardiac cycle, i.e. as a function of time (Abscissa). The black arrows emphasize the 'infarcted' segment (2 left columns), while the white arrows point to the 'normal' contracting segments (2 upper segments in the 2 left columns, and the full segments at the 2 right columns).

3.3 Clinical data - Comparison with diagnosis performed by an expert echocardiographer

The qualitative 'regional analysis' of wall motion, that was performed by the echocardiographer for the 9 patients included in this study, yielded quantification of function of 162 segments: 83 were diagnosed as normal and 79 with different degrees of a-kinetics.

In Fig. 3, two examples are given of color mapping of peak systolic longitudinal and transversal strain values. In Fig. 3(a) there are strain maps of a healthy subject, and Fig. 3(b) there are strain maps of a patient with a large LAD AMI (as validated also by angiography). The color at each segment denotes the value of the peak systolic strain according to the color map on the right side of the figure. The color map chosen is such that enables a clear distinction between the contracting segments (red colors) in the longitudinal direction (left panels) and segments that are stretched by the neighboring segments (blue color). In the transversal direction the normal segments appear in blue, as they become thicker during systole. Visual comparison of the results for the two subjects illustrates that for the normal subject the peak systolic strain values are homogenous along the myocardium and that for the pathological case a region near the apex appears that does not contract at all.

3(a)

3(b)

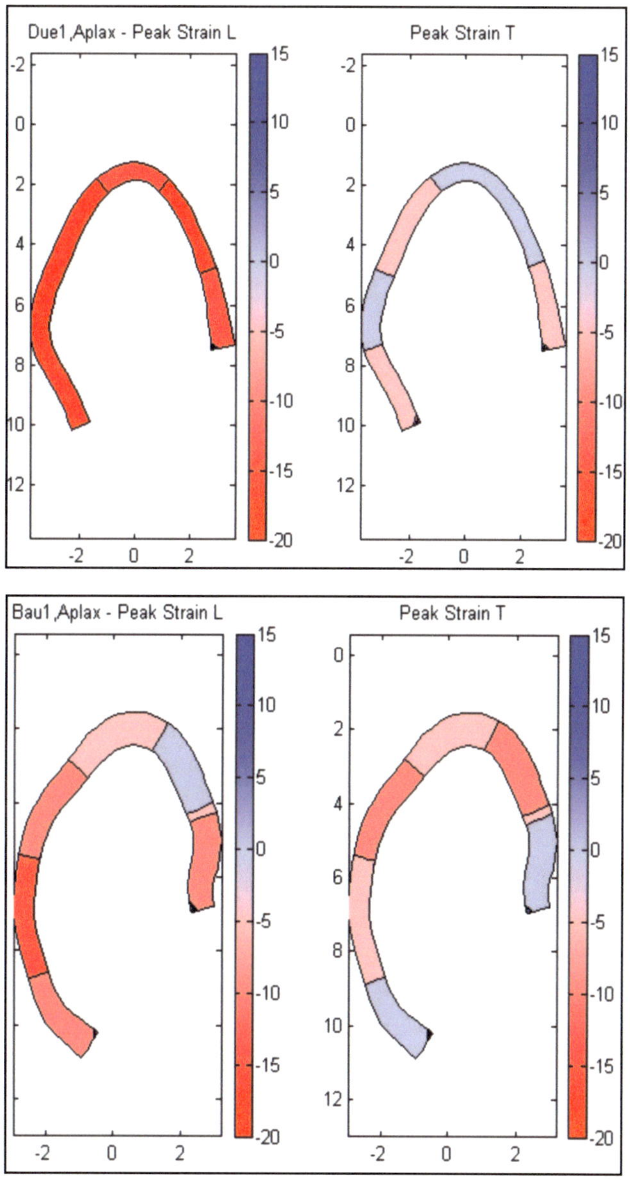

Fig. 3. Peak systolic strain values for each segment, calculated from data obtained from a normal subject (a) and from a patient with an infarct at the LAD (b). For each case: Left- peak systolic longitudinal strain (marked as 'Peak Strain L'), right - peak systolic transmural strain (marked as 'Peak Strain T').

Similarly, the results of the analysis of the peak systolic SR values at each segment, for the same two subjects, are depicted in Fig. 4. In Fig. 4(a) the results for a healthy subject are depicted, and in Fig. 4(b) for a patient with a large LAD AMI. The difference between the normal peak systolic SR maps and the pathological ones is clear.

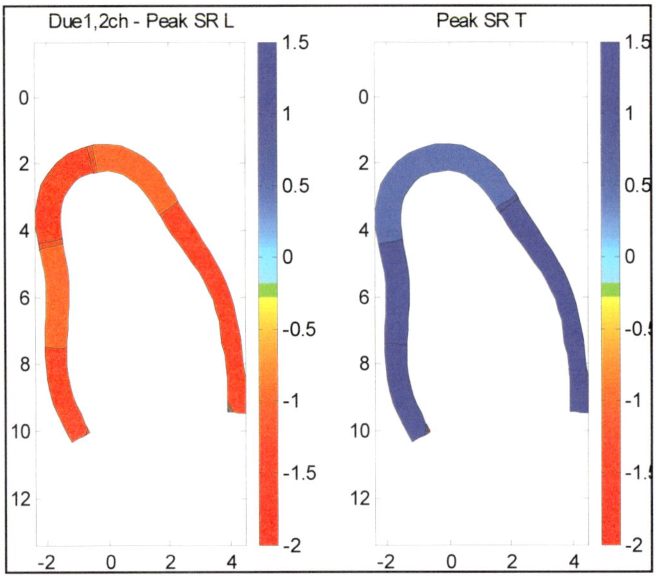

4(a)

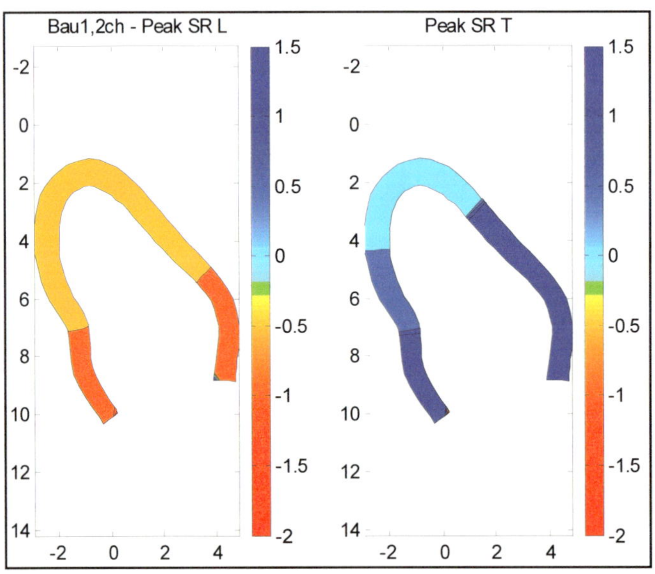

4(b)

Fig. 4. Peak systolic SR values for each segment, calculated from data obtained from a normal subject (a) and from a patient with an infarct at the LAD (b). For each case: Left - peak systolic longitudinal SR (marked as 'Peak SR L'), right - peak systolic transmural SR (marked as 'Peak SR T').

The statistical analysis of the results for all (9) subjects included calculation of the significance of the separation of the (162) segments into the four kinetic groups, according to the two motion parameters. The ANOVA analysis for the results of the smoothing performed by the wavelets method demonstrated that the peak systolic Strain results yielded a significant difference between the four groups: for the longitudinal peak Strain parameter, Slmax, $p<0.001$, and for the transversal peak Strain parameter, Stmax, $p<0.001$. The Scheffe test for Slmax showed significant differences between all groups except the diskinetic and the a-kinetic groups. The Scheffe test for Stmax found significant differences only between the normal group and the three pathological groups (Fig. 5, subplots (a) and (b)). Similarly, the ANOVA analysis of the peak systolic SR results yielded a significant difference between the four groups for the longitudinal peak SR parameter, SRlmax, $p<0.001$, and for the transversal peak SR parameter, SRtmax, $p<0.001$. The Scheffe test for SRlmax showed significant differences between all groups except the dis-kinetic and the a-kinetic groups. The Scheffe test for SRtmax found significant differences only between the normal group and the diskinetic and a-kinetic groups (Fig. 5, subplots (c) and (d)).

When comparing these results to the ANOVA analysis for the results of the polynomial smoothing - it is evident that for both the longitudinal peak Strain parameter, Slmax, and the longitudinal peak SR parameter, SRlmax, $p<0.001$, only the normal group can be separated from the 3 pathological groups (the hypo-kinetic, the diskinetic and a-kinetic groups) - Fig. 5, subplots (e) and (g), as well as (f) and (h). It is also evident that the entire peak systolic values are smaller (and the range narrower) when the smoothing is performed by the polynomial fitting (Abscissas of Fig. 5, subplots (e) to (h)) versus the wavelets smoothing (Abscissas of Fig. 5, subplots (a) to (d)).

3.4 Clinical data - Comparison with angiographic results – Qualitative study

This patient group consisted of 21 patients, of whom 5 were diagnosed by angiography as having no coronary obstruction and 16 diagnosed as patients who suffer from stenosis in one of their main coronary arteries. The standard echocardiographic examinations were post processed to produce the Strain and SR maps, as follows:

3.4.1 Healthy subjects - Homogenous strain and SR along the myocardium

M-mode maps of longitudinal SR and of longitudinal Strain are presented for two healthy subjects (Fig. 6) (b),(d). The upper row of maps depicts the results for the endocardial layer, the second from top row - midwall layer, the 3rd row from top - epicardial layer, the 4th row from top - the results of the 'AFI' method, which over-smoothes the data. In each map, the vertical axis represents the location along the anatomical M-mode line, starting from the septal base, through the apex and ending at the lateral base, while the horizontal axis depicts time. As can be seen in these maps, the pattern is homogenous along the myocardium (i.e. along the vertical axis). The red colors represent shortening, the blue colors stretching of the muscle.

3.4.2 Healthy subject - Normal strain in short axis views

The short axis views of healthy subjects demonstrated that circumferential strain is more significant at the endocardial layer than at the epicardial layer (Fig. 7). These differences were expected from geometric considerations and the assumption of tissue incompressibility, because concentric shells of myocardium must undergo proportionally greater changes in dimension for shells of smaller radius. The three subplots of Fig. 7 depict

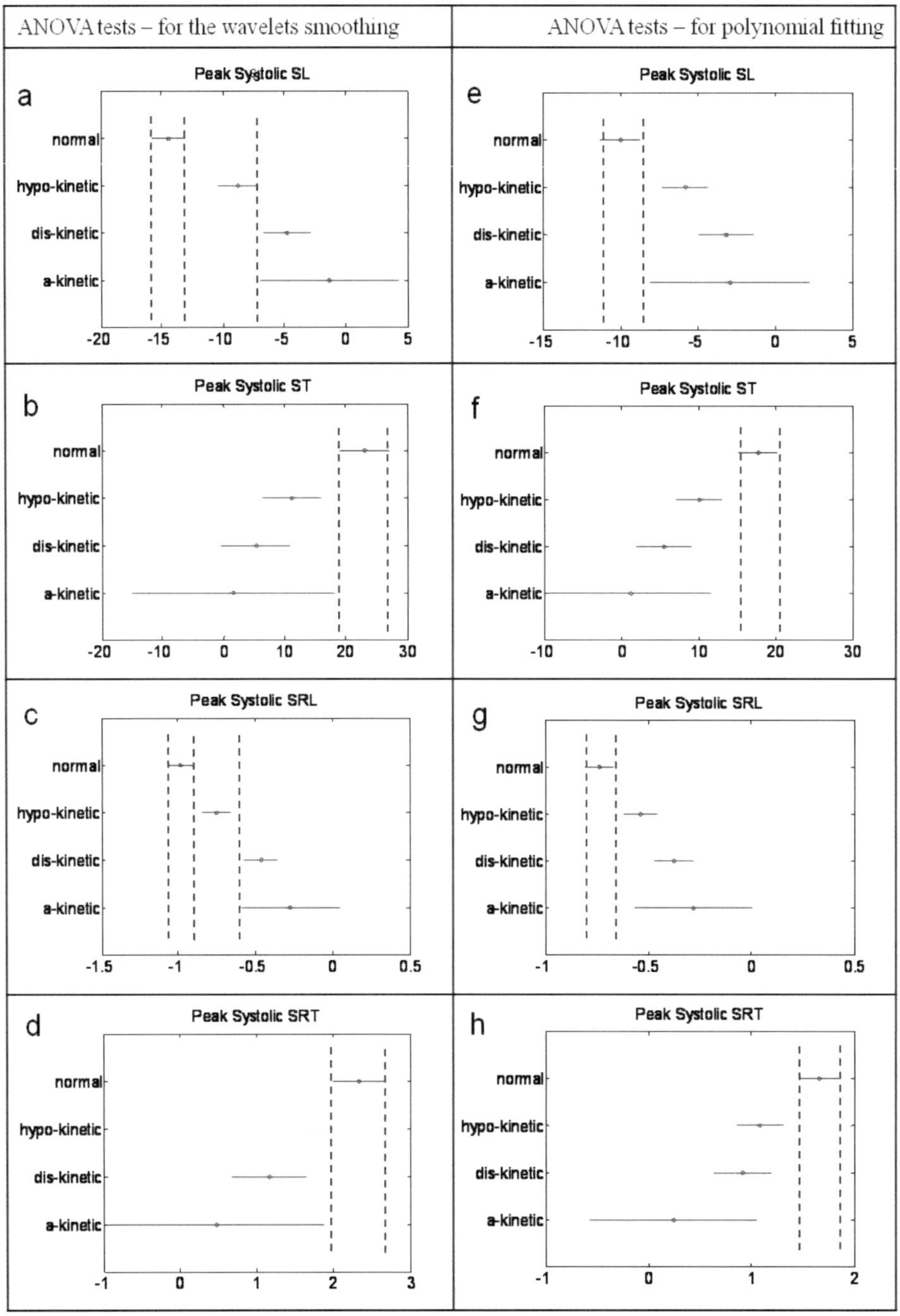

Fig. 5. Scheffe results for peak systolic longitudinal Strain (a, e), peak systolic transmural Strain (b, f), peak systolic longitudinal SR (c, g), peak systolic transmural SR (d, h). 162 segments are included in the analysis, 83 with normal contraction, 79 with different degrees of pathologies (45 segments hypo-kinetic; 29 diskinetic; 5 a-kinetic). Figures 5 (a-d) are results after wavelet smoothing, and figures 5 (e-h) are results after polynomial smoothing.

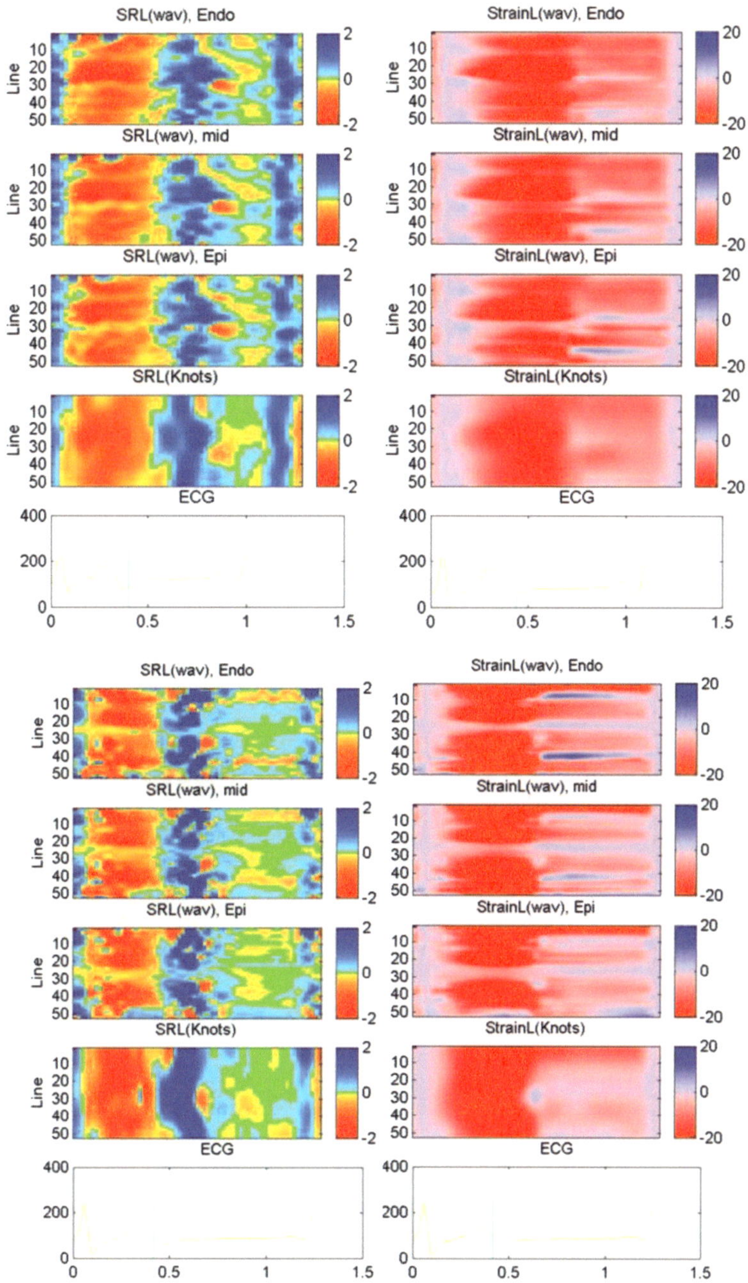

Fig. 6. Color-coded maps of results for 2 normal subjects that compare the wavelet analysis, which separates the 3 myocardial layers (1st row - subendocardium; 2nd row - midwall; 3rd row - epicardium), to the analysis that averages over the wall thickness (4th row). Columns 1 and 3: The longitudinal strain rate (SRL). Columns 2 and 4: longitudinal strain (StrainL). Each subplot is an M-mode plot (i.e. the ordinate depicts the longitudinal location), as a function of time (Abscissa - along the cardiac cycle).

3 presentations, at 3 different locations (different sets of TP's, at locations 14, 30, 38), of the Strain traces for a healthy subject. In each subplot, the graphs on the left show the circumferential and radial Strains, at the 4 TP's marked by crosses at the graph on the right. It can be clearly seen that in all locations the amplitude of the circumferential strain is larger at the sub-endocardium than at the sub-epicardium.

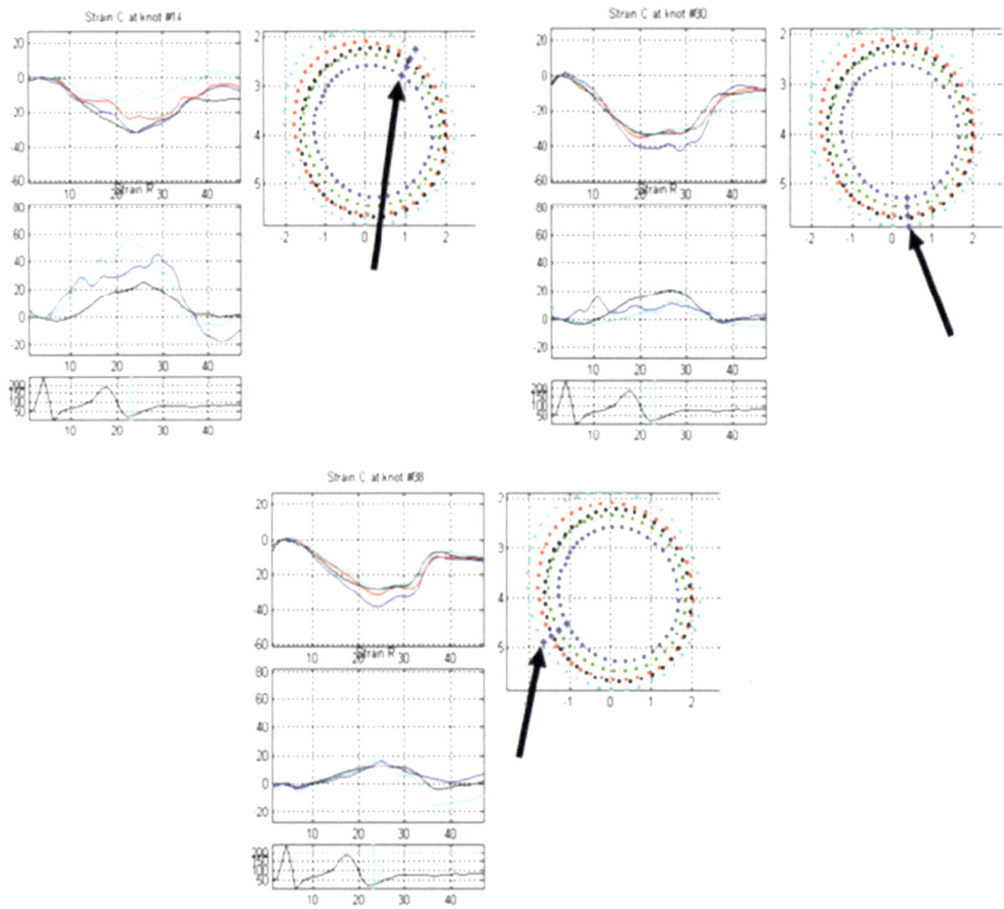

Fig. 7. Three examples of circumferential and Radial Strains, as measure from short-axis echocardiograms from a normal subject. In each example, the right subplot shows the 4 lines of TP's, with 4 specific points (marked by the arrow) that their time-dependant strains are depicted: The upper left subplot in each example depicts the circumferential strains, while the lower subplot depicts the radial strains.

3.4.3 Post-AMI patients - Strain/SR results vs. angiography findings

Out of the total of 21 subjects studied, 16 were post-AMI patients diagnosed with pathologies limited to a specific region. The detection of the location of each AMI, accomplished by using the M-mode Strain and SR maps, was validated by comparing the relevant segments with the segments predicted to be affected by the stenosis of the appropriate coronary artery, according to the AHA standard perfusion segmentation maps (Cerqueira et al., 2002).

Two examples are given here. Fig. 8 displays the results of the analysis for a patient with LAD stenosis, and Fig. 9 for a LCx stenosis patient. The left column in each figure is a set of M-mode maps of longitudinal strain, while the middle column is a set of maps of the transmural strain, where the upper row relates to the endocardial layer, the second from top relates to the midwall, the third from top relates to the epicardial layer, and the bottom row relates to the over-smoothed strain, calculated by the 'AFI' method. The region of reduced contractility is marked by the black arrow in the maps and by the red area superimposed on the B-mode gray scale image. Superimposed on this same B-mode image of the LV long axis are also the line of 'knots' (large color dots), calculated from the 4 lines of TP's by the 'AFI' method, as well as the Region of Interest in which the tracking and the analysis were performed.

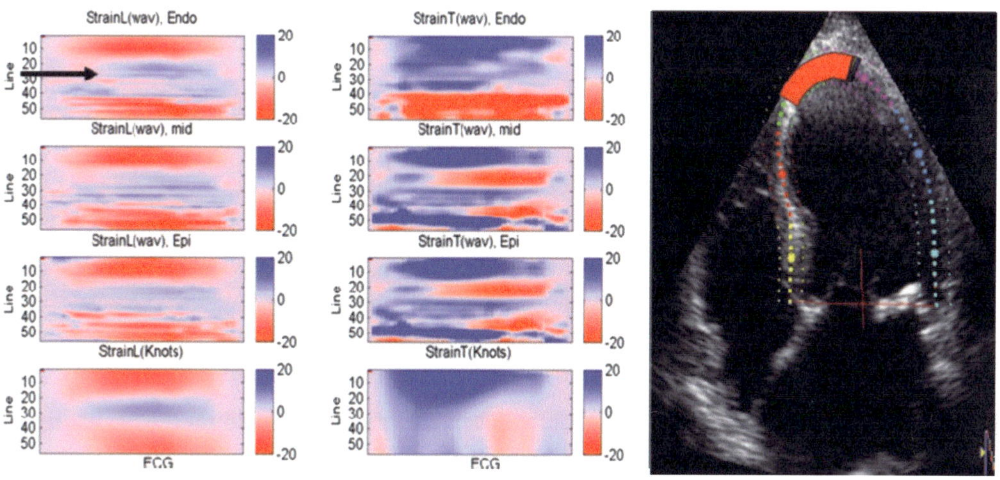

Fig. 8. Example of Strain results, as filtered by the wavelet method, calculated from long-axis echocardiogram of a patient with an AMI at the LAD. The left column subplots depict the longitudinal Strain, while the right column subplots depict the transverse Strain. Each subplot is an M-mode plot of Strain at different locations along the cross-section (i.e. the ordinate depicts the longitudinal location), along the cardiac cycle, i.e. as a function of time (Abscissa). The numbers (1-56) along the Ordinate reflect the TP number, as seen superimposed on the B-mode frame on the right hand-side, where point 1 is at the basal-septal location (lower-left), while point 56 is at the basal-freewall (lower right). Upper row - Strain at the subendocardium; 2nd row- Strain at the midwall; 3rd row - Strain at the epicardium; 4th row - Strain as calculated when values are first average across the wall (the AFI method). The black arrows on the left emphasize the infarcted region, also marked in red on the B-mode image on the right.

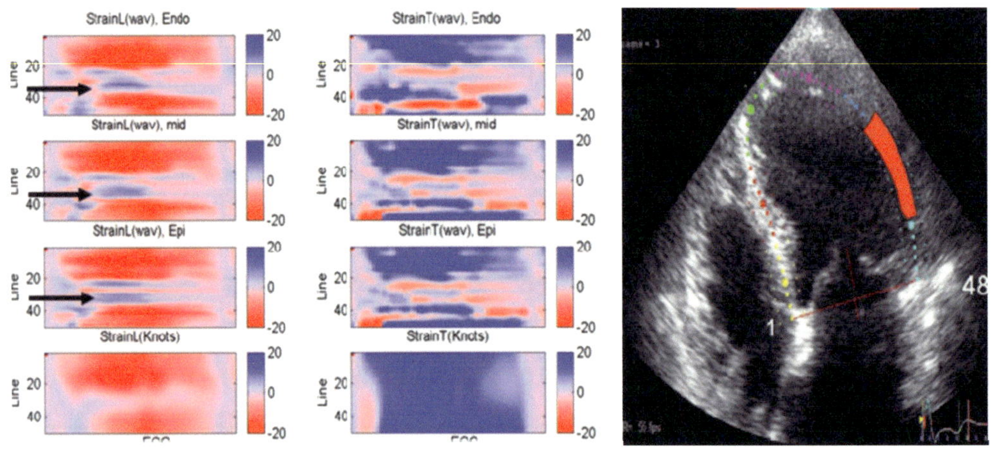

Fig. 9. Example of Strain results, as filtered by the wavelet method, calculated from long-axis echocardiogram of a patient with an AMI at the LCX. Details are similar to those given for Fig. 10 (except that here only 48 TP's have been assigned).

The total data set comprised of 63 sets (3 views acquired from 21 subjects: 5 healthy subjects, 2 patients suffering from RCA occlusion, 3 LCx and 11 LAD), which were graded according to the level of agreement with the angiography findings: matching of the coronary artery location - 1; partial matching - 2; no match - 3. Out of the 63 sets, 41 (65%) showed a good agreement, 19 (30%) partial matching, while in 3 (5%) there was no match at all.

Most of the cases of partial (or no) match between the diagnosis based on the Strain and SR maps and the diagnosis based on the angiography findings, were cases that were categorized as normal, and the Strain and SR maps showed a region with reduced contraction. This outcome may be either the result of low quality tracking in these regions (especially near the apex), or of true pathology, since all subjects were symptomatic and underwent an angiographic study, and were diagnosed according to its findings.

3.4.4 Ability to diagnose small AMIs

Since the method presented here produces maps that reveal motion and contraction at each of the three myocardial layers separately, it is now possible to detect smaller and non-transmural AMIs. Fig. 10 shows an example of a patient with a small LAD AMI, where its location is marked by a black arrow. The depressed contraction is mostly seen at the endocardial layer, while at the epicardial layer some contraction exists in nearly all regions. It can also be seen that while the depressed contraction caused by the occluded LAD artery is visible in the Strain maps produced by the new method, the maps produced by the 'AFI' method do not have the sufficient resolution to reveal the depressed Strain of the ischemic or infarcted region (bottom row).

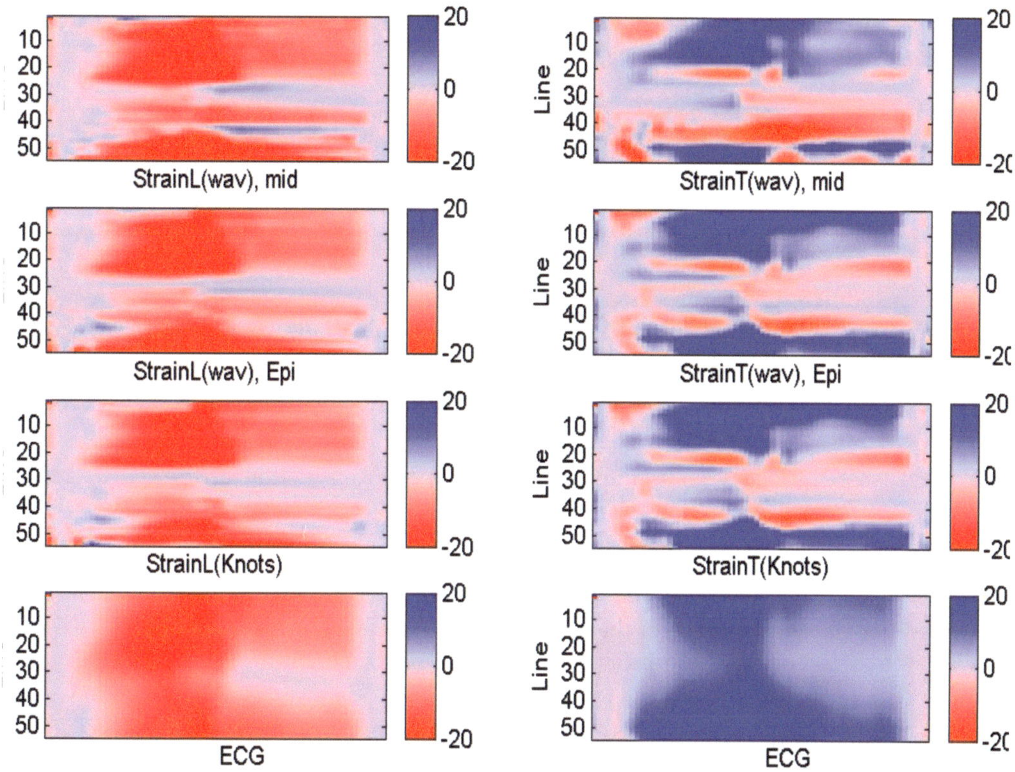

Fig. 10. Example of Strain results, as filtered by the wavelet method, calculated from long-axis echocardiogram of a patient with a small AMI at the LAD. Details are similar to those given for Fig. 10. This example demonstrates that the M-mode plot of Strain, as calculated by the AFI method (the lower row) - seems normal. (here 56 TP's have been assigned).

4. Discussion

The new method presented here, based on analysis of echocardiographic B-mode sequences, allows computing myocardial motion and contraction properties in all segments of the 2D myocardial cross-section, thus overcoming the intrinsic limitations of the clinically accepted Doppler-based techniques. Clinical experience confirms that the motion of even a normal heart is rarely along the direction of the myocardial wall, thus accurate results of Doppler-based techniques are obtained perhaps at the septum. Additionally, the Doppler-based techniques obviously do not provide both longitudinal and transverse measurements. They also cause reduction of the frame rate of the B-mode image acquisition, since the two measurements cannot be performed simultaneously. Therefore, Doppler data is usually acquired on a small set of image lines, (e.g. 16 samples in GE's Vivid3 and Vivid7), which increases the inaccuracy of the measurement.

The recently presented 'AFI' method (Rappaport et al. 2006; Leitman et al. 2004; Reisner et al. 2004) provides functional and clinically useful information throughout the imaged myocardial cross-section. This method, though, employs robust smoothing techniques and therefore the spatial resolution is relatively low. Moreover, since the motion information is represented for only one line of points along the longitudinal axis of the myocardium, variations between myocardial layers cannot be detected.

The accuracy of the high resolution method presented here, of measuring regional 2D strain, suffers from the same 2 inherent shortcomings as its earlier version (Reisner et al. 2004; Rappaport et al. 2006): it depends on tracking quality, and on the inability to follow the gross heart movement with the probe. The second shortcoming is specifically troublesome when 2D data is acquired by ultrasound 2D probe, held in place, while the motion of the heart is three-dimensional, causing acquisition of practically a different cross-section of tissue at each different instant. This causes reduction of the correlation of the speckle pattern in the analyzed 2-D sequences, and produces weaker relations between frames. Similar effects are observed for out-of-plane motion, which may cause intra-cardiac structures (for example, papillary muscles) to penetrate and exit the imaged plane, a limitation that is shared by other 2-D modalities.

Additional shortcoming is related to the calculation of SR, which is performed by spatial derivation of the velocities. Thus the error inherent in the velocity data is magnified. The other methods, however, also share this shortcoming.

While the above shortcomings are shared by all other ultrasound methods, the method presented here takes advantage of the basic data-set, the velocities at a set (4 by (50 to 60) by (50-70) time instants) of TP's, to provide 2D Strain and SR tensors at each myocardial point. This was demonstrated to provide analysis of local deformations (orientations and magnitudes) at different myocardial layers, including their variations in time, along and across the myocardial wall.

The performance of the method, using the wavelet shrinkage method, was found to be slightly better in terms of the sum of square errors, and much better in terms of computational load. A model was also used to demonstrate the feasibility of the method to detect a region comprising of 2 layers that do not contract, simulating a 'regional non-transmural AMI'. Both smoothing methods allowed discrimination between the two 'normal' layers and the two 'infarcted' layers at this region.

The preliminary clinical studies compared the diagnosis performed by the echocardiographer for the 162 segments with the set of parameters calculated during systole - the peak systolic Strain, and the peak systolic SR. The results obtained using the calculations of the longitudinal Strain and longitudinal SR have been found to be in good agreement with the expert's diagnosis, better than the agreement found for the transmural calculations. This result was expected since the width of the myocardium muscle is relatively small (only 4 TPs), and so the reliability of the calculations in the transmural direction is lower.

The comparison of the angiographic results with the regional Strain and SR of 63 data sets (21 subjects, 3 apical views for each subject) analyzed by the 2 smoothing methods, demonstrated that the 2 smoothing methods provide better spatial resolution than the AFI method, specifically among the different myocardial layers across the wall. The wavelet de-noising outperforms the polynomial fitting, as demonstrated in Fig. 5, allowing differentiation normal vs. pathological regions, but also between hypo-kinetic regions and diskinetic or a-kinetic regions. The separation into 3 groups was evident from the peak systolic Strain measurements, as well as from the peak systolic SR. The comparison to the angiographic study was done by observing the contraction patterns in M-mode maps of the Strain and SR of the four myocardial layers during the entire cardiac cycle. The results were also compared with the Strain and SR calculated by the 'AFI' method.

During systole, specifically during the ECG S-wave, the normal SR pattern reflects the myocardial shortening in the longitudinal direction and extension in the transversal direction. In most of the normal cases studied here, this contraction is apparent as a simultaneous shortening of all myocardial layers. In contrast, the contraction in the cases of the abnormal patients presented a different behavior: at the anomalous regions the myocardium did not contract at all in the longitudinal direction, or was even extended, while it shortened in the orthogonal direction. In some cases, diversity between the layers was observed, where some layers functioned normally and some abnormally. The normal SR pattern during the E wave was, as expected, of myocardial extension in the longitudinal direction and shortening in the transversal direction. In abnormal hearts, either the longitudinal extension did not occur or was weaker than the extension noticed in normal hearts.

A good agreement was found between the results of the present study, the results of the 'AFI' method and the areas supplied by the narrowed artery (as found by the angiography study). In those cases where there was no agreement or only partial agreement between the findings of the present study (based on the Strain - SR maps) and the angiography findings, the majority of the cases were those that were clinically categorized as normal, while the Strain - SR maps showed a region with reduced contraction. This outcome can be the result of either low quality of tracking in those regions (especially near the apex), or reduced functionality due to partial ischemia that the angiography failed to diagnose.

The examination of the circumferential strain of normal subjects (in short axis views) showed higher Strain values along the endocardial layer than the epicardial layer, similar to reported results (Helm et al. 2005), and as expected from geometrical considerations and tissue incompressibility. These results, therefore, demonstrate the reliability of the method of regional analysis.

Some of the smaller AMI's that were found by angiography and were also so diagnosed by the present method, but were not detected by the 'AFI' method. The method presented here has the potential to detect smaller AMI's and non-transmural AMI's better than currently available techniques, but this needs to be assessed in large-scale clinical studies.

The advantage of visualizing the Strain and SR as M-mode maps allows examining not only the peak Strain - SR, but also their temporal evolution. This visualization provides important information about the regional function of the left ventricle and yields semi-quantitative assessment of wall motion. Another advantage of visualizing Strain and not just motion information is its reduced sensitivity to translation of the whole heart.

In conclusion, the method presented here provides region information regarding the myocardial distribution of Strain and SR, which allows functional differentiation among the myocardial layers. The 2 smoothing methods provide good results, with the wavelet de-noising outperforming the polynomial fitting, allowing differentiating normal from pathological regions, but also between hypo-kinetic regions and diskinetic or a-kinetic regions. The higher spatial resolution may be useful in diagnosing transmural versus non-transmural AMI's, and due to the visualization methods used - dyssynchrony of activation and pathologies of Strain evolution, e.g. post systolic shortening.

5. Acknowledgments

This study was supported by the Magneton program, the Chief Scientist, Ministry of Industry and Trade, and by the Technion VPR Fund for the promotion of Research. The Authors are grateful for the generous support.

6. References

Behar, V., Adam, D., Lysyansky, P., Friedman, Z., The combined effect of nonlinear filtration and window size on the accuracy of tissue displacement estimation using detected echo signals. Ultrasonics 2004; 41:743-753.

Bertrand, M., Meunier, J., Doucet, M., Ferland, G., Ultrasonic biomechanical strain gauge based on speckle tracking, Proc. 1989 IEEE Ultrason. Symp.: 859 - 863.

Bachner-Hinenzon N Ertracht O, Lysiansky M, Binah O, Adam D. Layer-specific assessment of left ventricular function by utilizing wavelet de-noising: A validation study. Med Biol Eng Comput. 2011 Jan;49(1):3-13. Epub 2010 Jul 20.

Cerqueira, M.D., Weissman, N.J., Dilsizian, V., Jacobs, A.K., Kaul, S., Laskey, W.K., Pennell, D.J., Rumberger, J.A., Ryan, T., Verani, M.S., Standardized Myocardial Segmentation and Nomenclature for Tomographic Imaging of the Heart, Circulation, 2002; 105: 539-542.

De Boeck, B.W.L., Cramer, M-J.M., Loh, P., Doevendans, P.A.F.M., Two-Dimensional Strain Imaging to Assess the Origin and Extent of Ventricular Preexcitation Associated With an Accessory Bypass, Circulation 2006;113: 835-839.

Desco, M., Ledesma-Carbayo, M. J., et al., Assessment of normal and ischaemic myocardium by quantitative m-mode tissue Doppler imaging, Ultrasound in Med. & Biol., 2002; 28 (5): 561-569.

Donoho, D.L., De-Noising By Soft-Thresholding, IEEE Trans. on Information Theory, 1995; 41 (3): 613-627.

Donoho, D.L., Johnstone, I.M., Ideal spatial adaptation by wavelet shrinkage, Biometrika, 1994; 84 (3): 425-455.

Heimdal, A., Stoyen, A., Torp, H., Skjxrpe, T., Real-Time Strain Rate Imaging of the Left Ventricle by Ultrasound, J Am Soc Echocardiogr, 1998; 11 (11):1013-1019.

Helm, R.H., Leclercq, C., Faris, O.P., Ozturk, C., McVeigh, E., Lardo, A.C., Kass, D.A., Cardiac Dyssynchrony Analysis Using Circumferential Versus Longitudinal Strain Implications for Assessing Cardiac Resynchronization, Circulation, 2005;111: 2760-2767.

Herbots, L.,Maes, F., D'hooge, J, Claus, P., Dymarkowski, S., Martens, P., Mortelmans, L., Bijnems, B., Bogaert, J., Rademakers, F.E., Sutherland, G.R., Quantifying Myocardial Deformation Throughout the Cardiac Cycle: A Comparison of Ultrasound Strain Rate, Grey-Scale M-Mode and Magnetic Resonance Imaging, Ultrasound in Med. & Biol., 2004; 30 (5): 591-598.

Ledesma-Carbayo, M.J., Kybic, J., Desco, M., Santos, A., Sühling, M., Hunziker, P., and Unser, M., Spatio-temporal nonrigid registration for ultrasound cardiac motion estimation, IEEE Trans. Med. Imag., 2005; 24, (9), 1113-1126.

Leitman M, Lysyansky P, Sidenko S, Shir V, Peleg E, Binenbaum M, Kaluski E, Krakover R, Vered Z Two-dimensional strain-a novel software for real-time quantitative echocardiographic assessment of myocardial function, J Am Soc Echocardiogr, 2004; 17 (10):1021-1029.

Liel-Cohen N, Tsadok Y, Beeri R, Lysyansky P, Agmon Y, Feinberg MS, Fehske W, Gilon D, Hay I, Kuperstein R, Leitman M, Deutsch L, Rosenmann D, Sagie A, Shimoni S, Vaturi M, Friedman Z, Blondheim DS. A New Tool for Automatic Assessment of Segmental Wall Motion, Based on Longitudinal 2D Strain: A Multicenter Study by the Israeli Echocardiography Research Group. Circ Cardiovasc Imaging. 3(1):47-53, 2010.

Mallat, S., A Wavelet Tour of Signal Processing, Academic Press,1998.

Moore, C.C., Lugo-Olivieri, C.H., McVeigh, E.R., Zerhouni, E.A.: Three-dimensional systolic strain patterns in the normal human left ventricle: characterization with tagged MR imaging, Radiology, 2000; 214 (2): 453-466.

Nesto, R.W., and Kowalchuk, G.J., The Ischemic cascade: Temporal sequence of hemodynamic, electrocardiographic and symptomatic expressions of ischemia, American Journal of Cardiology, 1987; 59: 23C-30C.

O'Donnell, M., Skovoroda, A. R. and Shapo. B. M., Measurement of arterial wall motion using Fourier based speckle tracking algorithms, Proc. 1991 IEEE Ultrason. Symp., 1101-1104.

O'Donnell, M. Skovoroda, A.R.; Shapo, B.M.; Emelianov, S.Y.; Internal displacement and strain imaging using ultrasonic speckle tracking, IEEE Trans. Ultrason. Ferroelect. Frequency Contr., 1994, 41 (3): 314 -325.

Rappaport, D., Adam, D., Lysyansky, P., Riesner, S., Assessment of Myocardial Regional Strain and Strain Rate by Tissue Tracking in B-Mode Echocardiograms, Ultrasound in Med. & Biol., 2006; 32 (8): 1181–1192.

Reisner, S., Lysyansky, P., Agmon, Y., Mutlak, D., Lessick, J., Friedman, Z., Global longitudinal strain: A novel index of left ventricular systolic function. J Am Soc Echocardiogr, 2004;17: 630-633.

Suffoletto, M.S., Dohi, K., Cannesson, M., Saba, S., Gorcsan, J., Novel Speckle-Tracking Radial Strain From Routine Black-and-White Echocardiographic Images to Quantify Dyssynchrony and Predict Response to Cardiac Resynchronization Therapy, Circulation. 2006;113: 960-968.

Sutherland, G.R., Di Salvo, G., Claus, P., D'hooge, J., Bijnens, B., Strain and Strain Rate Imaging: A New Clinical Approach to Quantifying Regional Myocardial Function, J Am Soc Echocardiogr, 2004; 17 (7): 788-802.

Unser, M., A Review of Wavelets in Biomedical Applications, Proc. Of the IEEE, 1996; 84 (4): 626-638.

Voigt, J.U. and Flachskampf, F.A., Strain and Strain Rate Imaging - New and Clinically Relevant Echo Parameters of Regional Myocardial Function, Z. Kardiol, 2004; 93: 249-258.

Voigt JU, Nixdorff U, Bogdan R, Exner B, Schmiedehausen K, Platsch G, Kuwert T, Daniel WG, Flachskampf FA, Comparison of deformation imaging and velocity imaging for detecting regional inducible ischaemia during dobutamine stress echocardiography. Eur Heart J, 2004; 25 (17):1517-1525.

Weidemann, F., Dommke, C., Bijnens, B., Claus, P., D'hooge, J., Mertens, P., Verbeken, E., Maes, A., Van de Werf, F., De Scheerder, I., Sutherland, G.R., Defining the Transmurality of a Chronic Myocardial Infarction by Ultrasonic Strain-Rate Imaging, Circulation, 2003; 107: 883-888.

Yip, G., Abraham, T., Belohlavek, M., Khandheria, B., Clinical Applications of Strain Rate Imaging, J Am Soc Echocardiogr, 2003; 16 (12): 1334-1342.

Yip, G., Khandheria, B., Belohlavek, M., Pislaru, C., Seward, J., Bailey, K., Tajik, A.J., Pellikka, P., Abraham, T., Strain Echocardiography Tracks Dobutamine-Induced Decrease in Regional Myocardial Perfusion in Nonocclusive Coronary Stenosis, J Am Col Cardiol, 2004; 44:1664-1671.

Zwanenburg, J.J.M., Götte, M.J.W., Marcus, J.T., Kuijer, J.P.A., Knaapen, P., Heethaar, R.M., van Rossum, A.C., Propagation of Onset and Peak Time of Myocardial Shortening in Ischemic Versus Nonischemic Cardiomyopathy Assessment by Magnetic Resonance Imaging Myocardial Tagging, J Am Coll Cardiol 2005; 46: 2215-2222.

2

Strain Measurements Relative to Normal State Enhance the Ability to Detect Non-Transmural Myocardial Infarction

Noa Bachner-Hinenzon[1,*], Offir Ertracht[2,3,*], Zvi Vered[4,5], Marina Leitman[4,5], Nir Zagury[1], Ofer Binah[2,3] and Dan Adam[1]

[1]Faculty of Biomedical Engineering
[2]Department of Physiology
[3]Ruth and Bruce Rappaport Faculty of Medicine, Rappaport Family Institute for Research in the Medical Sciences Technion-Israel Institute of Technology, Haifa,
[4]Department of Cardiology, Assaf Harofeh Medical Center, Zerifin,
[5]Sackler School of Medicine Tel Aviv University
Israel

1. Introduction

Nowadays, diagnosis of heart pathologies in the clinic is mostly performed non-invasively by eyeballing the B-mode echocardiography cines and evaluating the ejection fraction and the regional wall motion. Yet, myocardial infarction (MI) usually causes reduced regional wall motion. During its diagnosis the echocardiographer grades the movement of each myocardial segment in order to estimate its function (Schiller et al., 1989). The disadvantage in this estimation is that it is subjective, and the echocardiographer must be experienced (Picano et al., 1991). As a result, echocardiographers provide different scoring to the same patient (Liel-Cohen et al., 2010). Hence, major efforts are invested in constructing automatic tools for wall motion estimation, as Speckle Tracking Echocardiography (STE).

The STE is an angle-independent, cost-effective and available tool, developed for automatic evaluation of left ventricular (LV) regional function (Leitman et al., 2004, Liel-Cohen et al., 2010, Reisner et al., 2004). The STE program processes standard echocardiographic two dimensional (2D) gray-scale cine loops and tracks the speckle movement frame-by-frame (Rappaport et al., 2006). Consequently, the regional myocardial velocities are calculated and local strain parameters are provided. During MI, these local strain parameters, calculated in the longitudinal, circumferential and radial orientations, were found to be strongly correlated to MI size (Fu et al., 2009, Gjesdal et al., 2007, 2008, Migrino et al., 2007, 2008). Furthermore, the detection of large MI was found to be very reliable (Gjesdal et al., 2008, Migrino et al., 2007). Yet, the detection of small non-transmural MI requires improvement. Since it is important to achieve early detection of non-transmural MI, in the present study we investigated the

---

[*]These authors contributed equally to the manuscript

hypothesis that taking into consideration the natural heterogeneity of the strain measurements among the different segments would enhance the differentiation between non-transmural MI and non-MI areas. This kind of measurement is particularly suitable for stress-echocardiography since this prevalent clinical study includes comparison of the echo results at stress to those at baseline, and is specified for the detection of minor ischemia.

In this study 13 rats in the acute phase of MI (24 hours) and 8 sham operated rats were scanned, and their short axis cines were analyzed by a STE program. Subsequently, the Radial Strain (S_R) and Circumferential Strain (S_C) were evaluated at 6 myocardial segments. The first step was to decipher the natural heterogeneity at normal state by measuring the peak systolic strain values for each segment averaged over the 21 rats. The second step was to measure the segmental peak systolic strain values conventionally and relatively to normal state. Subsequently, the strain values were compared to the MI size and location.

2. Methods

Animal experiments were conducted according to the institutional animal ethical committee guidelines (ethics number: IL-101-10-2007) in 3 month old adult male Sprague-Dawley rats weighing 310-340 gr. Rats were maintained at the Experimental Surgical Unit of the Technion, and fed on normal rodent chow diet, with tap water ad libitum, according to the Technion guidelines for animal care. The rats were housed at a constant temperature (21°C) and relative humidity (60%) under a regular light/dark schedule (light 6:00 AM to 6:00 PM).

In this study 21 adult male Sprague-Dawley rats were investigated. Thirteen rats underwent myocardial ischemia and reperfusion surgery and 8 rats served as a corresponding sham group.

2.1 Surgical procedure

Male Sprague-Dawley rats were randomly divided into 2 groups. All rats were anesthetized with a combination of 87 mg/kg ketamine and 13 mg/kg xylazine mixture. The animals were intubated and mechanically ventilated using a Columbus Instruments small-animal mechanical respirator (Columbus Instruments 950 North Hague Av. Columbus, OH. USA) at a rate of 80-90 cycles per minute with a tidal volume of 1-2 ml/100 gr. Using a left thoracotomy, the chest was opened, the pericardial sac dissected, and the heart exposed. A single stitch was placed through the myocardium at a depth slightly greater than the perceived level of the left anterior descending artery (LAD) while taking care not to puncture the ventricular chamber (Bhindi et al., 2006, Hale et al., 2005). In the first group, which included 13 rats, the suture was tightened by a loop that allowed its rapid opening. Half an hour after the occlusion the suture was rapidly opened in order to resume blood flow through the LAD. In the second group, which included 8 rats, the thread was placed through the myocardium but it was not tied up; however, the chest remained opened for half an hour. Finally, the chest was closed and the animal was allowed to recover.

2.2 Echocardiographic measurements

Echocardiographic transthoratic scans were performed at baseline and at 24 hours of reperfusion. For the baseline and 24 hours post-MI echocardiographic scans, animals were lightly sedated by an intraperitoneal injection of 29 mg/kg ketamine and 4.3 mg/kg xylazine mixture. Their chest was shaved and the scan was performed. During the scan, rats were placed in a left lateral decubitus position. The scan was performed via a commercially available echo-scanner - Vivid™ *i* ultrasound cardiovascular system (GE Healthcare Inc. Israel) using a 10S phased array pediatric transducer and a cardiac application. The transmission frequency was 10 MHz, the depth was 2.5 cm and the frame rate was 225-350 frames per second. The measurements included 2 short axis cross-sections at the Apical (AP) level and the Papillary Muscles (PM) level.

2.3 Speckle tracking echocardiography

The short axis ultrasound cines were post-processed by an enhanced STE program that measures the regional LV function at 6 segments with high spatial resolution (Bachner-Hinenzon et al., 2010, 2011). The program utilizes a commercial STE program called '2D-strain' (EchoPAC Dimension '08, GE Healthcare Inc., Norway). The commercial program requests the user to mark the endocardial border and to choose the width of the myocardium, imposes a grid of points in the assigned region, and tracks the speckles near the points and evaluates their velocities at each frame (Rappaport et al., 2006). The myocardial velocities were not processed by the built-in smoothing of the commercial program, but were de-noised by a 3D wavelet representation (MATLAB software, MathWorks Inc. USA), thereby increasing the spatial resolution of the calculated functional measurements (Bachner-Hinenzon et al., 2010). Subsequently, the Radial Strain (S_R) and Circumferential Strain (S_C) were evaluated at 6 segments. The strain parameters were measured from the de-noised velocities of each point on the grid. The S_R was calculated from the de-noised radial velocity, and the S_C and LV rotation were calculated from the de-noised circumferential velocity. Thereafter, the peak systolic values of the LV rotation S_R and S_C were calculated. The LV rotation is the rotation in degrees from the diastolic state. The S_C and S_R were measured in % from the diastolic state. End diastole is defined as the time just before the QRS complex in the ECG signal. The S_C and S_R were also calculated for each segment relatively to the normal values, as % of difference from the average baseline value divided by the average baseline value for each segment separately to create the 'S_C rel' and 'S_R rel'. For example, if the average normal strain was 14% at a specific segment, and the value decreased to 7%, the relative value was -50%.

2.4 Determination of MI size

The method used here for the assessment of the tissue viability, includes the use of two stains: (1) Evan's blue is used to delineate the Area At Risk (AAR), which is the area that was physically ligated 24 hours previously. (2) Triphenyltetrazolium Chloride (TTC), which delineates the MI area. Twenty four hrs post-surgery, the animals were re-anesthetized, intubated, and ventilated according to the protocol used in the surgery. The chest was opened to expose the heart. 1.5% Evan's blue solution (in PBS) was retrogradely injected through the aorta into the LV. The staining agent was then perfused through the open coronary arteries into the cardiac muscle, but not through the ligated artery and its downstream branches, delineating in dark blue the non-MI area of the heart. The heart was then removed and rinsed, in normal cold saline, of the excess Evan's blue and transferred to -80°C for 5-6 min and sliced manually into 7 transverse slices. The slices were dipped in 1% TTC solution (in DDW pH=7.4) at 37°C for 20 min, and then rinsed in PBS of the excess TTC solution, and weighted (Ojha et al., 2008, Reinhardt et al., 1993). To improve the delineation of the different colours, the slices were kept at 4°C in PBS + sodium azide (0.01%), as preservative, for 3 weeks (Pitts et al., 2007). Subsequently, the slices were placed on top of a light table and photographed on both sides. Using the ImageJ software (NIH, Bethesda, MD, USA http://rsb.info.nih.gov/ij) the pictures were analyzed, and the different areas were delineated. Using the weights of the slices and the percentages of the different colored areas of each slice, we calculated the percent of non-MI cardiac muscle (dark blue), area at risk (red and white) and infarcted area (white). The slices were numbered from 1 to 7 from apex to atria. The slices that matched the AP and PM levels of short axis scans were slices number 3 and 4, respectively. These slices were divided to 6 equal radial segments: inferior septum, anterior septum, anterior wall, lateral wall, posterior wall and inferior wall. Each segment was classified as normal or damaged with transmural or non-transmural MI, according to the TTC stain.

2.5 Statistical analysis

All variables were expressed by the mean ± SEM. Paired t-test was performed in order to compare the MI size at the AP and PM levels. One-way analysis of variance (ANOVA) for unequal variance was used to compare MI size (normal/transmural/non-transmural) to the peak systolic strains (S_C, S_R, S_C rel, S_R rel). One-way ANOVA for unequal variance was also used in order to compare between the peak systolic strain of the different segments for the baseline and 24 hours of reperfusion results. Two-way repeated measures ANOVA was used to compare the peak systolic strains (S_C, S_R) at different time points for the MI and sham groups. Receiver operating characteristics (ROC) method was used in order to predict transmural MI from all other segments (normal and non-transmural). The ROC method was also used in order to predict non-transmural MI from the normal segments. The area under the ROC curves was measured and compared in order to test whether the difference between the ROC curves was significant.

3. Results

3.1 MI size

In 156 segments of the AP and PM levels of the 13 MI rats the determination of MI size by the TTC staining yielded the following results: 91 normal segments, 22 non-transmural MI and 43 transmural MI segments. The transmural MI occurred mostly at the anterior and lateral walls (in 10 out of 13 rats), while non-transmural MIs were visualized at the posterior and inferior walls (in 9 out of 13 rats). The total MI size at the AP level was 23±13 % (min 0%, max 47%), and at the PM level was 19±8 % (min 7%, max 34%), while there was no significant difference in the MI size between the two levels. The results for the sham group showed 86 normal segments for the 8 sham rats.

3.2 Strain measurements at baseline

Heterogeneity of the peak systolic strains was defined as a significant difference between the measured values at the different segments. Typical strain maps at the normal state, which are presented in Fig. 1A, illustrate the heterogeneity of the S_R and S_C. The average baseline values of S_C and S_R for 21 rats are presented in Fig. 1B and Fig. 1C, respectively. One way ANOVA test for the normal peak systolic S_C values demonstrate that the heterogeneity of the peak systolic values at the AP level is significant (P<0.001), while this heterogeneity is no longer significant at the PM level (P=0.06, N.S). Yet, it can be seen that the pattern of the peak systolic S_C lines in Fig. 1B are similar for the AP and PM levels. One way ANOVA test for the peak systolic S_R values demonstrate that the heterogeneity of the peak systolic S_R is significant at both AP and PM levels (P<0.001). Both AP and PM levels show lower S_R at the inferior septum and anterior septum, and the values are higher for the lateral wall (P<0.05).

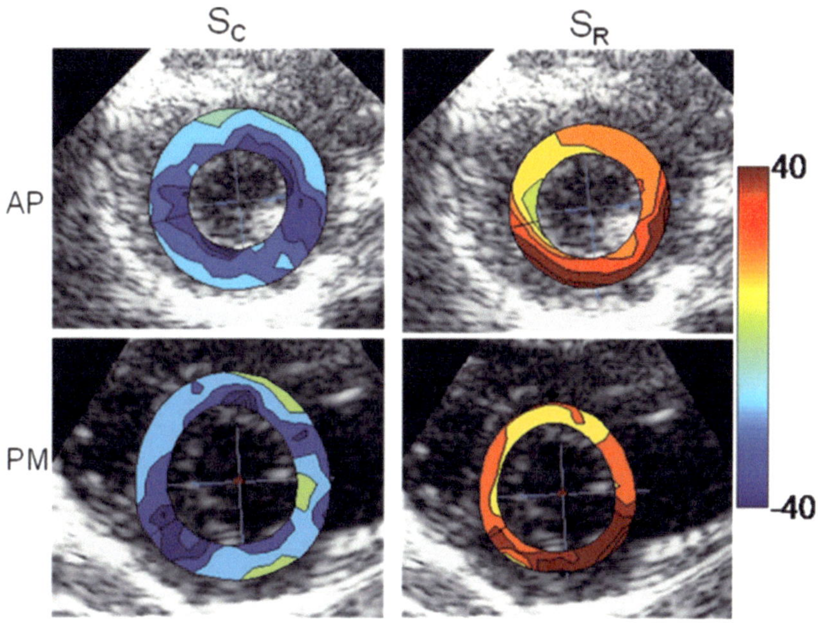

1A.

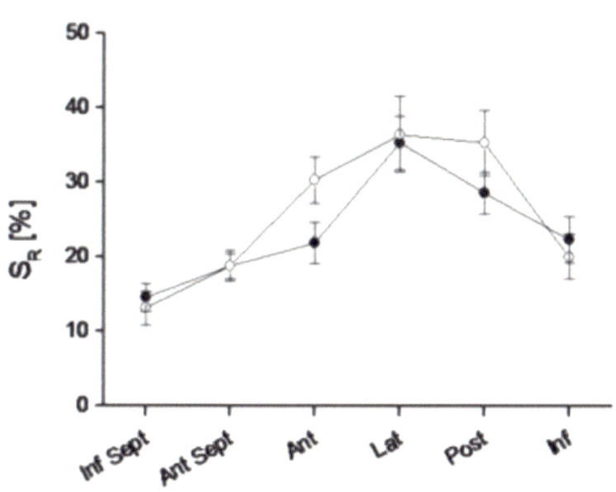

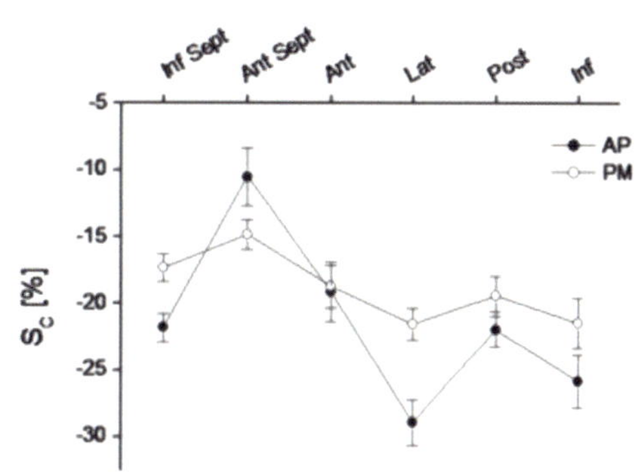

1B. 1C.

Fig. 1. The heterogeneity of normal strain values in % from diastolic state. Typical maps of end-systolic circumferential (S_C) and radial (S_R) strains at the apical (AP) and papillary muscles (PM) levels (1A). Blue color is defined as negative and red as positive. Peak systolic S_C (1B) and S_R (1C) at the different segments of the AP and PM levels averaged over 21 rats.

The global LV rotation was 4.9±0.5 deg counterclockwise at the AP level and 1.6±0.6 deg counterclockwise at the PM level.

3.3 Segmental strain measurements as function of time post-MI

Examples of strain maps of peak systolic values of S_C and S_R are depicted in Fig. 2 for slices of sham, non-transmural MI, and transmural MI. The changes in peak systolic S_C and S_R of both MI and sham groups at baseline and 24 hours of reperfusion are demonstrated in Fig. 3A-D. Twenty four hours after reperfusion, the peak systolic S_C and S_R were significantly decreased at the free wall in both AP and PM levels (Figs. 3A-D, $P<0.05$), while the septum maintained normal values.

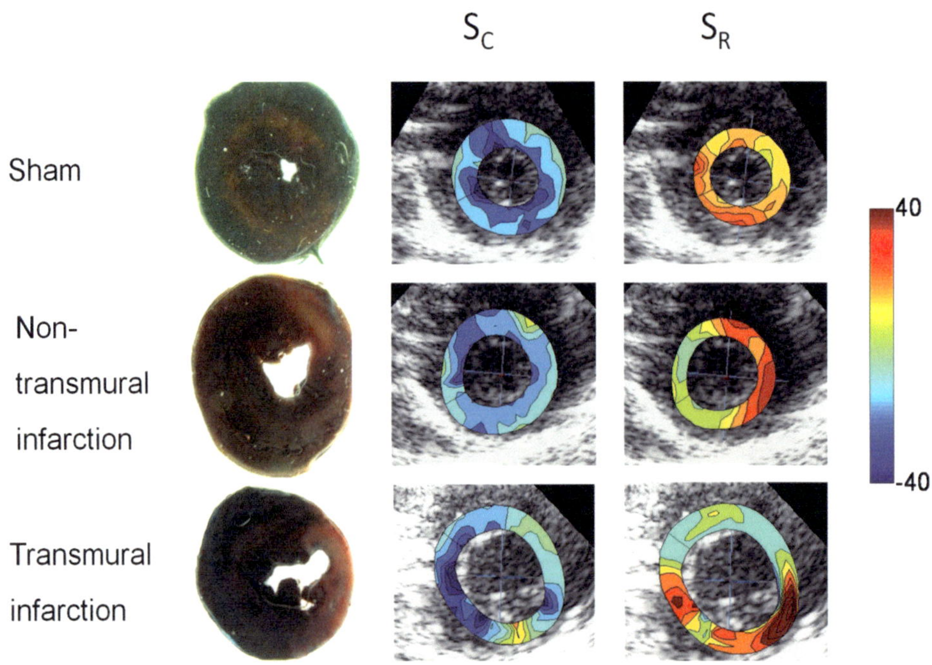

Fig. 2. Examples of TTC staining and end-systolic strain maps (% from diastolic state) for sham, non-transmural MI and transmural MI rats. Blue color is defined as negative and red as positive. In the example of sham rat it is well seen that the papillary muscles (PM) level is injured even though there was no LAD occlusion. In the non-transmural example, the yellow positive S_C is the MI area. This area looks rather normal in the S_R map. In the transmural example, green color of S_C is zero, and light blue of S_R is the thinning of the myocardium.

3.4 Strain measurements of MI rats versus sham rats

The peak systolic S_C values of the MI group decreased from normal values at the free wall of the AP and PM levels (Fig. 3A, 3C ,$P<0.05$). However, the peak systolic S_C values of the sham group decreased only at the lateral wall of the AP level (Fig. 3A, $P<0.05$), and posterior wall of the PM level (Fig. 3C, $P<0.01$), while there was no significant difference in the peak systolic S_C values between the MI and sham rats in these segments. The peak systolic S_C at the PM level maintained normal values for the sham group except for a slight reduction at the posterior wall (Fig. 3C, $P<0.01$).

The values of peak systolic S_R for the MI rats at the AP level at the anterior and lateral walls were smaller at 24 hours of reperfusion than baseline (Fig. 3B, $P<0.001$); however, the same reduction was noticed at the anterior wall of the sham group (Fig. 3B). Thus, only the peak systolic S_R of the lateral wall was significantly lower for the MI rats ($P<0.05$). At the PM level no significant difference was found in the peak systolic S_R between the sham group and the MI group (Fig. 3D). In both groups the peak systolic S_R became smaller at the lateral, posterior and inferior walls (Fig. 3D , $P<0.01$).

In both MI and sham groups, the LV rotation was depressed after surgery. Ten minutes after reperfusion, the LV apical rotations of the MI and sham groups were 0.2±0.4 deg and -1.1±1.4 deg, respectively. Twenty four hours after reperfusion, the LV rotations at the AP level of the MI and sham groups were 0.0±0.5 deg and -0.3±0.6 deg, respectively.

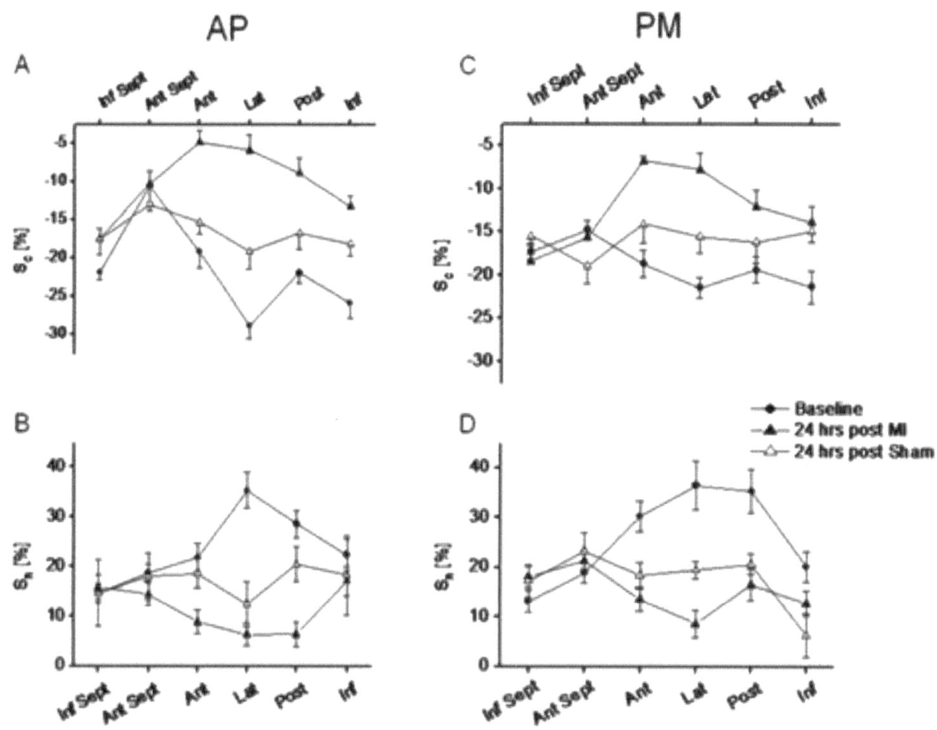

Fig. 3. Segmental circumferential strain (S_C) at the apical and papillary muscles levels as function of time (baseline and 24 hours of reperfusion) for the MI group and for the sham group (3A, 3C). Segmental radial strain (S_R) at the apical and papillary muscles levels as function of time for the MI group and for the sham group (3B, 3D).

3.5 Strain measurements versus MI size

Linear regression was performed between the MI size and the peak systolic S_C and S_R for both AP and PM levels. The linear regression was performed between the size of the MI (as % of area from the total area of the cross-section) and the peak systolic S_C and S_R averaged over the anterior, lateral and posterior segments of the same cross-section (MI area). Subsequently, the linear regression was performed between the cross-sectional MI size and the peak systolic S_C and S_R averaged over the inferior septum, anterior septum and inferior wall (non-MI area). This analysis revealed high correlation between the MI size and the peak systolic strains of the MI area (Fig. 4). The correlation was higher at the AP level (S_C R2=0.89, S_R R2=0.73) than at the PM level (S_C R2=0.73, S_R R2=0.67) as seen in Fig. 4. In contrast, no correlation was found between the peak systolic S_C and S_R of the non-MI area and the MI size (AP: S_C R2=0.25, S_R R2=0.02, PM: S_C R2=0.00, S_R R2=0.05) (data not shown). Finally, there was no correlation between the peak systolic S_C and S_R of the MI area and the non-MI area (AP: S_C R2=0.27, S_R R2=0.06, PM: S_C R2=0.24, S_R R2=0.06); see discussion.

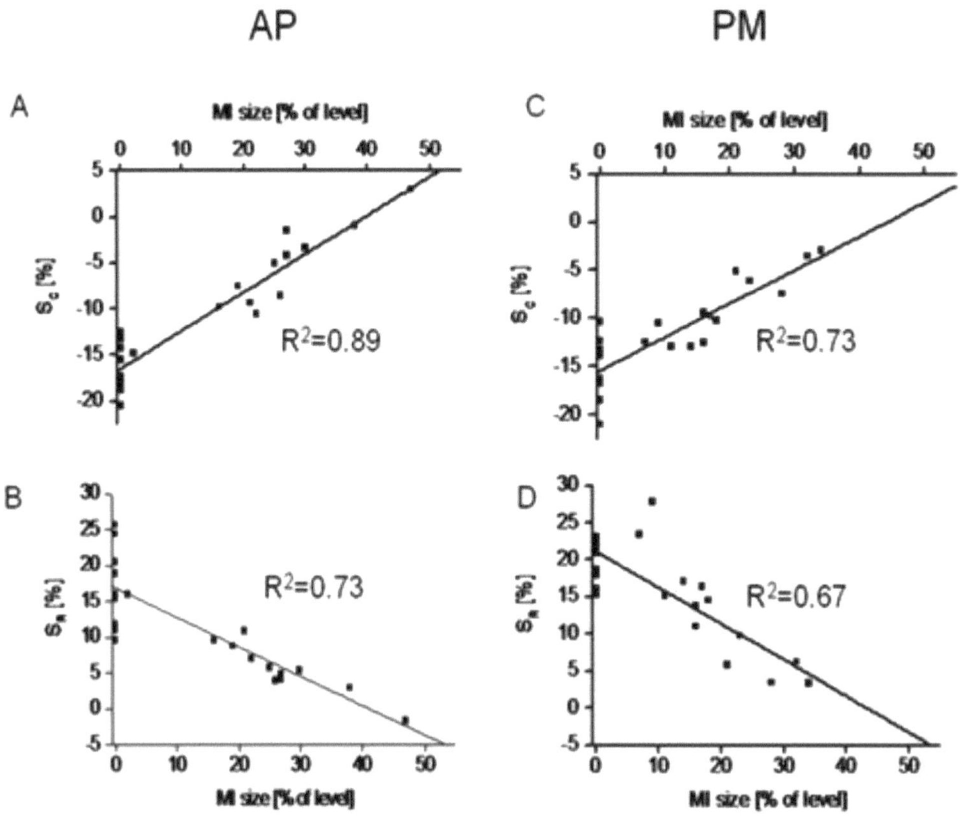

Fig. 4. Scatter plot and linear regression of apical peak systolic circumferential (S_C, 4A) and radial (S_R, 4B) strains versus MI size. Scatter plot and linear regression of peak systolic circumferential (S_C, 4C) and radial (S_R, 4D) strains at the papillary muscles level versus MI size. The strains are averaged over the anterior, lateral and posterior walls, and the MI size is measured per level.

Next, statistical analysis was performed to see whether there is a significant difference between the strain measurements of normal, non-transmural and transmural MI. As expected, segments with transmural MI demonstrated significantly lower peak systolic strain values than the normal segments in both AP and PM levels (Fig. 5, P<0.001). Furthermore, the segments with transmural MI could be distinguished from non-transmural MI segments by utilizing peak systolic S_C values as seen in Fig. 5A and Fig. 5E (AP P<0.01,

PM P<0.001). However, it was possible to do so with S_R values only at the PM level, as seen in Fig. 5F (P<0.01). The non-transmural MI segments could be distinguished from the normal segments at the PM level only by using peak systolic S_C values as seen in Fig. 5E (P<0.001), and not by using peak systolic S_R values (Fig. 5F). At the AP level it was impossible to distinguish the non-transmural MI segments from the normal segments by using peak systolic S_C and S_R as seen in Figs. 5A and 5B, respectively.

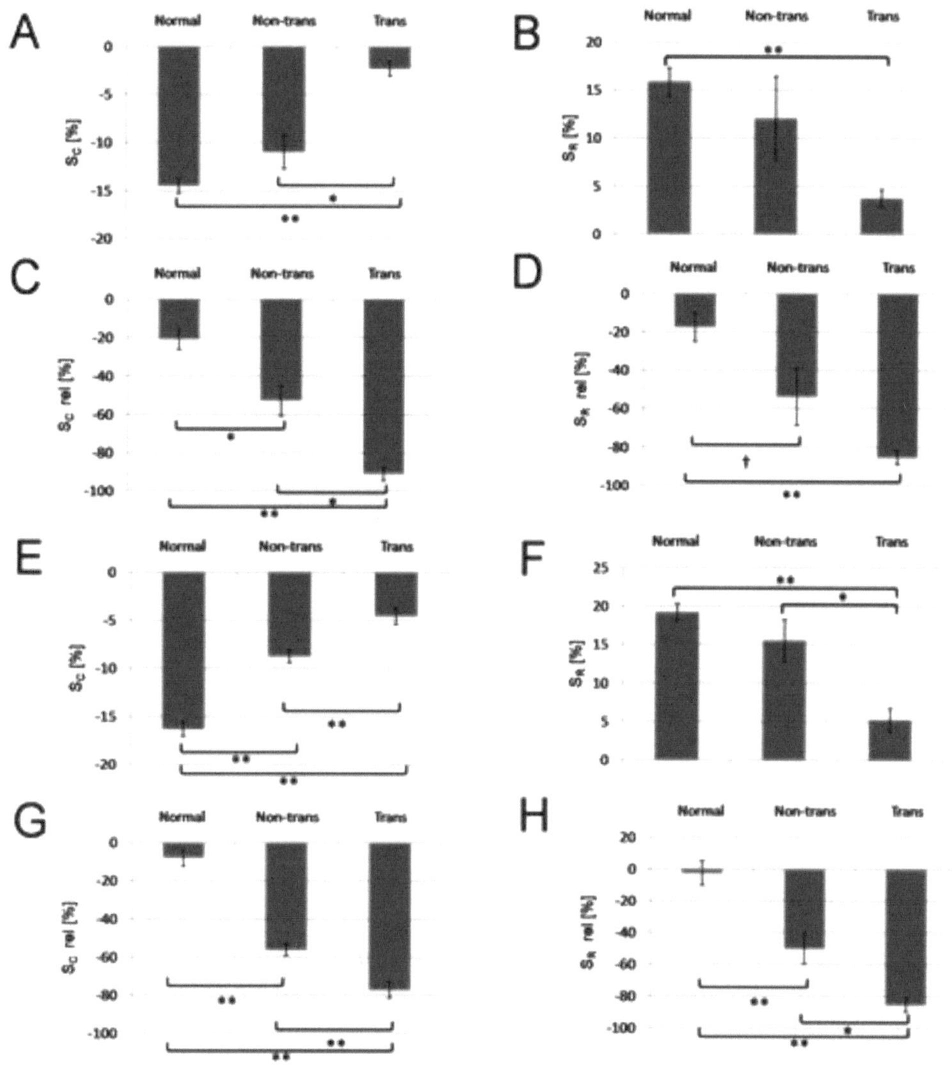

Fig. 5. Apical peak systolic circumferential (S_C, 5A) and radial (S_R, 5B) strains versus MI size (normal, transmural and non-transmural). Apical peak systolic circumferential (S_C rel, 5C) and radial (S_R rel, 5D) strains relative to normal state versus MI size. Peak systolic circumferential (S_C, 5E) and radial (S_R, 5F) strains at the papillary muscles level versus MI size. Peak systolic circumferential (S_C rel, 5G) and radial (S_R rel, 5H) strains relative to normal state at the papillary muscles level versus MI size. *P<0.01, **P<0.001, †P<0.05.

3.6 Strain measurements relative to normal state values

The peak systolic S_C and S_R relative to normal state values distinguished non-transmural MI from normal segments at the AP (Fig. 5C and Fig. 5D) and PM (Fig. 5G and Fig. 5H) levels (S_C rel P=0.01, S_R rel P<0.05, PM: S_C rel P<0.001, S_R rel P<0.001), while it was impossible at the AP level (Figs. 5A and 5B), and was possible at the PM level only by peak systolic S_C (Fig. 5E).

In order to compare between the peak systolic S_C and S_R and their values relative to normal state (peak systolic S_C rel and S_R rel) a ROC method was utilized and the areas under the curves were compared (Fig 6). The results are summarized in Table 1. In all cases the S_C relative to its normal state values provided the best results; however, in the detection of transmural MI, there is no significant difference between S_C relative to normal state and peak systolic S_C. The comparison between ROC curves, analyzing the detection of transmural MI at the AP level, appears in Fig. 6A. When studying the capabilities of detecting non-transmural MI, the S_C relative to its normal state values provided better results at the apex as seen in Fig. 6B (P<0.01), however, there was no significant difference in the capability of detection at the PM level. The detection of non-transmural MI by peak systolic S_R was enhanced by utilizing the measurement of peak systolic S_R relative to its normal state in both AP and PM levels. Nevertheless, at the PM level this detection was significantly less effective than the detection by peak systolic S_C as seen in Table 1 (P<0.05).

		Transmural MI		Non-transmural MI	
Parameter		AP	PM	AP	PM
S_C	Sensitivity	96 %, -7.5 %	100%, -9.4%	88%, -13.4%	100%, -13.4%
	Specificity	90%, -7.5 %	80%, -9.4%	65%, -13.4%	84%, -13.4%
S_R	Sensitivity	84%, 7.7%	81%, 7.5%	100%, 11.1%	57%, 10.3%
	Specificity	80%, 7.7%	98%, 7.5%	72%, 11.1%	89%, 10.3%
S_C rel	Sensitivity	**100%, -68.5%**	**100%, -56.9%**	**88%, -50.7%, ***	**100%, -41.1%**
	Specificity	**96%, -68.5%**	**83%, -56.9%**	**84%, -50.7%, ***	**87%, -41.1%**
S_R rel	Sensitivity	77%, -77.3%, †	82%, -77.3%	100%, -58.1%, *	64%, -48.5%, †
	Specificity	92%, -77.3%, †	97%, -77.3%	81%, -58.1%, *	84%, -48.5%, †

S_C and S_R are the peak systolic values. S_C rel and S_R rel are the peak systolic values relative to normal state. Specificity and sensitivity values appear on the left and their cut-off value appears on the right. Significant difference of ROC curves between the parameter and the parameter relative to normal state appears in the table as *P<0.01, † P<0.05.

Table 1. Specificity and sensitivity of peak systolic S_C and S_R

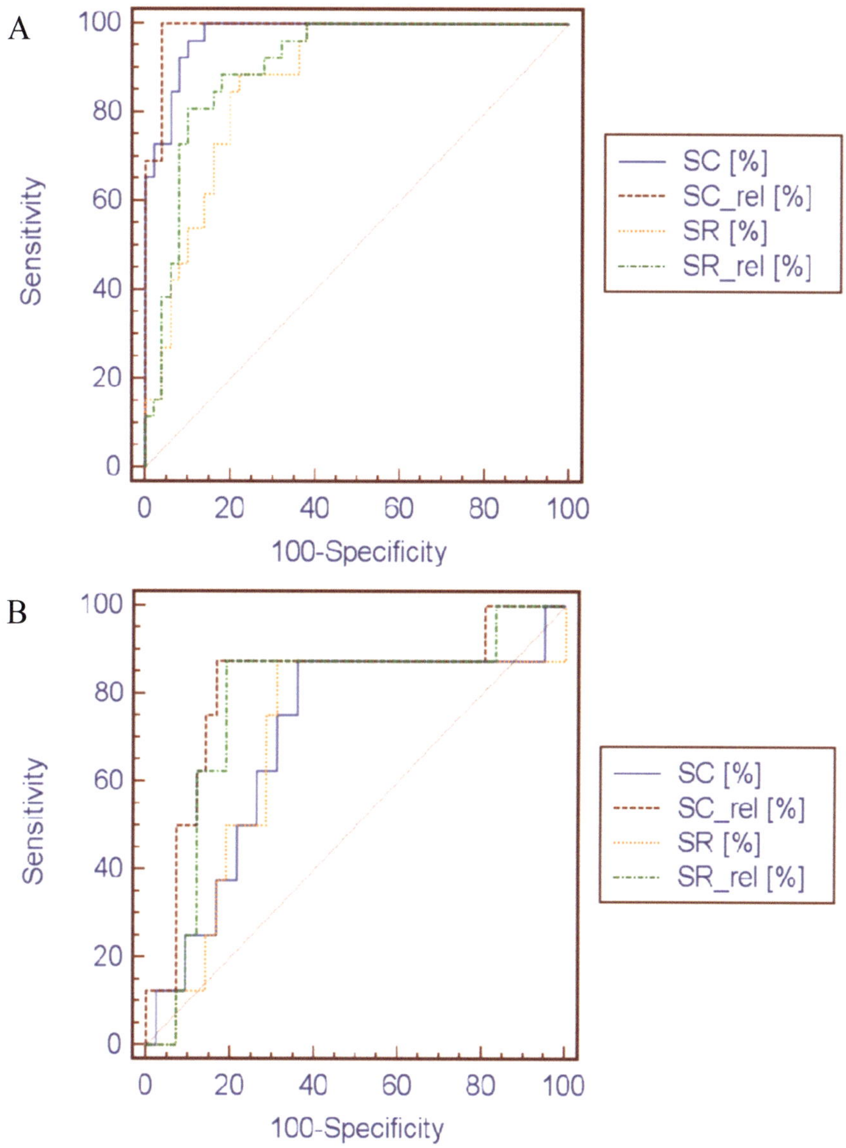

Fig. 6. Receiver operating characteristics curve of apical circumferential (S_C) and radial (S_R) strains and apical circumferential and radial strains relative to normal state (S_C rel, S_R rel) in the detection of transmural MI (6A) and non-transmural MI (6B). In the detection of non-transmural MI there is a significant difference between the S_C and S_R curves and the S_C rel and S_R rel curves ($P<0.01$).

4. Discussion

In the present study we tested the hypothesis that taking into consideration the natural heterogeneity of the strain measurements among the different segments would enhance the differentiation between non-transmural MI and non-MI areas. Our main findings were: 1) In normal rats, while peak systolic S_C is heterogeneous at the AP level, the heterogeneity is not statistically significant at the PM level. 2) In normal rats, peak systolic S_R is heterogeneous at both AP and PM short axis levels. 3) Peak systolic S_C is more sensitive to the presence of MI than peak systolic S_R. 4) Peak systolic S_C value, when calculated relatively to normal values (% of reduction from normal value) is more sensitive to the presence of non-transmural MI than the conventional peak systolic S_C value. 5) Peak systolic strains (S_C and S_R) at the MI areas have high correlation to MI size. 6) Peak systolic strains (S_C and S_R) at remote areas from the MI do not correlate to MI size. 7) Sham operated rats demonstrated lower strain values mostly at the anterior and lateral walls probably due to stunning of the myocardium due to the insertion of the needle (The needle was inserted and the thread was placed through the myocardium but it was not tied up). 8) LV apical rotation was severely depressed in both MI and sham rats.

In this study the heterogeneity of the peak systolic S_C and S_R was demonstrated in normal rats. Moreover, it was shown that this heterogeneity should be taken into account when attempting to detect non-transmural MI. When the normal heterogeneity of the strain values was not taken into consideration, normal segments with lower strain values were classified as non-transmural MI (false positive), and thus the specificity of the classification of non-transmural MI was only 65% and 69%, when using peak systolic S_C and S_R, respectively (Table 1). Measuring the peak systolic S_C and S_R values relatively to normal values caused an increase of the correct classification of the non-transmural MI, and the specificity was increased to 84% and 79%, when using peak systolic S_C and S_R relative to normal values, respectively. It is important to mention that the peak systolic strain for each segment was measured relatively to the average normal value of 21 rats and not relatively to its own baseline value, which may allow a more general implementation of the technique. Such a sensitive regional analysis of the strain measurements was possible due to the utilization of a novel wavelet de-noising process, which was applied to the myocardial velocities after the speckle tracking, instead of the built-in smoothing process of the commercial STE program.

Detection of MI by STE was previously reported by Gjesdal et al., who analyzed the global longitudinal and circumferential strains of patients with chronic ischemic heart disease (Gjesdal et al., 2007, 2008). The detection of MI mass was found to be precise when by utilizing global longitudinal and circumferential strains (Gjesdal et al., 2008). However, in the present study, we propose to enhance the detection, specifically of non-transmural MI, by taking into consideration the normal segmental heterogeneity. The normal segmental heterogeneity of the longitudinal strain was studied by Marwick et al., who performed the measurements over 250 normal subjects (Marwick et al., 2009). Marwick et al. found peak systolic longitudinal strain of -13.7±4.0 % at the basal septum, while the global longitudinal strain value of -15.3±1.9% was considered by Gjesdal et al. as a value signifying a medium sized MI. Thus, normal segments with lower strain values might be classified by mistake as an infarcted area. It is important to note that taking into consideration the heterogeneity of the normal values is relevant only if the heterogeneity is significant. The heterogeneity of the peak systolic S_C at the PM level is not statistically significant. Thus, taking into consideration the normal values influences only the measurement peak systolic S_C values of the AP level.

The detection of transmural MI does not require normalization to baseline. The strain values are severely reduced, and in some cases the myocardium even undergoes stretching instead of contraction during diastole, as seen in the transmural MI example in Fig. 2 and in the study of Migrino et al. (Migrino et al., 2007). In this study we found that the peak systolic S_C is a better detector of transmural MI than peak systolic S_R ($P<0.05$). Gjesdal et al. (Gjesdal et al., 2008)and Popović et al. (Popović et al., 2007)) also reported better detection of transmural MI by S_C than by S_R (Gjesdal et al., 2008); however Migrino et al. reported that S_R is a better predictor of transmural MI (Migrino et al., 2007, 2008). The S_R cannot be a better predictor of transmural MI since the STE commercial program contains stronger spatial smoothing at the radial direction than that at the circumferential direction. This phenomenon is demonstrated by comparing Figs. 2B and 2C in Popović et al. In their Fig. 2B there was heterogeneity in the segmental peak systolic S_C in normal and MI states. In contrast, no heterogeneity was seen by the S_R in Fig. 2C (Popović et al., 2007). The normal heterogeneity of the peak systolic S_R that was measured in our present study (Fig. 1C) can be seen by eyeballing the short-axis scans. Another influence of the smoothing process is the correlation between the strain at the MI areas and the non-MI areas. Migrino et al. reported a correlation of 0.82 between end systolic S_R of the MI and periinfarct areas. Moreover, they reported a correlation of 0.64 between end systolic S_R of the MI and remote areas (Migrino et al., 2008). These strong correlations, which occur due to the smoothing process of the commercial program, do not occur when using the wavelet de-noising process that we propose in this study. The correlation between the non-MI area and the MI area in this study was 0.24 for the S_C and 0.06 for the S_R at the PM level. This result demonstrates that the peak systolic S_R of the remote areas at 24 hours of reperfusion do not correlate to the MI size. This result was not surprising since a previous Doppler echocardiography study has already reported that remote areas can show normal contractility (Vartdal et al., 2007).

4.1 Study limitations

The main limitation of the wavelet de-noising process used here is its sensitivity to artifacts at the B-mode cines. The commercial program compensates for artifacts, such as areas in which the myocardium is shaded by the ribs (black area), by imposing there the averaged values. The wavelet de-noising shows no movement in these areas while the commercial program depicts normal movement. Thus, when applying the wavelet de-noising algorithm used here, it is important to include only ultrasound cines with good image quality.

5. Conclusions

Based on our results we concluded that in the rat model a natural heterogeneity among the strain values exists. Taking into consideration this normal heterogeneity, by measuring the strains relatively to the normal values, improves the detection of non-transmural MI. This kind of measurement is particularly suitable for stress-echocardiography, which includes comparison of the echo results at stress to those at baseline, and is specified for the detection of minor ischemia.

In humans, this kind of study should be performed in the future by normalizing the longitudinal strain relative to baseline and not the circumferential strain as performed here, since the heterogeneity of the strain in humans mostly exists at the longitudinal direction from base to apex (Bachner-Hinenzon et al., 2010).

6. Acknowledgments

This work was supported by the Chief Scientist, the Ministry of Industry and Commerce Magneton project, the Technion VP for Research and the Alfred Mann Institute at the Technion (AMIT).

7. References

Bachner-Hinenzon N Ertracht O, Lysiansky M, Binah O, Adam D. Layer-specific assessment of left ventricular function by utilizing wavelet de-noising: A validation study. Med Biol Eng Comput. 2011 Jan;49(1):3-13. Epub 2010 Jul 20.

Bachner-Hinenzon N, Ertracht O, Leitman M, Vered Z, Shimoni S, Beeri R, Binah O, Adam D. Layer-specific strain analysis by speckle tracking echocardiography reveals differences in left ventricular function between rats and humans. Am J Physiol Heart Circ Physiol. 2010 Sep;299(3):H664-72. Epub 2010 Jul 2.

Bhindi R, Witting PK, McMahon AC, Khachigian LM, Lowe HC. Rat models of myocardial infarction. Pathogenetic insights and clinical relevance. Thromb Haemost. 96(5):602-10, 2006.Review.

Fu Q, Xie M, Wang J, Wang X, Lv Q, Lu X, Fang L, Chang L. Assessment of regional left ventricular myocardial function in rats after acute occlusion of left anterior descending artery by two-dimensional speckle tracking imaging. J Huazhong Univ Sci Technolog Med Sci. 29(6):786-90, 2009.

Gjesdal O, Helle-Valle T, Hopp E, Lunde K, Vartdal T, Aakhus S, Smith HJ, Ihlen H, Edvardsen T. Noninvasive separation of large, medium, and small myocardial infarcts in survivors of reperfused ST-elevation myocardial infarction: a comprehensive tissue Doppler and speckle-tracking echocardiography study. Circ Cardiovasc Imaging. 1(3):189-96, 2008.

Gjesdal O, Hopp E, Vartdal T, Lunde K, Helle-Valle T, Aakhus S, Smith HJ, Ihlen H, Edvardsen T. Global longitudinal strain measured by two-dimensional speckle tracking echocardiography is closely related to myocardial infarct size in chronic ischaemic heart disease. Clin Sci (Lond). 113(6):287-96, 2007.

Hale SL, Sesti C, Kloner RA. Administration of erythropoietin fails to improve long-term healing or cardiac function after myocardial infarction in the rat. J Cardiovasc Pharmacol. 46(2):211-5, 2005.

Leitman M, Lysyansky P, Sidenko S, Shir V, Peleg E, Binenbaum M, Kaluski E, Krakover R, Vered Z. Two-dimensional strain-a novel software for real-time quantitative echocardiographic assessment of myocardial function. J Am Soc Echocardiogr. 17(10):1021-9, 2004.

Liel-Cohen N, Tsadok Y, Beeri R, Lysyansky P, Agmon Y, Feinberg MS, Fehske W, Gilon D, Hay I, Kuperstein R, Leitman M, Deutsch L, Rosenmann D, Sagie A, Shimoni S, Vaturi M, Friedman Z, Blondheim DS. A New Tool for Automatic Assessment of Segmental Wall Motion, Based on Longitudinal 2D Strain: A Multicenter Study by the Israeli Echocardiography Research Group. Circ Cardiovasc Imaging. 3(1):47-53, 2010.

Marwick TH, Leano RL, Brown J, Sun JP, Hoffmann R, Lysyansky P, Becker M, Thomas JD. Myocardial strain measurement with 2-dimensional speckle-tracking echocardiography: definition of normal range. JACC Cardiovasc Imaging. 2(1):80-4, 2009.

Migrino RQ, Zhu X, Morker M, Brahmbhatt T, Bright M, Zhao M. Myocardial dysfunction in the periinfarct and remote regions following anterior infarction in rats quantified by 2D radial strain echocardiography: an observational cohort study. Cardiovasc Ultrasound. 6:17, 2008.

Migrino RQ, Zhu X, Pajewski N, Brahmbhatt T, Hoffmann R, Zhao M. Assessment of segmental myocardial viability using regional 2-dimensional strain echocardiography. J Am Soc Echocardiogr. 20(4):342-51, 2007.

Notomi Y, Lysyansky P, Setser RM, Shiota T, Popovic ZB, Martin- Miklovic MG, Weaver JA, Oryszak SJ, Greenberg NL, White RD, Thomas JD. Measurement of ventricular torsion by two-dimensional ultrasound speckle tracking imaging. J. Am. Coll. Cardiol. 45: 2034–2041, 2005.

Ojha N, Roy S, Radtke J, Simonetti O, Gnyawali S, Zweier JL, Kuppusamy P, Sen CK. Characterization of the structural and functional changes in the myocardium following focal ischemia-reperfusion injury. Am J Physiol Heart Circ Physiol. 294(6):H2435-43, 2008.

Picano E, Lattanzi F, Orlandini A, Marini C, L'Abbate A. Stress echocardiography and the human factor: the importance of being expert. J Am Coll Cardiol. 17(3):666-9, 1991.

Pitts KR, Stiko A, Buetow B, Lott F, Guo P, Virca D, Toombs CF. Washout of heme-containing proteins dramatically improves tetrazolium-based infarct staining. J Pharmacol Toxicol Methods. 55(2):201-8, 2007.

Popović ZB, Benejam C, Bian J, Mal N, Drinko J, Lee K, Forudi F, Reeg R, Greenberg NL, Thomas JD, Penn MS. Speckle-tracking echocardiography correctly identifies segmental left ventricular dysfunction induced by scarring in a rat model of myocardial infarction. Am J Physiol Heart Circ Physiol. 292(6):H2809-16, 2007.

Rappaport D, Adam D, Lysyansky P, Riesner S. Assessment of myocardial Regional Strain and Strain Rate by Tissue Tracking in B-Mode Echocardiograms. Ultrasound in Med. & Biol., 32(8): 1181–1192, 2006.

Reinhardt CP, Weinstein H, Wironen J, Leppo JA. Effect of triphenyl tetrazolium chloride staining on the distribution of radiolabeled pharmaceuticals. J Nucl Med. 34(10):1722-7, 1993.

Reisner SA , Lysyansky P, Agmon Y, Mutlak D, Lessick J, Friedman Z. Global longitudinal strain: a novel index of left ventricular systolic function. J. Am. Soc. Echocardiogr. 17(6): 630-633. 2004.

Schiller NB, Shah PM, Crawford M, DeMaria A, Devereux R, Feigenbaum H, Gutgesell H, Reichek N, Sahn D, Schnittger I, et al. Recommendations for quantitation of the left ventricle by two-dimensional echocardiography. American Society of Echocardiography Committee on Standards, Subcommittee on Quantitation of Two-Dimensional Echocardiograms. J Am Soc Echocardiogr. 2(5):358-67, 1989.

Vartdal T, Brunvand H, Pettersen E, Smith HJ, Lyseggen E, Helle-Valle T, Skulstad H, Ihlen H, Edvardsen T. Early prediction of infarct size by strain Doppler echocardiography after coronary reperfusion. J Am Coll Cardiol. 24;49(16):1715-, 2007.

3

Speckle Reduction in Echocardiography: Trends and Perceptions

Seán Finn, Martin Glavin and Edward Jones
National University of Ireland, Galway
Republic of Ireland

1. Introduction

Speckle is the fine-grained texture-like pattern seen in echocardiography, and indeed in all modalities of clinical ultrasound. The application of various image processing techniques to ultrasonography has been explored in the literature, and a common goal is the reduction or removal of the speckle component while preserving image structure. This assumes that speckle is a form of noise which is best removed; a view that is not always shared by those in clinical practice. This chapter presents a thorough overview of current trends in ultrasonic speckle reduction techniques, with an emphasis on echocardiography.

The phenomenon of speckle formation is described in Section 2 below. A review of the statistical methods used to model speckle is also presented in this chapter. Section 3 then details the main approaches for speckle reduction, covering the most recent of both compounding and post-acquisition techniques. Section 4 of this chapter presents a review and analysis of the methods of evaluation used to rate the performance of various speckle reduction approaches for clinical ultrasound. A particular focus is given to those which include consultation with practising clinicians in the field. The relationship between subjective clinical opinion and some objective image quality metrics on the quality of speckle filter echocardiographic video will be detailed. Details will be presented of a comprehensive evaluation methodology, which aims to combine clinical expertise and numerical assessment. Finally, Section 5 will conclude the chapter.

2. Speckle formation and statistics

While the term *ultrasound* can technically be used to refer to all acoustics of frequency greater than the upper threshold of human audibility ($f > 20$ kHz), clinical imaging is generally in the 1-20 MHz range (Rumack et al., 2004). Imaging is based on the transmission of acoustic pulses into the body, which interact with the tissue medium. Echoes are reflected by interfaces between tissue of differing acoustic properties, which are detected by a receiver. If the propagation velocity of sound waves in the imaged medium is known, the depth of interactions giving rise to the echoes can be determined. Characteristics of the returned signal (e.g. amplitude, phase) provide information on the interaction, and indicate the nature of the media involved. The amplitude of the reflected signal is used to produce ultrasound images, while the frequency shifts provide information on moving targets such as blood. Fig. 1 displays examples of clinical echocardiograms containing speckle.

The propagation speed in tissue varies with tissue type, temperature and pressure. Assuming constant temperature and pressure in the body, only the tissue type is considered (Quistgaard, 1997). The mean speed of sound propagation in human soft tissue is generally taken as 1540 m/s. Acoustic pulses transmitted into the body can experience:

Reflection: Also known a backscatter, reflection occurs when an acoustic pulse encounters an interface between tissues of differing acoustic impedances.

Refraction: When sound waves pass through an interface between media of different propagation speeds, a change in the direction of propagation occurs.

Absorption: Energy from the acoustic pulse is absorbed into the tissue, by conversion to thermal energy.

The acoustic impedance of a medium (Z) is the product of its density, ρ, and the speed of acoustic propagation in that medium, c ($Z = \rho c$).

The strength of reflection at an interface depends on the difference in acoustic impedance on each side of the boundary, as well as the size of the interface, its surface characteristics, and the angle of insonification. (Middleton & Kurtz, 2004; Rumack et al., 2004). The reflection coefficient at the interface is given in the same manner as the analogous case of electromagnetic propagation:

$$\Gamma = \frac{Z_2 - Z_1}{Z_2 + Z_1} \tag{1}$$

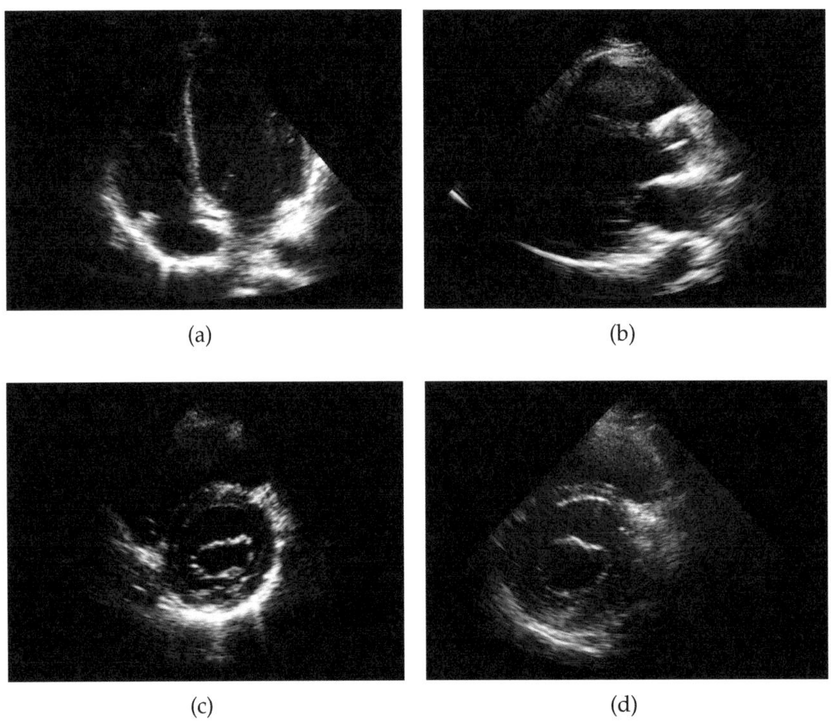

Fig. 1. Clinical ultrasound images, used in speckle filter evaluation.

Depending on the nature of the interface, two types of reflection are observed: *Specular Reflection* occurs when the interface is large and smooth with respect to the ultrasound pulse wavelength, e.g. the diaphragm and a urine filled bladder (Rumack et al., 2004). Strong clear reflections are produced, in the same fashion as for a mirror. Detection of these echoes is highly dependent on the angle of insonification (Rumack et al., 2004). *Scattering* results from interfaces much smaller than the wavelength of the ultrasound pulse. A volume of small scattering interfaces such as blood cells or a non smooth organ surface produce echoes which are scattered in all directions. This collection of scatterers are said to act as a diffuse reflector. The constructive and destructive interference of these scattered echoes results in a granular artefact known as *speckle*. Refraction is governed by Snell's law:

$$\frac{\sin\theta_1}{\sin\theta_2} = \frac{c_1}{c_2} \tag{2}$$

where the quantities θ_1, θ_2, c_1, and c_2 are respectively the angles of incidence and refraction, and the corresponding speeds of propagation. Attenuation of the acoustic pulse is mainly due to absorption and scattering (Quistgaard, 1997), and can be modelled as: $A(x,t) = A(x,0)e^{-\alpha f 2x}$ (Thijssen, 2003). where $A(x,t)$ is the amplitude at depth x and time t, f is the frequency and α is the attenuation coefficient. Generally attenuation is quite severe: in (Quistgaard, 1997), a halving of intensity every 0.8 cm at 5 MHz operation is described.

The interference experienced by reflections from diffuse scatterers result in a granular pattern known as speckle. Speckle is common to all imaging systems using coherent waves for illumination, including laser and radar imagery. In echocardiography, speckle noise is prominent in all cross-sectional views (Massay et al., 1989), and its effect is far more significant than additive noise sources such as sensor noise (Zong et al., 1998).

The basic description of ultrasound speckle in the literature is based on the characterisation of laser speckle by Goodman (Goodman, 1975; 1976). This approach is extended to acoustic imagery by a number of authors (Burckhardt, 1978; Wagner et al., 1988; 1983). Burckhardt (Burckhardt, 1978) notes that despite its random appearance, speckle is essentially deterministic: scans under identical situations produce the same speckle pattern. This behaviour is in contrast to that of true stochastic processes such as electrical noise. There is no direct relationship between the imaged medium and the observed speckle pattern however. If the same object is imaged with different imaging parameters, the speckle pattern produced is quite different. Burckhardt thus concludes that the speckle pattern has only a tenuous relationship to the imaged medium, and is instead dependant on the parameters of the imaging system. The size of the speckle granules are of similar size to the resolution of the scanner, in both axial and lateral directions. Burckhardt justifies the treatment of pulsed acoustics as a coherent wave source in the situation where the each pulse contains a number of cycles of the carrier wave.

Each ultrasound pulse encloses a three dimensional volume which defines the smallest resolvable structure, which is known as the resolution cell. The nature of the speckle at an image location is determined by the number of diffuse scatterers which are present in the resolution cell at the relevant position in the imaged medium. If the number of scatterers is large and randomly positioned, the resulting pattern is known as fully formed (or fully developed) speckle. In this case the speckle pattern depends only on the imaging system.

Wagner *et al.* (Wagner et al., 1983) show that in the case of a mixture of diffuse and specular scattering, the speckle pattern is related to the underlying texture of the medium.

The randomly scattered echoes from the scatterers are summed within each resolution cell. These echoes are sinusoidal in nature. Expressed as phasors, the summation is described as a random walk of the real and imaginary components. In the case of fully developed speckle, and with uniformly distributed phase values between 0 and 2π, these components have a circular Gaussian distribution (Wagner et al., 1983):

$$p(a_r, a_i) = \frac{1}{2\pi\sigma^2} \exp\left(-\frac{a_r^2 + a_i^2}{2\sigma^2}\right) \tag{3}$$

where (a_r, a_i) are the real and imaginary components. The amplitude within each resolution cell, $A = \sqrt{a_r^2 + a_i^2}$, is then given by a Rayleigh distribution:

$$p(A) = \frac{A}{\psi} \exp\left(-\frac{A^2}{2\psi}\right), \quad A \geq 0 \tag{4}$$

The Rayleigh parameter ψ depends on the mean square scattering amplitude of the medium (Goodman, 1975). Burckhardt defined an SNR measure for the amplitude as $SNR_A = \bar{A}/\sigma_A$. i.e. the ratio of mean to standard deviation. It can be shown that $SNR_A = 1.91$ for the Rayleigh distribution of fully developed speckle. Burckhardt explores the statistics of image compounded from multiple individual scans, and demonstrates a method of simulating a theoretically maximally speckle free image from a known structure. Alternative distributions to Rayleigh have been proposed for situations not meeting the requirements of fully developed speckle, such as insufficient numbers of scatterers per resolution cell, or non random positioning. These include the Rician, Nakagami and *K* distributions (Shankar et al., 2001; Shankar, 1995; Smolíovái et al., 2004).

The number of scatterers required for fully formed speckle varies in the literature. Ten or greater is a common figure (Krissian et al., 2007; Lizzi et al., 1997; Thijssen, 2003), although it is stated in (Ng et al., 2006) that at least thirty scatterers should be present for the central limit theorem to hold. It has also been shown that neither the number of scatterers or their random positioning are required for fully developed speckle governed by Rayleigh statistics (Dantas et al., 2005): a sparse set of uniformly positioned equivalent scatters can also produce a fully formed speckle pattern.

3. Techniques for reducing speckle

The reduction of speckle while preserving image structure is a challenging image processing problem, due to the multiplicative-like behaviour of speckle. This can is evident from the relatively large volume of literature dedicated methods of reducing or eliminating speckle. The common justifications for the removal of speckle in these works are the general reduction in image quality due to the presence of speckle. However, the question of whether or not to remove speckle as noise in clinical imagery is an open one, and depends largely on the application. A number of specific negative effects of speckle, and benefits of its removal in clinical ultrasonography have been noted:

- Speckle introduces spurious 'false-fine' structures, which give the appearance of resolution beyond that of the imaging system (Dantas et al., 2005).
- Small grey level differences can be masked (Burckhardt, 1978), which can obscure tissue boundaries (Dantas & Costa, 2007; Dantas et al., 2005).
- Image contrast is reduced (Dantas & Costa, 2007; Zhang et al., 2007).
- Human interpretation of ultrasonography can be negatively impacted (Abd-Elmoniem et al., 2002; Zhang et al., 2007; Zong et al., 1998), introducing a degree of subjectivity (Dantas & Costa, 2007). The presence of speckle has been determined to be the cause of an eight-fold reduction in lesion detectability (Bamber & Daft, 1986). Reduction of echocardiographic speckle has been shown to positively affect subjective image quality and improve boundary definition (Massay et al., 1989).
- The effectiveness (speed and accuracy) of automated processing tasks is also reduced by speckle (Abd-Elmoniem et al., 2002; Yu & Acton, 2002; Zhang et al., 2007; Zong et al., 1998), such as edge detection, segmentation and registration.
- While speckle can be viewed as deterministic (Dantas et al., 2005), it does not contain information on the imaged structure in the fully developed speckle case.

Approaches to speckle reduction can be broadly grouped into compounding and postacquisition methods.

3.1 Compounding approaches

These techniques combine two or more images of the same area. The measurements from image structure will be partially correlated, while the speckle pattern will differ. Compounding these images (e.g. by averaging) results in an image with enhanced structure and a reduced speckle pattern. A number of different scanning methods can be used to produce the images to be compounded. Frequency compounding uses images with separate frequency ranges within the transducer bandwidth (Galloway et al., 1988; Gehlbach & Sommer, 1987; Magnin et al., 1982; Trahey, Allison, Smith & von Ramm, 1986). A common technique is spilt spectrum processing (SSP) (Bamber & Phelps, 1991; Newhouse et al., 1982; Stetson et al., 1997), in which the wideband RF signal is split into a number of subbands using bandpass filters. Envelope detection of these RF subbands yields amplitude data, which is combined to produce an image with enhanced structure and reduced speckle component. The recent method of Dantas and Costa (Dantas & Costa, 2007) is applied to the entire 2D RF image. This is in contrast to some SSP methods, which are applied to each 1D RF scan line individually. The RF image was decomposed into a number of orientation specific subbands by use of a bank of modified log Gabor filters. Each subband RF image was used to generate an amplitude image, and the final speckle reduced image was produced by compounding these amplitude images. The technique was tested by application to simulated images and comparison to maximally speckle free reference images generated using the method of Burckhardt (Burckhardt, 1978).

Other compounding approaches include spatial compounding, which combine multiple images from different scan directions (O'Donnell & Silverstein, 1988; Pai-Chi & O'Donnell, 1994; Trahey, Smith & von Ramm, 1986). Burckhardt (Burckhardt, 1978) showed that in order for these scans to be independent of each other (and so having uncorrelated speckle patterns), the transducer must be translated by approximately half its element width.

Temporal compounding (frame averaging) operates as the name suggests by combining scans performed over time. This approach suffers from a dependence on motion: in a still medium the speckle pattern will not change. Conversely, fast moving organs such as the heart may appear smeared with this method. Some modern ultrasound system are capable of performing spatial compounding by sweeping the scan beam over the medium, while the transducer is held statically (Jespersen et al., 2000). A recent transducer design makes use of a particular arrangement of receive elements to acquire multiple independent images simultaneously (Behar et al., 2003).

3.2 Postacquisition speckle reduction

Postacquisition methods operate on the image after it has been envelope detected, and have the advantage of not requiring a specific mode of scanning, or access to the RF data. Aa simulation study comparing postacquisition filters to spatial compounding reported better image improvement for filtering, in terms of speckle reduction and image quality (Adam et al., 2006). The number of postacquisition speckle reduction methods in the literature is large, and the selection detailed here are grouped according to their general approach.

3.2.1 Adaptive filters

Adaptive filters attempt to adjust the level of filtering at each image location. The Lee filter (Lee, 1980; 1981), Kuan filter (Kuan et al., 1987) and Frost filter (Frost et al., 1982) were proposed for the task of speckle removal in synthetic aperture radar (SAR), and assume a multiplicative model for speckle noise. Enhanced versions of the Lee and Frost filter were also proposed (Lopes et al., 1990). These are improved by the classification of image pixels into a number of classes, and filtering accordingly. The method of Bamber and Daft (Bamber & Daft, 1986) extended this adaptive approach to ultrasound images by varying the degree of smoothing according to a local estimate of the level of speckle.

Median filtering was extended to the case of speckle removal by Loupas *et al.* (Loupas et al., 1989). This approach replaced pixels with the weighted median of a dynamically sized window, and is known as the adaptive weighted median filter (AWMF). Region growing techniques such as (Chen et al., 2003; Huang et al., 2003; Karaman et al., 1995; Koo & Park, 1991) have been applied to ultrasonography. Pixels are grouped in these methods, according to similarity of intensity and connectivity. Spatial filtering is performed to extend these regions, and the challenge is the selection of appropriate similarity criteria.

A recently proposed method by Tay *et al.* (Tay et al., 2006a;b) used an iterative technique of speckle reduction by the removal of outliers. The locale around each pixel is examined, and local extrema are replaced with a local average. This process is repeated until no further outliers are found. Thus the filter reduces the local variance around each pixel, and is referred to by the authors as the "Squeeze Box" filter.

The non-local means filter of Coupé *et al.* (Coupé et al., 2009) estimates the true value of each pixel as the weighted sum of the windowed averages of within a search volume centred at the pixel of interest. This technique was adapted to speckled ultrasonography by incorporation of a multiplicative noise model by Bayesian estimation.

Massay *et al.* (Massay et al., 1989) proposed a method of speckle reduction using local statistics: the level of smoothing is determined by an estimate of local speckle level.

3.2.2 Diffusion filtering

Perona and Malik (Perona & Malik, 1990) introduced the first anisotropic diffusion method for additive noise. This is an iterative method of smoothing an image, similar in concept to heat diffusion.

A diffusion function is calculated at each iteration, with the aim of inhibiting smoothing across image edges and permitting it in homogeneous areas. Diffusion takes place according to the following Partial Differential Equation (PDE):

$$\frac{\partial I(x,y;t)}{\partial t} = \nabla \cdot \{c(|\nabla I_\sigma(x,y;t)|).\nabla I(x,y;t)\}, \quad I(x,y;0) = I_0(x,y) \tag{5}$$

where $I(x,y;t)$ is the image under diffusion, t is an artificial time dimension representing the progress of diffusion, I_0 is the observed image, ∇ and $\nabla \cdot ()$ are the gradient and divergence operators, and $|\cdot|$ represents magnitude. The diffusion function $c(\cdot)$ controls the level of diffusion at each image position. Smoothing is inhibited across image edges by choosing a monotonically decreasing function of gradient magnitude for $c(|\nabla I(x,y;t)|)$, such as $c(x) = e^{-(x/k)^2}$. Here k is an edge threshold, set to 90% of the absolute gradient histogram integral. A number of extensions to this method have been proposed, most notably that of Catté *et al.* (Catté et al., 1992), who regularised the calculation of $c(\cdot)$. This makes (5) mathematically well-posed, having a unique solution. While this method is capable of intra-region smoothing with edge preservation for images corrupted with additive noise, its effect on images corrupted with multiplicative noise is less than satisfactory (Yu & Acton, 2002).

To address the unsiutablility of Perona and Malik's diffusion for multiplicative speckled situations, Yu and Acton (Yu & Acton, 2002) proposed a diffusion function based on the coefficient of variation used in synthetic aperture radar:

$$\frac{\partial I(x,y,t)}{\partial t} = \nabla.[c(q).\nabla I(x,y,t)], \quad I(x,y,0) = I_0(x,y) \tag{6}$$

In contrast to (5), the diffusion function $c(.)$ is not a function of the gradient magnitude, but rather of the Instantaneous Coefficient of Variation (ICOV) q. The ICOV is based on the variation coefficient used in SAR filtering as a signal/edge discriminator, and is defined as:

$$q(x,y,t) = \sqrt{\frac{(0.5)\left(|\frac{\nabla I}{I}|\right)^2 - (0.25)^2\left(\frac{\nabla^2 I}{I}\right)^2}{[1 + (0.25)\left(\frac{\nabla^2 I}{I}\right)]^2}} \tag{7}$$

where ∇^2 is the Laplacian operator. The diffusion function $c(.)$ used here is:

$$c\left[q(x,y,t), q_0(t)\right] = \left(1 + \frac{q^2(x,y,t) - q_0^2(t)}{q^2(x,y,t)(1 + q_0^2(t))}\right)^{-1} \tag{8}$$

where q_0 is the 'speckle scale function', a diffusion threshold controlling the level of smoothing, equivalent to the noise variation coefficient C_n of the SAR filters.

The work of Aja-Fernandez and Alberola-Lopez (Aja-Fernandez & Alberola-Lopez, 2006) proposed a number of improvements to the SRAD technique, known as detail preserving anisotropic diffusion (DPAD). Noting that (8) is derived from the Lee filter, this is replaced with the following derived from the Kuan filter:

$$c\left[q(x,y,t), q_0(t)\right] = \frac{1 + 1/q^2(x,y,t)}{1 + 1/q_0^2(t)} \tag{9}$$

The second alteration concerns the calculation of the ICOV, showing that (7) is equivalent to the ratio of local standard deviation and mean estimators. In (7), these local estimators were calculated in using the four nearest neighbours of each pixel, while in DPAD a larger neighbourhood is used for more accurate estimates:

$$q(x,y,t) = \sqrt{\frac{\sigma_I^2(x,y,t)}{\bar{I}(x,y,t)^2}} = \sqrt{\frac{\frac{1}{|\eta_{x,y}| - 1} \sum_{p \in \eta_{x,y}} \left(I_p - \bar{I}(x,y,t)\right)^2}{\bar{I}(x,y,t)^2}} \tag{10}$$

where $\eta_{x,y}$ is a square $Z \times Z$ neighbourhood, and $\bar{I}(x,y,t) = (1/|\eta_{x,y}|) \sum_{p \in \eta_{x,y}} I_p$. This is shown to be more accurate than the formulation of (7). The third contribution of (Aja-Fernandez & Alberola-Lopez, 2006) related to the estimation of $q_0(t)$, calculated as $median\{q(x,y;t)\}$. This approach requires less computation than the previously proposed method of (Yu & Acton, 2004), and produced similar results.

Tensor valued schemes, proposed by Weickert (Weickert, 1998; 1999), allow the strength of diffusion to vary directionally at each location. Denoted Coherence Enhancing Diffusion (CED), Weickert's method aims to enhance the enhance the smooth curves within an image, such as those often present in medical images. The structure tensor T is used to describe the image gradient:

$$T \quad = \nabla I \otimes \nabla I^T = \begin{pmatrix} I_x^2 & I_{xy} \\ I_{xy} & I_y^2 \end{pmatrix} \tag{11}$$

where I_x, I_y are the x and y gradients of the image: $\nabla I = (I_x, I_y)$. To make the gradient description robust to small noise fluctuations, local averaging of the observed image is performed as $I_\sigma = K_\sigma * I$, where $*$ represents convolution, and K_σ is a Gaussian kernel of variance σ^2. The gradient ∇I_σ represents only information from image details larger than $O(\sigma)$. Thus σ is referred to as the *noise scale*. The structure tensor is formed using a second level of Gaussian smoothing:

$$T_\rho = K_\rho * (\nabla I_\sigma \nabla I_\sigma^T) = \begin{pmatrix} T_{11} & T_{12} \\ T_{21} & T_{22} \end{pmatrix} \tag{12}$$

The values of T_ρ then represent image information from a neighbourhood defined by ρ, the *integration scale*. While the structure tensor is simply another representation of the image gradient ∇I, and contains no more information than ∇I, it has the advantage of allowing local averaging as in (12) without cancellation.

The eigenvectors of T_ρ are denoted by $(\vec{\omega}_1, \vec{\omega}_2)$, and the corresponding eigenvalues by (μ_1, μ_2). If the eigenvalues are ordered so that $\mu_1 \geq \mu_2$, then $(\vec{\omega}_1, \vec{\omega}_2)$ give the directions of maximum and minimum local variation, respectively. These are the directions normal and tangent to the local image gradient, the gradient and contour directions. The corresponding eigenvalues give the strength of the gradient in these directions, and also provide information on the local coherence or anisotropy. A measure of local coherence is defined as $\kappa = (\mu_1 - \mu_2)^2$ (Weickert, 1999). The CED diffusion process is described by the PDE:

$$\frac{\delta I(x,y,t)}{\delta t} = \nabla.(D \nabla I(x,y,t)) \tag{13}$$

where D is the diffusion matrix, constructed with the same eigenvectors as T_ρ ($\vec{e}_1 = \vec{\omega}_1, \vec{e}_2 = \vec{\omega}_2$) and eigenvalues (λ_1, λ_2) given by:

$$\lambda_1 = c_1, \quad \lambda_2 = \begin{cases} c_1, & \text{if } \mu_1 = \mu_2 \\ c_1 + (1 - c_1) \exp\left(\frac{-c_2}{\kappa}\right), & \text{otherwise} \end{cases} \tag{14}$$

where c_1 and c_2 are parameters constrained by $0 < c_1 \ll 1$ and $c_2 > 0$.

The nonlinear coherent diffusion (NCD) method of Abd-Elmoniem *et al.* (Abd-Elmoniem et al., 2002) is a tensor valued anisotropic diffusion scheme for the removal of speckle. The eigenvalues of the diffusion tensor define the directional strength of diffusion at each image location, and these are chosen to reflect an estimate of the strength of speckle at that location. Image regions closely resembling fully developed speckle are mean filtered, while those dissimilar remain unaltered. Similar to the CED method, this approach uses a tensor-valued diffusion function, calculated as a component-wise convolution of a Gaussian kernel with the structure tensor:

$$J_\rho = K_\rho * (\nabla I \, \nabla I^T) = \begin{pmatrix} K_\rho * I_x^2 & K_\rho * I_{xy} \\ K_\rho * I_{xy} & K_\rho * I_y^2 \end{pmatrix} \tag{15}$$

Here, the initial stage of smoothing performed in (12) is not used. As in the CED method, ρ is integration scale, the window size over which the orientation information is averaged. The PDE (13) again describes the diffusion, using a diffusion tensor constructed so as to have the same eigenvectors as J_ρ, but with eigenvalues λ_1, λ_2 defined as:

$$\lambda_1 = \begin{cases} \alpha\left(1 - \frac{\kappa}{s^2}\right), & \text{if } \kappa \leq s^2 \\ 0, & \text{otherwise} \end{cases}, \quad \lambda_2 = \alpha \tag{16}$$

where α is a parameter determining the level of smoothing in regions of fully developed speckle, and s^2 is a heuristically chosen 'stopping level'.

The orientated SRAD (OSRAD) proposed by Krissian *et al.* (Krissian et al., 2007) extended the SRAD method to a tensor diffusion scheme, so diffusion can vary with direction to speckle adaptive diffusion filtering. The improvements of the DPAD method are also used in this method, such as the use of a larger window to estimate $q(x,y;t)$, and the median estimation of $q_0(t)$. The OSRAD diffusion function $c(q)$ is based on the Kuan *et al.* filter, as in (9). It was shown that the local directional variance is related to the local geometry of the image.

This method can be implemented by the use of the structure tensor, as in (Weickert, 1999) and (Abd-Elmoniem et al., 2002), or by using the Hessian matrix as in (Krissian, 2002). In the 2-D case, $(\vec{\omega}_1, \vec{\omega}_2)$ are the eigenvectors of T_ρ from (12), and are used as the basis of the diffusion matrix, D. The eigenvalues of D, which determine the strength of diffusion in the gradient and curvature directions, are given as:

$$\lambda_1 = c_{srad} \quad , \quad \lambda_2 = c_{tang} \tag{17}$$

Where c_{srad} is the SRAD diffusion ($c(q)$), and c_{tang} is a constant. Diffusion is then performed as per (13).

3.2.3 Multiscale methods

Multiscale methods are common in image processing, and both the wavelet and pyramid (Burt & Adelson, 1983) transforms have been employed in the reduction of speckle. The well-known wavelet transform isolates local frequency subbands using a quadrature mirror pair of filters. The the pyramid transform does not require quadrature filters. More details on this method can be found in (Adelson et al., 1984).

Wavelet techniques can be grouped into those which operate by thresholding, Bayesian estimation, or correlation between coefficients. Many techniques use the soft thresholding approach of Donoho (Donoho, 1995), of which some of the first adoptions for speckle were proposed by (Guo et al., 1994) and (Moulin, 1993). These methods use a logarithmic transformation to allow treatment of the speckle as additive. The thresholding method of (Hao et al., 1999) operates on the output of the AWMF filter. The difference image between the AMWF output and the original image contains the high frequency information removed by the AWMF. Both images have speckle removed by soft thresholding in the wavelet domain, and after reconstruction the two images are summed together.

Using a multiplicative model for a speckled image, the method of Zong *et al.* (Zong et al., 1998) applies logarithmic and wavelet transforms as:

$$\begin{aligned} I(i,j) &= R(i,j)n(i,j) \\ I^l(i,j) &= R^l(i,j) + n^l(i,j) \\ W[I(i,j)] &= \{(W_k^d[I(i,j)])_{1 \le k \le J}^{d=1,2}, S_K[I(i,j)]\} \end{aligned} \tag{18}$$

where R and n are the speckle free and speckle noise components, (i,j) are the pixel indecies, and $I^l = log(I)$. Here $n^l(i,j)$ is approximated as additive white noise. The K-level discrete Dyadic Wavelet Transform (DWT) of (Mallat & Zhong, 1992) generates $W_k^d\{I(i,j)\}$, the set of wavelet coefficients at scale 2^k (level k) and spatial orientation d ($d = 1$ for horizontal and $d = 2$ for vertical). The approximation coefficients at the coarsest scale K are denoted by $S_K\{I(i,j)\}$. Soft thresholding is applied to the finer scales (levels one and two), with coefficient dependent thresholds.

A nonlinear function is applied to the other, coarser, scales. This incorporates hard thresholding and a nonlinear contrast enhancement term:

$$E(v) = \begin{cases} 0, & \text{if } |v| < T_1 \\ sign(v)T_2 + \bar{u}, & \text{if } T_2 \leq |v| \leq T_3 \\ 1, & \text{otherwise} \end{cases} \tag{19}$$

where $v \in [-1, 1]$ represents each wavelet coefficient, and the three thresholds are related as $0 \leq T_1 \leq T_2 \leq T_3 \leq 1$. The value of $\bar{u}$ is determined according to $\bar{u} = a(T_3 - T_2)\{f[c(u-b)] - f[-c(u+b)]\}$. The sigmoid function is represented by f, and

$$u = \frac{sign(v)(|v| - T_2)}{T_3 - T_2}, \quad a = \frac{1}{f[c(1-b)] - f[-c(1+b)]} \tag{20}$$

Thus the operator $E(v)$ is dependant on five parameters: b, c, T_1, T_2, T_3.

Noise removal in the wavelet domain is also performed using Bayesian denoising techniques, which model the distributions of the wavelet coefficients. This a priori information is used to infer the noise free coefficients. Gupta *et al.* (Gupta et al., 2005) modelled the wavelet coefficients of the underlying speckle free image using a generalised Laplacian distribution, simultaneously removing speckle and performing compression using a quantisation function. This function adapts to the estimated level of speckle.

Achim *et al.* (Achim et al., 2001) modelled the wavelet coefficients of $I^l(i,j)$ as the convolution of a symmetric α stable (SαS) distribution (as $R(i,j)$), and a zero mean Gaussian distribution for $n(i,j)$. The variance of the Gaussian noise is estimated using the median absolute deviation (MAD) method, while the parameters of the SαS distribution are estimated by least squares fitting of the observed density function spectrum to the empirical characteristic function. After estimation of the parameters of the statistical model, a shrinkage function is found by numerical calculation of the maximum a posteriori (MAP) estimation curve. The wavelet coefficients are modified by the shrinkage function, and the inverse wavelet transform produces the denoised image.

The technique of Rabani *et al.* (Rabbani et al., 2008) models the distribution of the noise free wavelet coefficients using a local mixture of either Gaussian or Laplacian distributions. The speckle noise is assumed to be either Gaussian or Rayleigh in nature. For all combinations of local mixture distributions and speckle noise distributions, both the MAP and minimum mean squared error (MMSE) estimators are derived analytically. A recently proposed method by Fu *et al.* (Fu et al., 2010) accomplishes bivariate shrinkage of the wavelet coefficients. This approach models the joint density of the coefficients in each scale with their parents in the next coarser scale.

The third type of wavelet noise removal uses the correlation of useful wavelet coefficients across scales (Pižurica et al., 2003). This technique does not rely on a model for the image noise, but rather locates the signals of interest based on their interscale persistence. This initial classification step is followed by empirical estimates of the signal and noise probability density functions (PDFs). These are used to define a shrinkage map which suppress those wavelet coefficients resulting from noise.

The NMWD method (Yue et al., 2006) aims to combine wavelet analysis with anisotropic diffusion. Wavelet based signal/noise discrimination is employed to overcome the shortcomings of the image gradient (as used in the PMAD, CED and NCD methods) for discrimination in speckled images. The gradient cannot always precisely separate the image and noise in ultrasound images, as variations due to speckle noise may be larger than those corresponding to underlying image (Yue et al., 2006). The image is decomposed using the DWT of Mallat and Zhong, as in the Zong *et al.* method. The modulus of the wavelet coefficients at each scale is defined as:

$$M_k\{I(i,j)\} = \sqrt{\sum_{d=1}^{2} |W_k^d\{I(i,j)\}|^2_{k=1,2,..,K}} \tag{21}$$

The normalised wavelet modulus was found to be large in edge-related regions and small for noise and texture, and so is used for signal/noise discrimination in this method. For amplitude images the wavelet modulus is normalised by:

$$\tilde{M}_k I = \frac{M_k\{I(i,j)\}}{\mu_Z}, \quad k = 1,2,..,K \tag{22}$$

Here μ_Z is a local mean calculated using a widow size $Z \times Z$. The histogram of $\tilde{M}_k I$ is modelled as a Rayleigh mixture distribution, composed of the sum of edge and noise pixels as:

$$\tilde{M}_k I \simeq n_k p_{n,k}(x, \lambda_n) + (1 - n_k) p_{e,k}(x, \lambda_e) \tag{23}$$

where $p_{n,k}$ is a Rayleigh distribution with parameter λ_n, representing the noise pixels. Similarly, $p_{e,k}$ are the edge pixels, Rayleigh distributed with parameter λ_e. The proportion of the mixture distribution resulting from noise-related values is given as n_k. The parameters of the normalised modulus distribution ($\sigma_{n,k}$, $\sigma_{e,k}$ and n_k) are estimated using the Expectation-Maximisation (EM) method (Dempster et al., 1977). These parameters are used to determine the strength of n anisotropic diffusion process. After diffusion, the wavelet coefficients are used the synthesize the speckle reduced image. This process is repeated for a number of iterations.

As well as wavelet based methods, multiresolution pyramid methods of speckle reduction have been proposed. The approach of Aiazzi *et al.* (Aiazzi et al., 1998) extends the approach of the Kuan filter to process each layer in the multiscale pyramid decomposition. Sattar *et al.* (Sattar et al., 1997) presented a method which both reduces speckle and enhances image edges. Multiscale decomposition is performed using a pyramid transform. An edge detector is applied to the lowpass image, the output of which determines the coefficients from the high pass image which are included in reconstruction. The success of this method is therefore dependant on accurate operation of the edge detector, and a number of different techniques are tested.

The approach of Zhang *et al.* (Zhang et al., 2007) combines the approaches of multiscale analysis and anisotropic diffusion, and so is similar in approach to the NMWD method above.

4. Evaluation of speckle reduction

As shown above, a large variety of speckle reduction filters have been proposed. Evaluating the relative performance of these filters has been performed by a number of different methods.

The majority of the papers proposing these filters contain a comparison of the proposed method with some others from the literature. Common techniques for evaluating relative performance are quantitative image quality metrics, and qualitative inspection, often by the authors themselves. Test data for evaluation includes clinical and phantom images, as well as simulated ultrasound which allows evaluation of filtering relative to an ideal speckle free reference. A select number of independent reviews have also been published, which vary in the nature and depth of the investigation performed.

Thakur and Anand (Thakur & Anand, 2005) compared the suitability of a number of different wavelets for the reduction of speckle in ultrasound imagery. Adam *et al.* (Adam et al., 2006) looked at the effect of a combination of spatial compounding and postacquisition filtering. Different methods of compounding these images were evaluated in this work, in combination with a number of postacquisition filters. These were applied to simulated kidney images generated using the Field II software package (Jensen, 1996). It was shown that postacquisition filtering improved the images to a greater degree than compounding alone, and that the SRAD filter was the better of the two considered. A recent comparison by Mateo and Fernández-Caballero (Mateo & Fernández-Caballero, 2009) evaluated median filtering, the AWMF filter, two low-pass filters, and a simple wavelet filter. Lowpass filtering with the Butterworth filter was deemed by the authors to be the best of the methods considered. A comprehensive comparison of a large number of speckle reduction filters for application to clinical carotid ultrasonography was presented by Loizou *et al.* (Loizou et al., 2005). Evaluation was performed both by automated analysis, and also using classification by experts. In both cases, the focus was on the diagnosis of atherosclerosis (thickened artery walls due to plaque deposit). A set of clinical images from patients deemed to be at risk of this condition was used in filter evaluation, and these were divided into a symptomatic set (from patients who have displayed symptoms of this condition, such as stroke incidents), and an symptomatic set. For the test by automated analysis, 440 images were used, divided equally between the two sets. Automated analysis proceeded by calculating a large number (56) of texture features for each filtered image. The level of separability between the symptomatic and symptomatic sets was then analysed using a number of approaches, using a distance metric an the statistical Wilcoxon rank sum test. A set of image quality metrics were also applied, comparing the filtered image to the unfiltered version in each case. The expert test was performed with 100 images, split evenly between symptomatic and symptomatic groups. The filtered and unfiltered images were shown to two experts at random, and each expert rates the quality of the image on a scale of one to five. Only one method (the Geometric filter) was seen to improve the image quality as perceived by both experts across the entire dataset. A difference in the evaluations between the experts was noted, although this was not investigated statistically. The authors accounted for this by reference to the differing clinical specialities of the experts.

The present author conducted and reported on a study which compared clinical and computational evaluation of speckle filtering in echocardiographic images (Finn et al., 2009). Subjective visual assessment was performed by a group of six clinical experts, all of whom are experienced cardiac physicians or technicians. The majority of the evaluation strategies described in the literature review of the previous chapter report results of visual inspection by the authors themselves, rather than the opinion of clinical experts (exception include (Loizou et al., 2005; Zong et al., 1998)). The basic qualities which are generally held to constitute favourable speckle filtering (homogeneous variance reduction, mean intensity preservation and edge preservation) can be readily determined visually, and do not require clinical expertise or training. However, the assessment of clinical images for diagnostic purposes does require such training and expertise. This study explored the clinical opinion of the quality of speckle filtered echocardiographic images, as judged by experts in the field. A large set of speckle filtered echocardiographic videos were produced by application of a number of speckle reduction filters: The SRAD filter (Yu & Acton, 2002), the NCD filter (Abd-Elmoniem et al., 2002), and the GLM filter proposed by Pižurica *et al.*. Example echocardiographic images processed by these filters are displayed in Fig. 2. A total set of forty eight filtered videos were produced in this fashion, showing differing levels of speckle reduction and image characteristics.

The clinical experts assessed subjective video quality in three criteria, chosen based on the opinion of a senior clinical expert of important clinical factors:

Speckle Level The expert's assessment of the level of speckle in each video.

Detail Clarity Quantifies the subjective resolvability of diagnostically important details.

Overall Quality This quantifies the overall quality of the video, including any other clinical considerations not covered by the other criteria.

A large set of quantitative image quality metrics, commonly used in the literature for evaluation of speckle reduction, were also applied. Statistical analysis was performed in order to determine:

1. If there were any significant differences between the expert scores
2. If there were any statistically significant relationships between the three scoring categories for each expert.

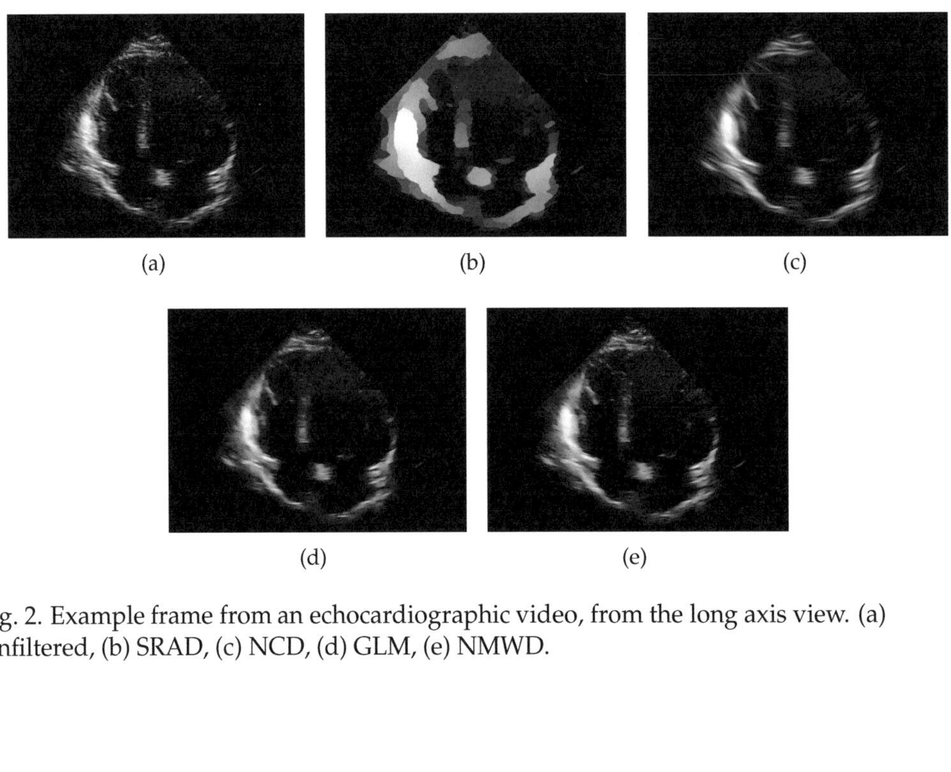

Fig. 2. Example frame from an echocardiographic video, from the long axis view. (a) Unfiltered, (b) SRAD, (c) NCD, (d) GLM, (e) NMWD.

3. If there were significant relationships between the subjective expert scores and the image quality metrics.

The expert scores are an ordinal categorical data set, and so the non-parametric Kruskal-Wallis test (Kruskal & Wallis, 1953) was used to investigate inter-expert differences. For the second and third analyses above, correlations were quantified using Spearman's rank correlation coefficient (ρ) (Spearman, 1904). All tests were performed using the SPSS software package, and the level of significance was chosen as 1% ($p = 0.01$) throughout.

Filtering resulted in a reduction in perceived Speckle Level in almost two thirds of cases. However, the aggregate Overall Quality and Detail Clarity scores were negative in over half of cases, indicating that the experts did not view speckle reduction as beneficial for manual analysis. This is in general agreement with the results of Loizou *et al.* (Loizou et al., 2005). The results of Dantas and Costa (Dantas & Costa, 2007) appear to be relevant: while speckle reduction does not necessarily lead to a loss of clarity, it does remove 'false-fine' structures (spurious fine detail, beyond the scanning resolution). While these details do not represent tissue structure, its removal can lead to a perceived reduction in sharpness. The assessment of the experts here was not universally negative however.

The Kruskal-Wallis test resulted in no no statistically significant differences between the experts in the Overall Quality scores at a 1% level of significance, but that a significant difference exists between experts in both the Speckle Level and Detail Clarity scores. For all of the experts, the relationship between Overall Quality and Detail Clarity is strongly positive and statistically significant. The ρ values for the relationship between Overall Quality and Speckle Level show positive relationships in all cases, but is only significant at the 1% level for four of the six experts. The relationship between the Detail Clarity and Speckle Level scores again indicate a positive relationship, and are significant for all but one of the experts.

The relationship between the expert scores and the objective image quality metrics is shown in Table 1 to be significant for three metrics:

Pratt's Figure of Merit (FoM) (Pratt, 1977) measures edge pixel displacement between each filtered image I_{filt} and the original image I_{orig}:

$$FoM(I_{filt}, I_{orig}) = \frac{1}{max(N_{filt}, N_{orig})} \sum_{i=1}^{\hat{N}} \frac{1}{1 + d_i^2 \alpha} \tag{24}$$

where N_{filt} and N_{orig} are the number edge pixels in edge maps of I_{filt} and I_{orig}. Parameter α is set to a constant $\frac{1}{9}$ (Yu & Acton, 2002), and d_i is the Euclidean distance between the ith detected edge pixel and the nearest ideal edge pixel. The FoM metric measures how well the edges are preserved through out the filtering process. This metric is shown to have a significant relationship with the Overall Quality expert score at the 1% significance level.

Mean Squared Error (MSE) The MSE measures the average absolute difference between two the original and filtered images (average intensity change due to filtering):

$$MSE(I_{filt}, I_{orig}) = \frac{1}{XY} \sum_{i=1}^{Y} \sum_{j=1}^{X} (I_{filt}(i,j) - I_{orig}(i,j))^2 \tag{25}$$

where both images are of size $X \times Y$. This metric is shown to have a significant inverse relationship with the Speckle Level expert score at the 1% significance level.

Edge Region MSE This is the same as the MSE above, but only pixels in the vicinity of image edges are considered.

This metric is shown to have a significant relationship with the Detail Clarity expert score at the 1% significance level.

	Expert 1	Expert 2	Expert 3	Expert 4	Expert 5	Expert 6
Overall Quality/ FOM	ρ=0.74 p=176.5×10^{-11}	ρ=0.59 p=123.0×10^{-7}	ρ=0.53 p=124.1×10^{-6}	ρ=0.72 p=607.0×10^{-11}	ρ=0.55 p=452.7×10^{-7}	ρ=0.82 p=992.7×10^{-15}
Detail Clarity/ Edge Region MSE	ρ=-0.67 p=164.0×10^{-9}	ρ=-0.62 p=240.0×10^{-8}	ρ=-0.49 p=402.0×10^{-6}	ρ=-0.76 p=346.8×10^{-12}	ρ=-0.49 p=332.9×10^{-6}	ρ=-0.83 p=205.6×10^{-15}
Speckle Level/ MSE	ρ=-0.69 p=531.1×10^{-10}	ρ=-0.47 p=726.0×10^{-6}	ρ=-0.85 p=306.8×10^{-16}	ρ=-0.47 p=710.1×10^{-6}	ρ=-0.64 p=992.1×10^{-9}	ρ=-0.87 p=214.3×10^{-17}

Table 1. Intra-expert association between scoring categories and metrics, using Spearmans correlation (ρ), with significance.

Having established relationships between objective image quality metrics and subjective expert opinion, the present author recently conducted a comprehensive review of speckle filtering methods as applied to echocardiography (Finn et al., 2010). A comprehensive evaluation of a wide range of techniques was performed, taking into account both clinical and simulated ultrasound images, and also the computational requirements of each method. Fifteen recent filtering approaches, including anisotropic diffusion, wavelet denoising and local statistics, were evaluated. These are summarised in Table 2.

Method	Type	Refrences	Abbreviation
Perona and Malik Diffusion	AD	Perona & Malik (1990)	PMAD
Speckle Reducing Anisotropic Diffusion	AD	Yu & Acton (2002)	SRAD
Detail Preserving Anisotropic Diffusion	AD	Aja-Fernandez & Alberola-Lopez (2006)	DPAD
Coherence Enhancing Diffusion	AD	Weickert (1999)	CED
Nonlinear Coherent Diffusion	AD	Abd-Elmoniem et al. (2002)	NCD
Oriented Speckle Reducing Anisotropic Diffusion	AD	Krissian et al. (2007)	OSRAD
Zong *et al.* Filter	W	Zong et al. (1998)	Zong
Generalized Likelihood Method	W	Pižurica et al. (2003)	GLM
Nonlinear Multiscale Wavelet Diffusion	W	Yue et al. (2006)	NMWD
Lee Filter	SAR	Lee (1980)	Lee
Frost *et al.* Filter	SAR	Frost et al. (1982)	Frost
Kuan *et al.* Filter	SAR	Kuan et al. (1987)	Kuan
Enhanced Lee Filter	SAR	Lopes et al. (1990)	EnhLee
Enhanced Frost *et al.* Filter	SAR	Lopes et al. (1990)	EnhFrost
Geometric Filter	-	Crimmins (1985)	Geo

Table 2. Despeckle Filter Summary. *AD* = Anisotropic Diffusion, *W* = Wavelet.

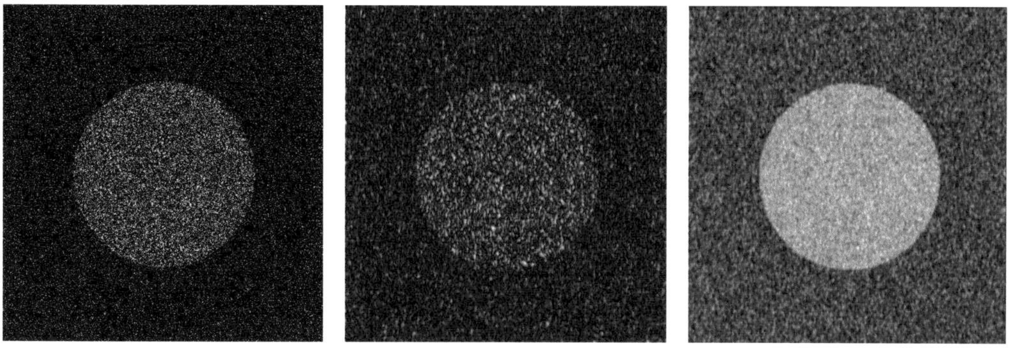

(a) (b) (c)

Fig. 3. Example simulated ultrasound image. (a) Echomap, (b) Speckled amplitude image, (c) Speckle free MW image.

Various approaches of varying simplicity have been employed in the literature to produce simulated images (Achim et al., 2001; Sattar et al., 1997; Yu & Acton, 2002). Ultrasound imaging can be treated as a linear process (Jensen, 1991; Ng et al., 2006), i.e. the filtering of an echogenicity map with a point spread function (PSF). An axially-varying PSF was used in (Ng et al., 2007), approximated as piecewise constant, similar to (Michailovich & Adam, 2005). This approach was also employed here, with PSFs at various depths generated using the Field II simulation software (Jensen, 1996) and demodulated to baseband.

While the PSF models the imaging system, the imaged medium is modelled as an echogenicity map $h(x,y)$ composed of complex point scatterers, similar to (Dantas & Costa, 2007). Scatterers are positioned randomly within regions of varying density. The phase values of the scatterers follows a uniform distribution, varying from $0 \rightarrow 2\pi$ rad, while scatterer magnitude follows a Gaussian distribution with unity mean and $\sigma = 0.1$. Fig. 3(a) shows an example of an echomap with two regions of differing scatterer densities, with density values of 40% and 10%. Echogenicity maps are filtered to generate a simulated image as $RF(x,y) = h(x,y) * p(x,y), I(x,y) = |RF(x,y)|$. where p is the analytic form of the PSF function at the correct depth, and $*$ denotes convolution. Examples of the granular speckle pattern produced can be seen in Fig. 3(b).

The Maximum Writing (MW) technique (Burckhardt, 1978) is used to generate a maximally speckle free version of each of the twenty simulated images. The above convolution is performed multiple times, randomly varying scatterer phase. This produces a series of images with the same structure but differing speckle patterns, the maximum of which is the speckle free image: $I_{MW} = \max\{|p(x,y) * (|h(x,y)|\exp[\phi_n])|\}$ (ϕ_n is the phase of the nth set of scatterers generated). In practice, this technique is applied until the contribution of the nth amplitude image is smaller than 0.1% of average image brightness, similar to the approach of (Dantas & Costa, 2007). Fig. 3(c) displays the MW output. A total of twenty simulated images are used in speckle filter evaluation. Fig. 4 displays typical results of filter application to the simulated images.

The output of the local statistics filters vary in the speckle suppression level: the Lee, Frost and enhanced Frost remove most of the speckle pattern with some blurring. The Kuan and

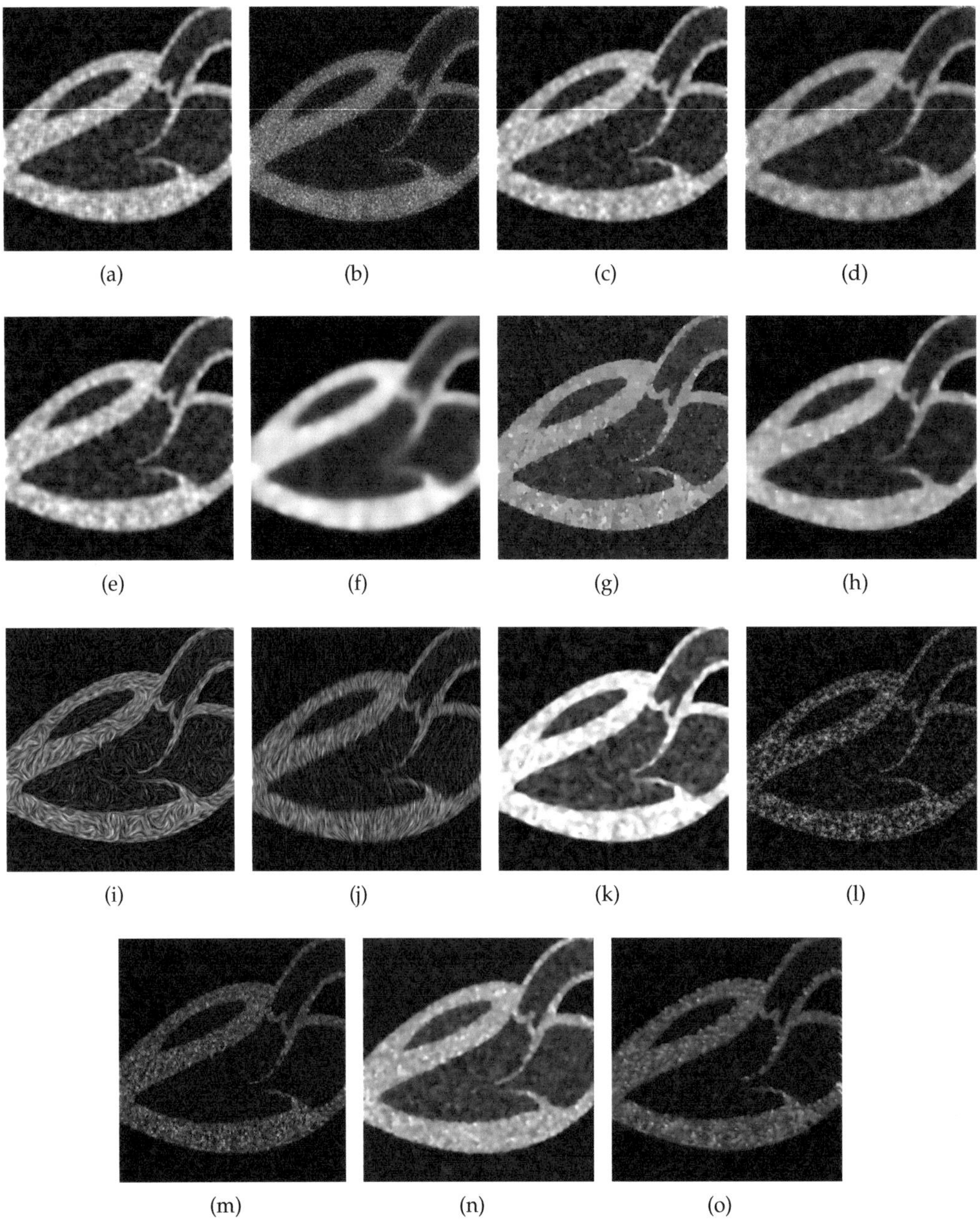

Fig. 4. Sample speckle filter output for a simulated image. (a) Lee, (b) Kuan, (c) Frost, (d) EnhLee, (e) EnhFrost, (f) PMAD, (g) SRAD, (h) DPAD, (i) CED, (j) NCD, (k) OSRAD, (l) Zong, (m) GLM, (n) NMWD, (o) Geo.

ehhanced Lee filter remove considerably less of the speckle pattern. The anisotropic diffusion filters also exhibit a range of output quality. The PMAD filter required many iterations to remove speckle, resulting in a blurred output. The SRAD and DPAD filters both display strong speckle suppression. Due to a larger window size, the DPAD filter remove more of the speckle, producing images which are more uniform. The CED method and the NCD filter both display artefacts, introduced by the enhancement of image contours (including those of the speckle texture). This effect is more pronounced for the NCD filter. The OSRAD filter displays a strong degree of speckle suppression, and preserves the image borders. The Zong and GLM filter outputs both show a degree of speckle remaining. The NMWD filter is seen to produce output with most of the speckle pattern removed. Finally, the Geometric filters output displays a good level of speckle reduction, however some of the speckle pattern does still remain.

A set of clinical images are used in evaluation. A total of 500 frames are used to evaluate filtering performance, taken from 100 videos from 40 patients. They were scanned using a General Electric Vivid 7 Series scanner (GE Healthcare, Piscataway, NJ, USA). The results of applying the filters to the image of Fig. 1(a) are shown in Fig. 5.

The local statistics filters output are quite similar in appearance, and still contain some speckle. As with the simulated images, the anisotropic diffusion filters produce output with a range of characteristics. The PMAD filter produces images which are extremely blurred. The SRAD and DPAD filters both show strong speckle suppression, however the SRAD output appears more distorted. As with the simulated images, the CED and NCD filters introduce small scale artefacts to the images. The OSRAD filter again shows strong speckle suppression. Frames processed with the Zong wavelet filter have a somewhat washed-out appearance, and not all of the speckle is removed. The GLM, NMWD and Geometric filtered frames have most of the speckle removed, however the GLM output appears slightly blurred.

Five image quality metrics are applied to both the simulated and clinical echocardiographic images. In addition to the FoM and the edge MSE are detailed above, the following are considered:

Structural Similarity (SSIM) The SSIM measure (Wang et al., 2004) to asses the preservation of structural information in the filtering process:

$$SSIM = \frac{1}{M}\sum \frac{(2\mu_1\mu_2 + C_1)(2\sigma_{12} + C_2)}{(\mu_1^2 + \mu_2^2 + C_1)(\sigma_1^2 + \sigma_2^2 + C_2)} \tag{26}$$

where μ_1, μ_2 and σ_1, σ_2 are the means and standard deviations of the images being compared, and σ_{12} is the covariance between them. These quantities are calculated using local statistics within a total of M windows, the average of which is taken in (26). Constants $C_1, C_2 \ll 1$ ensure stability (Wang et al., 2004), and M is chosen as 32. The SSIM has values in the $0 \rightarrow 1$ range, with unity representing structurally identical images.

Contrast to Noise Ratio (CNR) The CNR quantifies the level of contrast between a region of interest and the background, and is calculated as:

$$CNR = \frac{|\mu_1 - \mu_2|}{\sqrt{\sigma_1^2 + \sigma_2^2}} \tag{27}$$

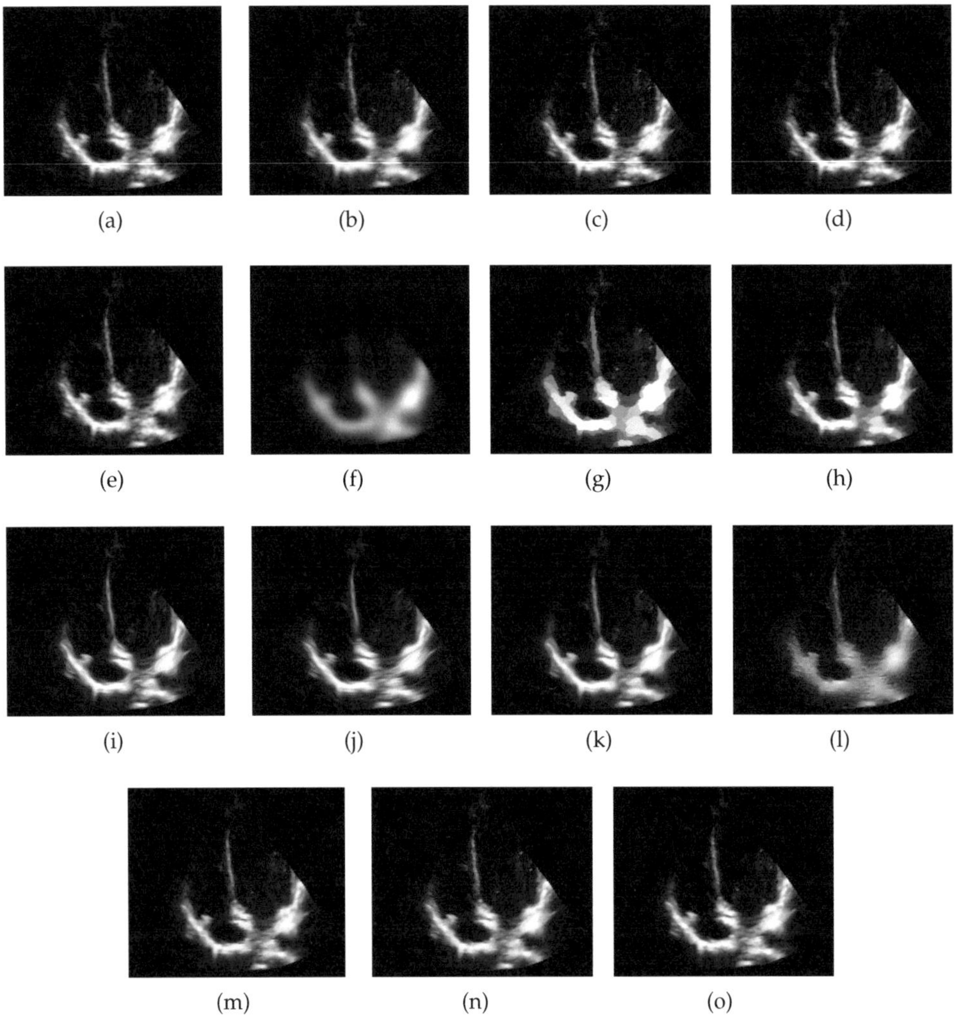

Fig. 5. Speckle filter output for the clinical image of Fig. 1(a). (a) Lee, (b) Kuan, (c) Frost, (d) EnhLee, (e) EnhFrost, (f) PMAD, (g) SRAD, (h) DPAD, (i) CED, (j) NCD, (k) OSRAD, (l) Zong, (m) GLM, (n) NMWD, (o) Geo.

where μ_1 and σ_1^2 are the mean and variance of a region of interest, and μ_2 and σ_2^2 are the mean and variance of a similar sized region in the image background.

$\mathbf{SNR_A}$ Burckhardt's (Burckhardt, 1978) SNR_A quantifies the level of speckle as the ratio of mean to standard deviation of the amplitude values.

For the simulated images, the SNR_A metric shows that the level of speckle is reduced by all of the filters. The MW reference has a higher average SNR_A than the post processing filters as expected, although some post processing filters exceed or match the MW SNR_A in individual regions. The NMWD and OSRAD filters achieve the highest average SNR_A values of the speckle reduction filters. The SRAD filter also performs well in this measure of speckle reduction. The OSRAD filter exceeds the average SNR_A of the MW reference in one image region, and matches it in another. SRAD exceeds the MW reference average SNR_A in a single image region. The rest of the anisotropic diffusion methods have varying results as quantified by SNR_A. The NCD, DPAD and PMAD filters are rated highly, however the CED method performs poorly. Of the SAR filters, the Lee filter achieves the highest SNR_A score. Apart from the NMWD filter, the wavelet based methods perform quite poorly in this test.

Application of the other image quality metrics to the simulated images shows that the OSRAD, CED and NCD filters have the lowest edge region MSE, i.e. the smallest difference in the intensity of pixels close to image edges. By contrast, the FoM metric quantifies the average distortion in edge pixel locations between each filtered image and the MW reference image. The filters which perform best here are the Zong wavelet filter and the SAR filters. The filters with output most similar to the MW edges, as measured by the edge region MSE, perform poorly in the FoM. The SSIM metric compares the average structural similarity of filtered output with the MW reference. Calculated values are quite low, with the CED filter having the highest average of 0.22. Thus the speckle filters output are not structurally similar to the MW reference images. The CNR metric quantifies the average difference in contrast between each filtered output and the corresponding MW reference. Negative CNR values here indicate a lower contrast value than the MW reference. Over one third of the filters show improved average contrast relative to the MW image, the greatest of which are for the PMAD and OSRAD filters.

Applying metrics to the output of the clinical image set shows that the filters which remove the most speckle are the same as in the simulated case, although the level of improvement in the SNR_A metric is lower than for the simulated images. The smaller SNR_A increase can be explained by the differences in image content between the simulated and clinical images. Unlike the simulated images, the clinical images contain specular as well as scattered reflections. In addition they contain deviations from Rayleigh statistics (Molthen et al., 1995). The OSRAD filter achieves the highest average FoM value. The diffusion filters in general achieve mixed FoM scores, while some of the SAR filters achieve quite high scores. The Enhanced Lee, Frost and Zong filters are on average the most similar to the speckled input according to the SSIM metric. For the Enhanced Lee and Frost filters, the SNR_A values indicate that this may be due to a low level of overall filtering. The CNR shows that the contrast increases for all post processing filters, with the OSRAD, SRAD and NMWD attaining the greatest improvement. The lowest average difference in edge region pixel intensity due to filtering is observed for the NMWD and OSRAD filters. The Frost, CED and Kuan filters also preserve the content of edge region pixels quite well as measured by this metric.

The computational requirements for each of the filtering methods are determined by calculation of the number of multiplications, additions, and look-up table operations. A number of considerations are detailed here. For the anisotropic diffusion filters, the choice of discretization method has a large impact on computational requirements. A discretization scheme which allows the choice of a larger timestep (τ) can achieve a given level of diffusion with less iterations. Three discretization methods were compared: a simple explicit scheme, the Additive Operator Splitting (AOS) scheme of (Weickert et al., 1998), and the Jacobi scheme of (Krissian et al., 2007). For each of these methods the error is found relative to a reference diffusion (explicit discretization with a very small τ) for the diffusion methods of (Perona & Malik, 1990) and (Aja-Fernandez & Alberola-Lopez, 2006). The error for all discretisation schemes increases with larger τ. The error measured for the explicit scheme is small as expected, but the valid range of τ is constrained to small values. The error for the AOS scheme and the Jacobi method are higher than the explicit method. It is observed that the AOS scheme performs similarly for both the PMAD and DPAD diffusion methods, while the Jacobi discretization results in a significantly higher error for one of the diffusion functions. Further details can be found in (Finn et al., 2010). In the analysis of computational requirements, various other implementational details are considered, which are also detailed in this paper.

After quantification of the filter complexity for each filter, it was found that the most computationally intensive method is the NMWD filter, for typical filtering scenarios. This filter required almost five times as many multiplications as the next most demanding. The DPAD and SRAD filters have higher requirements than the other diffusion methods, but this is due to the large number of iterations required. The DWT used in the GLM filter requires much more computation than the DWT of the Zong filter. The efficiency of the semi-implicit scheme for the anisotropic diffusion filters is demonstrated by the similarity between their requirements and the SAR filters.

The use of simulated images permits comparison of speckle reduced filtered output with a maximally noise free reference. Quantification of speckle reduction capabilities using the SNR_A has shown that anisotropic diffusion based methods have in general the strongest suppression of speckle. The application of objective metrics such as the FoM, Edge MSE, CNR and SSIM quantifies other aspects of the filtering process. The improvement in CNR values of the SRAD, OSRAD and NMWD filters shows that these methods can achieve greater contrast than other methods.. Average edge pixel distortion due to filtering was lowest in the matrix diffusion and SAR filters, as seen by both the high FoM and low edge region MSE values. This indicates that these methods distort image boundaries the least amount. In the case of the SAR filters however, this is due to a low overall level of filtering.

Based on analysis of computational complexity, it is clear that there is a large disparity in the requirements of the speckle reduction methods considered here. The SAR and geometric filters have the lowest computational overhead, but this comes at the expense of lower speckle reduction capability. The wavelet based approaches are hindered from a performance perspective by the requirements of implementing wavelet analysis and reconstruction. In particular, the NMWD filter performs wavelet analysis and reconstruction for each iteration, leading to the largest requirement of all considered methods. The anisotropic diffusion methods all have similar processing needs, and these fall between those of the SAR methods and the wavelet based filters. Efficient implementation of these methods is only possible by the use of a discretisation method which allows a large timestep.

This study concluded by noting that the optimal filtering method for echocardiography depends on the scenario: If the main concern is a constraint on available processing capability, the SAR filters are the best due to their low requirements. In particular the Lee filter is a reasonable choice given its speckle suppression ability and low overhead. If however the main objective is to remove as much speckle as possible, the NMWD filter has the strongest speckle suppression capabilities. This comes at the expense of the highest computational complexity however, and the preservation of edges is not optimal. The OSRAD method represents the best trade-off between both of these situations. The level of speckle suppression achievable using this approach is very close to that of the NMWD, with the advantage of a much smaller processing overhead. The OSRAD method was therefore considered the best compromise.

5. Conclusion

This chapter has presented an overview of the speckle artefact from ultrasound, with a focus on echocardiography. A description of nature and modelling of speckle was presented. The reduction or removal of speckle from clinical ultrasound and echocardiography is a common goal of image processing in the literature, and many of the recent approaches are detailed in Section 3 above.

The assessment of the quality of speckle reduced video is not a straightforward task. In the literature, many methods of review focus on numerical metrics and visual analysis without consideration of clinical opinion. For the case of clinical echocardiography, the extension of assessment technique to include expert physician opinion allows a more realistic evaluation. Image quality metrics are still of high importance however, due to their ease of computation and their objective nature.

This chapter has described a study in which the relationships between such metrics and objective expert opinion are explored, and it was found that certain metrics are strong indicators of physicians assessment. An extensive study of a large number of speckle reduction filters is also described above, focusing on real world application. A large number of speckled images, both clinical and simulated, are used as test data. Assessment includes image quality metrics (some of which are indicators of physicians evaluation) and also a computational requirement analysis.

An important aspect of evaluating the quality of speckle reduced echocardiography is that there are often differences between clinical and image processing perspectives. In particular, clinical experts do not appear to prefer the use of speckle filtered images for diagnostic analysis. It should be noted that there are situations where speckle preservation is desired. In particular, clinicians may prefer the original speckled images in some situations (Zhang et al., 2007). Dantas and Costa (Dantas & Costa, 2007) noted that when speckle is removed, the loss of false fine detail can lead to a perceived reduction in image sharpness, even if the boundaries of anatomical structures are not blurred. The speckle pattern is seen as having diagnostic utility in specific conditions, such as diffuse liver diseases (Kadah et al., 1996) in abdominal imaging and hypertrophic cardiomyopathy in echocardiography (Massay et al., 1989). Some automated processing tasks take advantage of the speckle pattern, such as feature tracking (Trahey et al., 1987) and tissue characterisation, some recent examples of which can be found in (De Marchi et al., 2006; Maurice et al., 2005; Tsui et al., 2005). So while some particular applications are best served by preserving speckle, others benefit from its removal. Perhaps the most pragmatic approach was taken by Zhang *et al.* (Zhang et al., 2007), who promote the idea of the speckle reduced image as a complementary addition to the original image, rather than a replacement.

6. References

Abd-Elmoniem, K., Youssef, A.-B. & Kadah, Y. (2002). Real-time speckle reduction and coherence enhancement in ultrasound imaging via nonlinear anisotropic diffusion,

49(9): 997–1014.
Achim, A., Bezerianos, A. & Tsakalides, P. (2001). Novel Bayesian multiscale method for speckle removal in medical ultrasound images, 20(8): 772–783.
Adam, D., Beilin-Nissan, S., Friedman, Z. & Behar, V. (2006). The combined effect of spatial compounding and nonlinear filtering on the speckle reduction in ultrasound images, *Ultrasonics* 44(2): 166–181.
Adelson, E., Anderson, C., Bergen, J., Burt, P. & Ogden, J. (1984). Pyramid methods in image processing, *RCA Engineer* 29(6).
Aiazzi, B., Alparone, L. & Baronti, S. (1998). Multiresolution local-statistics speckle filtering based on a ratio Laplacian pyramid, 36(5): 1466–1476.
Aja-Fernandez, S. & Alberola-Lopez, C. (2006). On the estimation of the coefficient of variation for anisotropic diffusion speckle filtering, 15(9): 2694–2701.
Bamber, J. C. & Daft, C. (1986). Adaptive filtering for reduction of speckle in ultrasonic pulse-echo images., *Ultrasonics* pp. 41–44.
Bamber, J. & Phelps, J. (1991). Real-time implementation of coherent speckle suppression in B-scan images, *Ultrasonics* 29(3): 218–224.
Behar, V., Adam, D. & Friedman, Z. (2003). A new method of spatial compounding imaging, *Ultrasonics* 41(5): 377–384.
Burckhardt, C. (1978). Speckle in ultrasound B-Mode scans, 25(1): 1–6.
Burt, P. & Adelson, E. (1983). The Laplacian pyramid as a compact image code, 31(4): 532–540.
Catté, F., Lions, P.-L., Morel, J.-M. & Coll, T. (1992). Image selective smoothing and edge detection by nonlinear diffusion, *SIAM J. Numer. Anal.* 29(1): 182–193.
Chen, Y., Yin, R., Flynn, P. & Broschat, S. (2003). Aggressive region growing for speckle reduction in ultrasound images, *Pattern Recogn. Lett.* 24(4-5): 677–691.
Coupé, P., Hellier, P., Kervrann, C. & Barillot, C. (2009). Nonlocal means-based speckle filtering for ultrasound images, 18(10): 2221–2229.
Crimmins, T. (1985). Geometric filter for speckle reduction, *Appl. Opt.* 24: 1438–1443.
Dantas, R. & Costa, E. (2007). Ultrasound speckle reduction using modified Gabor filters, 54(3): 530–538.
Dantas, R. G., Costa, E. T. & Leeman, S. (2005). Ultrasound speckle and equivalent scatterers, *Ultrasonics* 43(6): 405–420.
De Marchi, L., Testoni, N. & Speciale, N. (2006). Prostate tissue characterization via ultrasound speckle statistics, *IEEE Int. Symp. Signal Processing Information Technology*, pp. 208–211.
Dempster, A. P., Laird, N. M. & Rubin, D. B. (1977). Maximum likelihood from incomplete data via the EM algorithm, *J. R. Stat. Soc. B* 39(1): 1–38.
Donoho, D. L. (1995). De-noising by soft-thresholding, 41(3): 613–627.
Finn, S., Glavin, M. & Jones, E. (2010). Echocardiographic speckle reduction comparison, 58(1): 82–101.
Finn, S., Jones, E. & Glavin, M. (2009). Objective and subjective evaluations of quality for speckle reduced echocardiography, *Proc. IEEE Intl. Annu. Conf. Engineering Medicine and Biology Society*, pp. 503–506.
Frost, V. S., Stiles, J. A., Shanmugan, K. S. & Holtzman, J. C. (1982). A model for radar images and its application to adaptive digital filtering of multiplicative noise, 4(2): 157–166.
Fu, X.-W., Ding, M.-Y. & Cai, C. (2010). Despeckling of medical ultrasound images based on quantum-inspired adaptive threshold, *Electron. Lett.* 46(13): 889–891.

Galloway, R. L., McDermott, B. A. & Thurstone, F. L. (1988). A frequency diversity process for speckle reduction in real-time ultrasonic images, pp. 45–49.

Gehlbach, S. M. & Sommer, F. G. (1987). Frequency diversity speckle processing, *Ultrasonic Imaging* 9: 92–105.

Goodman, J. (1975). Statistical properties of laser speckle patterns, *in* J. Dainty (ed.), *Laser Speckle and Related Phenomena*, Vol. 9 of *Topics in Applied Physics*, Springer, Berlin, pp. 9–75.

Goodman, J. W. (1976). Some fundamental properties of speckle, *J. Opt. Soc. Am.* 66(11): 1145–1150.

Guo, H., Odegard, J., Lang, M., Gopinath, R., Selesnick, I. & Burrus, C. (1994). Wavelet based speckle reduction with application to SAR based ATD/R, *Proc. IEEE Int. Conf. Image Processing*, Vol. 1, pp. 75–79.

Gupta, N., Swamy, M. & Plotkin, E. (2005). Despeckling of medical ultrasound images using data and rate adaptive lossy compression, 24(6): 743–754.

Hao, X., Gao, S. & Gao, X. (1999). A novel multiscale nonlinear thresholding method for ultrasonic speckle suppressing, 18(9): 787–794.

Huang, H.-C., Chen, J.-Y., Wang, S.-D. & Chen, C.-M. (2003). Adaptive ultrasonic speckle reduction based on the slope-facet model, *Ultrasound Med. Biol.* 29(8): 1161–1175.

Jensen, J. (1991). A model for the propagation and scattering of ultrasound in tissue, *J. Acoust. Soc. Am.* 89: 182–190.

Jensen, J. A. (1996). FIELD: A program for simulating ultrasound systems, *Proc. 10th NordicBaltic Conference Biomedical Imaging*, Vol. 4, pp. 351–353.

Jespersen, S., Wilhjelm, J. & Sillesen, H. (2000). In vitro spatial compound scanning for improved visualization of atherosclerosis, *Ultrasound Med. Biol.* 26(8): 1357–1362.

Kadah, Y., Farag, A., Zurada, J., Badawi, A. & Youssef, A.-B. (1996). Classification algorithms for quantitative tissue characterization of diffuse liver disease from ultrasound images, 15(4): 466–478.

Karaman, M., Kutay, M. & Bozdagi, G. (1995). An adaptive speckle suppression filter for medical ultrasonic imaging, 14(2): 283–292.

Koo, J. I. & Park, S. B. (1991). Speckle reduction with edge preservation in medical ultrasonic images using a homogeneous region growing mean filter (HRGMF), *Ultrasonic Imaging* 13(3): 211–237.

Krissian, K. (2002). Flux-based anisotropic diffusion applied to enhancement of 3-d angiogram, 21(11): 1440–1442.

Krissian, K., Westin, C.-F., Kikinis, R. & Vosburgh, K. (2007). Oriented speckle reducing anisotropic diffusion, 16(5): 1412–1424.

Kruskal, W. H. & Wallis, W. A. (1953). Errata: Use of ranks in one-criterion variance analysis, *J. Am. Stat. Assoc.* 48(264): 907–911.

Kuan, D., Sawchuk, A., Strand, T. & Chavel, P. (1987). Adaptive restoration of images with speckle, ASSP-35(3): 373–383.

Lee, J.-S. (1980). Digital image enhancement and noise filtering by use of local statistics, PAMI-2(2): 165–168.

Lee, J.-S. (1981). Speckle analysis and smoothing of synthetic aperture radar images, *Comput. Vision Graph.* 17(1): 24–32.

Lizzi, F. L., Astor, M., Liu, T., Deng, C., Coleman, D. J. & Silverman, R. H. (1997). Ultrasonic spectrum analysis for tissue assays and therapy evaluation, *Int. J. Imag. Syst. Tech.* 8(1): 3–10.

Loizou, C. P., Pattichis, C. S., Christodoulou, C. I., Istepanian, R. S. H., Pantziaris, M. & Nicolaides, A. (2005). Comparative evaluation of despeckle filtering in ultrasound imaging of the carotid artery, 52(10): 1653–1669.

Lopes, A., Touzi, R. & Nezry, E. (1990). Adaptive speckle filters and scene heterogeneity, 28(6): 992–1000.

Loupas, T., McDicken, W. & Allan, P. (1989). An adaptive weighted median filter for speckle suppression in medical ultrasonic images, 36(1): 129 –135.

Magnin, P. A., von Ramm, O. T. & Thurstone, F. L. (1982). Frequency compounding for speckle contrast reduction in phased array images, *Ultrasonic Imaging* 4: 267–281.

Mallat, S. & Zhong, S. (1992). Characterization of signals from multiscale edges, 14(7): 710–732.

Massay, R. J., Logan-Sinclair, R. B., Bamber, J. C. & Gibson, D. G. (1989). Quantitative effects of speckle reduction on cross sectional echocardiographic images., *Br. Heart J.* 62(4): 298–304.

Mateo, J. L. & Fernández-Caballero, A. (2009). Finding out general tendencies in speckle noise reduction in ultrasound images, *Expert Syst. Appl.* 36(4): 7786–7797.

Maurice, R. L., Brusseau, E., Finet, G. & Cloutier, G. (2005). On the potential of the Lagrangian speckle model estimator to characterize atherosclerotic plaques in endovascular elastography: In vitro experiments using an excised human carotid artery, *Ultrasound Med. Biol.* 31(1): 85–91.

Michailovich, O. & Adam, D. (2005). A novel approach to the 2-d blind deconvolution problem in medical ultrasound, 24(1): 86–104.

Middleton, W. D. & Kurtz, A. B. (2004). *Ultrasound: The Requisites (Requisites in Radiology Series)*, 2 edn, Elsevier Mosby, Philadelphia, PA.

Molthen, R. C., Shankar, P. M. & Reid, J. M. (1995). Characterization of ultrasonic B-scans using non-Rayleigh statistics, *Ultrasound Med. Biol.* 21(2): 161–170.

Moulin, P. (1993). A wavelet regularization method for diffuse radar-target imaging and speckle-noise reduction, 3(1): 123–134.

Newhouse, V., Bilgutay, N., Saniie, J. & Furgason, E. (1982). Flaw-to-grain echo enhancement by split-spectrum processing, *Ultrasonics* 20(2): 59–68.

Ng, J., Prager, R., Kingsbury, N., Treece, G. & Gee, A. (2006). Modeling ultrasound imaging as a linear, shift-variant system, 53(3): 549–563.

Ng, J., Prager, R., Kingsbury, N., Treece, G. & Gee, A. (2007). Wavelet restoration of medical pulse-echo ultrasound images in an em framework, 54(3): 550–568.

O'Donnell, M. & Silverstein, S. (1988). Optimum displacement for compound image generation in medical ultrasound, 35(4): 470–476.

Pai-Chi, L. & O'Donnell, M. (1994). Elevational spatial compounding, *Ultrasonic imaging* 16(3): 176–189.

Perona, P. & Malik, J. (1990). Scale-space and edge detection using anisotropic diffusion, 12(7): 629–639.

Pižurica, A., Philips, W., Lemahieu, I. & Acheroy, M. (2003). A versatile wavelet domain noise filtration technique for medical imaging, 22(3): 323–331.

Pratt, W. K. (1977). *Digital Signal Processing*, Wiley, New York.

Quistgaard, J. (1997). Signal acquisition and processing in medical diagnostic ultrasound, 14(1): 67–74.

Rabbani, H., Vafadust, M., Abolmaesumi, P. & Gazor, S. (2008). Speckle noise reduction of medical ultrasound images in complex wavelet domain using mixture priors, 55(9): 2152–2160.

Rumack, C., Wilson, S., Charboneau, J. & Johnson, J. (2004). *Diagnostic ultrasound*, 3rd edn, Elsevier Mosby, Philadelphia, PA.

Sattar, F., Floreby, L., Salomonsson, G. & Lovstrom, B. (1997). Image enhancement based on a nonlinear multiscale method, 6(6): 888–895.

Shankar, P., Dumane, V., Reid, J., Genis, V., Forsberg, F., Piccoli, C. & Goldberg, B. (2001). Classification of ultrasonic b-mode images of breast masses using nakagami distribution, 48(2): 569–580.

Shankar, P. M. (1995). A model for ultrasonic scattering from tissues based on the K distribution, *Phys. Med. Biol.* 40(10): 1633–1649.

Smolíovái, R., Wachowiak, M. P. & Zurada, J. M. (2004). An information-theoretic approach to estimating ultrasound backscatter characteristics, *Comput. Biol. Med.* 34(4): 355–370.

Spearman, C. (1904). The proof and measurement of association between two things, *Amer. J. Psychol.* 15: 72–101.

Stetson, P., Sommer, F. & Macovski, A. (1997). Lesion contrast enhancement in medical ultrasound imaging, 16(4): 416–425.

Tay, P., Acton, S. & Hossack, J. (2006a). A stochastic approach to ultrasound despeckling, *Proc. 3rd IEEE Int. Symp. Biomedical Imaging: Nano to Macro*, pp. 221–224.

Tay, P., Acton, S. & Hossack, J. (2006b). Ultrasound despeckling using an adaptive window stochastic approach, *Proc. IEEE Int. Conf. Image Processing*, pp. 2549–2552.

Thakur, A. & Anand, R. (2005). Image quality based comparative evaluation of wavelet filters in ultrasound speckle reduction, *Digit. Signal Process.* 15(5): 455–465.

Thijssen, J. M. (2003). Ultrasonic speckle formation, analysis and processing applied to tissue characterization, *Pattern Recogn. Lett.* 24(4-5): 659–675.

Trahey, G. E., Allison, J. W., Smith, S. W. & von Ramm, O. T. (1986). A quantitative approach to speckle reduction via frequency compounding, *Ultrasonic Imaging* 8: 151–164.

Trahey, G. E., Allison, J. W. & von Ramm, O. T. (1987). Angle independent ultrasonic detection of blood flow, BME-34(12): 965–967.

Trahey, G. E., Smith, S. W. & von Ramm, O. T. (1986). Speckle reduction in medical ultrasound via spatial compounding, *Proc. SPIE Medicine XIV PACS*, Vol. 4, pp. 629–637.

Tsui, P.-H., Wang, S.-H. & Huang, C.-C. (2005). The effect of logarithmic compression on estimation of the nakagami parameter for ultrasonic tissue characterization: a simulation study, *Phys. Med. Biol.* 50(14): 3235–3244.

Wagner, R., Insana, M. & Smith, S. (1988). Fundamental correlation lengths of coherent speckle in medical ultrasonic images, 35(1): 34–44.

Wagner, R., Smith, S., Sandrik, J. & Lopez, H. (1983). Statistics of Speckle in Ultrasound B-Scans, 30(3): 156–163.

Wang, Z., Bovik, A., Sheikh, H. & Simoncelli, E. (2004). Image quality assessment: from error visibility to structural similarity, 13(4): 600–612.

Weickert, J. (1998). *Anisotropic Diffusion in Image Processing*, Teubner-Verlag, Stuttgart, Germany. Out of print.

Weickert, J. (1999). Coherence-enhancing diffusion filtering, *Int. J. Comput. Vision* 31(2-3): 111–127.

Weickert, J., Romeny, B. & Viergever, M. (1998). Efficient and reliable schemes for nonlinear diffusion filtering, 7(3): 398–410.

Yu, Y. & Acton, S. (2002). Speckle reducing anisotropic diffusion, 11(11): 1260–1270.

Yu, Y. & Acton, S. (2004). Edge detection in ultrasound imagery using the instantaneous coefficient of variation, 13(12): 1640–1655.

Yue, Y., Croitoru, M., Bidani, A., Zwischenberger, J. & Clark, J. J. (2006). Nonlinear multiscale wavelet diffusion for speckle suppression and edge enhancement in ultrasound images, 25(3): 297–311.

Zhang, F., Yoo, Y. M., Koh, L. M. & Kim, Y. (2007). Nonlinear diffusion in Laplacian pyramid domain for ultrasonic speckle reduction, 26(2): 200–211.

Zong, X., Laine, A. & Geiser, E. (1998). Speckle reduction and contrast enhancement of echocardiograms via multiscale nonlinear processing, 17(4): 532–540.

4

Speckle Detection in Echocardiographic Images

Arezou Akbarian Azar, Hasan Rivaz and Emad M. Boctor
The Russell H. Morgan Department of Radiology and Radiological Science
The Johns Hopkins University School of Medicine, Baltimore
USA

1. Introduction

B-scan Echocardiographic images unlikely carry unlikely images by scattering of ultrasound beams backed from structures within the body organ that is being scanned. Two major types of scatterings are diffused and coherent scatterings. Diffuse scatterings are caused when there are a large number of scatterers is with random phase within the resolution cell of the ultrasound beam and causes speckles in the reconstructed image; whereas the e coherent scattering arises when the scatterers in the resolution cell are in phase and causes light or dark spots in the image. Rayleigh distribution is the most common statistical model for the envelope signal and assumes that a large number of scatterers per resolution cell exist. However in some ultrasonic imaging fields such as echocardiography, Rayleigh distribution fits to reflect properties of reflections from blood but fails with complex structures such as myocardial tissue. The K distribution , on the other hand, was initially designed for the envelope signal and have been proposed to model different kinds of tissue in ultrasound envelope imaging. This distribution also has the advantage to model both fully and partially developed speckle. The first-order envelope statistics have been thought to follow a Rayleigh distribution, but recent work has shown that more general models, such as the Nakagami, K, and homodyned K distributions better describe envelope statistics.

With the current digital ultrasound imaging, the radio-frequency (RF) signal has gained more interest as it may contain more information than the envelope echo. When there are a large number of scatterers per range cell it yields Gaussian statistics for the RF signal, but the statistics of the RF signal in the case of partially developed speckle don't follow the Gaussian distribution. Therefore, in this study to model statistical behaviour of the RF data, we used K distribution framework, described in and for such statistics applied them to the RF data. By splitting the ultrasound image to image patches, statistical features for image patches can be extracted using the statistical modelling of the RF signal. These features could overlap for some tissues and the pattern classification approaches should be utilized to classify tissues based on the extracted statistical features. Over past decades, several supervised and unsupervised classification and segmentation algorithms have been proposed to process the medical images. Some of these techniques are listed in. Because of above mentioned problems (overlap between statistical features of tissues) and the fact that in our application (speckle classification), we cannot have enough training material and the data size (=number of image patches) is finite and small, we only focused on the unsupervised clustering techniques in this study.

2. Methods

2.1 Speckles artifact

One of inherent characteristics of coherent imaging techniques including ultrasound imaging is the presence of speckle-type- noise. Speckle is a random and deterministic pattern in the image formed by the use of the coherent radiation of a medium containing many scatterers. Although the texture of the speckle pattern does not correspond to under-scanning structure, the local brightness of the speckle pattern reflects the local echogenicity of the under-scanning scatterers. As can be seen in figure 1, each pixel in an ultrasound image is formed by the back scattered echoes from an approximately ellipsoid called the resolution cell. If each resolution cell in an image patch has many scatterers, the corresponding patch is called fully developed speckle (FDS). Speckle has a negative impact on ultrasound imaging. It has been shown that the detectability of lesion reduced approximately by a factor of eight due to the presence of speckle in the image. To track speckles as well as to estimate probe movement and improve performance of algorithms for adaptive speckle suppression and the elevational separation of B-scans by speckle decorrelation, we needed to model both fully speckle (blood pool) and partially developed speckle (tissue area). To this end, in the next subsections we investigated the ability of various statistical modelling of the RF signal and different unsupervised clustering techniques.

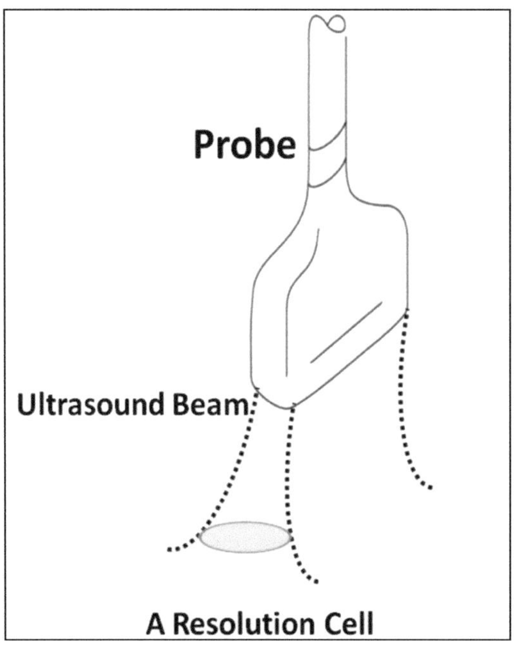

Fig. 1. Ultrasound beam and resolution cell.

2.2 Statistical features for speckle classification

2.2.1 Rayleigh distribution

Given the assumption of fully developed speckle, the envelope RF image patch, $Y = \{y_{i,j}\}$, is modeled by Rayleigh statistics, where the probability density function (pdf) is given by:

$$p(y_{i,j}) = \frac{y_{i,j}}{\sigma_{i,j}^2} e^{-\frac{y_{i,j}^2}{2\sigma_{i,j}^2}} \tag{1}$$

The underlying parameter of the Rayleigh distribution, Σ={σi,j}, associated with each pixel intensity of the RF image, $y_{i,j}$, is related to the acoustic properties at the corresponding location (i, j), in particular, the so-called echogenicity. Let $Z=\{z_{i,j}\}$ be a N ×M B-mode image corrupted by speckle where each pixel is generated according to the following Log-Compression law:

$$zi,j = a \log(yi,j + 1) + b \tag{2}$$

where (a, b) are unknown parameters which account for the contrast and brightness respectively. Given (1), the distribution of the observed pixels z,

$$p(z_{i,j}) = \left\{ \left| \frac{dy}{dx} \right| p(y) \right\}_{z=z_{i,j}} = \frac{y_{i,j}(y_{i,j}+1)}{a\sigma_{i,j}^2} e^{-\frac{y_{i,j}^2}{2\sigma_{i,j}^2}} \tag{3}$$

where $y = e^{\frac{z-a}{b}} - 1$. As pointed out in , (3) defines a double exponential distribution with known standard deviation (SD) analytical expression, yielding an estimate for a:

$$\hat{a}_{i,j} = \sqrt{24}\frac{\sigma_z(i,j)}{\pi} \tag{4}$$

where $\sigma_z(i, j)$ is the SD of the observations inside the window w, centred at the (i, j)th pixel.

To estimate the parameter b, we first consider the minimum of the observed pixels $z_{i,j}$ given by:

$$\begin{aligned} s = \min\{i,j\} &= a\log(\min\{y_{i,j}\}+1)+b \\ &= a\log(t+1)+b \end{aligned} \tag{5}$$

which means that:

$$b = s(Z) - a\log(t(\sigma, L)+1) \tag{6}$$

with $Z = \{z_{i,j}\}$. The distribution of b, derived in , is:

$$p(b \mid s(Z), \sigma) = \frac{L}{a\sigma^2} t(t+1) e^{-\frac{L}{2\sigma^2}t^2} \tag{7}$$

where $t = e^{\frac{s-b}{a}} - 1$. An estimator of b is found by computing the expected value of $b_{i,j}$ using a numerical approach, such that:

$$\hat{b}_{i,j} - \sum_{k=1}^{L} b_{i,j}(k) p(b_{i,j}(k) \mid s, \beta_{i,j}) \tag{8}$$

where $b_{i,j}(k) = k\, s/(L-1)$ and $k = 0, 1, ..., L-1$ are L uniformly distributed values in the interval [0, s], since $b \geq 0$ and from (6), $b \leq s$. In (8),

$$\beta_{i,j} = \sqrt{\frac{1}{2nm}\Omega_{k,l} q_{k,l}^2} \tag{9}$$

is Maximum Likelihood (ML) estimation of σi,j from the pixels inside the window $[w, q_{k,l}]$.

The estimators of a and b, considered constant across the image, are obtained by averaging the estimates $\hat{a}_{i,j}$ and $\hat{b}_{i,j}$, such that: $\hat{a} = \frac{1}{NM}\sum_i^N \sum_j^M \hat{a}_{i,j}$ and $\hat{b} = \frac{1}{NM}\sum_i^N \sum_j^M \hat{b}_{i,j}$.

These parameters ($\hat{a}, \hat{b}$) are used to retrieve the envelope RF image according to:

$$y_{i,j} = e^{\frac{z_{i,j} - b}{a}} - 1 \tag{10}$$

In some ultrasonic imaging fields such as echocardiography Rayleigh distribution fits to reflect properties of t model reflections from blood but fails with complex structures such as myocardial tissue. Another statistical model named K distribution have been proposed to model different kinds of tissue in ultrasound envelope imaging.

2.2.2 K distribution

The K distribution has been developed for the envelope signal. The interest of such distribution in ultrasonic images relies on its ability to model both fully speckle (blood pool) and partially developed speckle (tissue area) situations. In this section, we briefly describe the K distribution and the corresponding pdf for the RF signal. The backscattered ultrasonic signal results from the individual energy contributions of each scatterer embedded in the resolution cell. This situation can mathematically be described as a random walk in the complex plane. From this random flight model, the analytic signal can be expressed as a random process depending on the number of scatterers present inside the resolution cell, their relative position and contribution. Thus, a joint density function of the envelope and phase can be obtained by expressing both statistical properties of the phase and amplitude of each scatterer. This results in a K distribution when the scatterers phase is assumed to be uniformly distributed and when their amplitude is modelled as a K distribution itself.

The RF signal corresponds to the real part of the analytic signal. The power density function (pdf) of the RF signal thus corresponds to the marginal distribution obtained by integrating the pdf corresponding to the analytic signal with respect to its imaginary part, which yields the following expression (see for details):

$$pdf^{RF}(x) = \frac{b}{\sqrt{\pi}.\Gamma(\nu)} \left(\frac{b|x|}{2}\right)^{\nu - 0.5} K_{\upsilon-0.5}(b|x|) \tag{11}$$

where Γ is the Gamma function and $K_{\upsilon-0.5}$ is the modified Bessel function of the second kind of order $\upsilon - 0.5$.

This expression is completely specified by its two parameters υ & b, such that n controls the shape and b the scale of the pdf.

The corresponding distribution is called KRF distribution in the following. This pdf may thus provide the basis for segmentation of ultrasonic images in the case of partially developed speckle. However, KRF distribution has the following disadvantages based on the literature:

Numerical simulation show that estimation bias grows rapidly as parameter n increases, yielding unreliable estimates in blood regions (i.e. $\upsilon >> 1$);

Equation (2) implies repeated evaluation of a Bessel function, increasing the computational cost of the algorithm.

2.2.3 Statistical features for speckle classification

The coherent signal to the diffuse signal energy ratio (r) for a patch in an ultrasound image and the effective number of scatterers per resolution cell (μ) could be used as statistical features to identify speckles and characterize tissues. Speckle detection is a useful input for adaptive speckle suppression algorithms and for use in decorrelation algorithms to estimate the elevational distance between neighbouring B-scans.

To find r and μ, we need to model envelope signal behaviour. Having found r and μ we can then label as speckle patches with high μ and low k. Based on we calculate these statistics on arbitrary powers v of the image patch A.

$$
\begin{aligned}
R &= \frac{mean}{Std} = \frac{\langle A^{\nu} \rangle}{\sqrt{\langle A^{2\nu} \rangle - \langle A^{\nu} \rangle^{2}}} \\
Skewness &= \frac{(A^{\nu} - \langle A^{\nu} \rangle)^{3}}{(\langle A^{2\nu} \rangle - \langle A^{\nu} \rangle^{2})^{3/2}} \\
Kurtosis &= \frac{(A^{\nu} - \langle A^{\nu} \rangle)^{4}}{(\langle A^{2\nu} \rangle - \langle A^{\nu} \rangle^{2})^{4/2}}
\end{aligned}
\qquad (12)
$$

Where Std means standard deviation, <. > =mean. Based on the results in , values of v more than one is suggested to perform well. As explained in the previous subsections, each statistical models for the RF signal has some advantages and some disadvantages. This suggests that we must consider both statistical models (Rayleigh and KRF) to better characterize statistical behaviour of the RF signal. Therefore for each image patch A, we propose to compute statistical features in (10) and Maximum Likelihood (ML) $\beta_{i,j}$ in (8) estimation of the data A following the Rayleigh distribution.

After extracting features for each image patch A, we can use the classification scheme shown in figure 2 to classify each image patch to FDS and non-FDS.

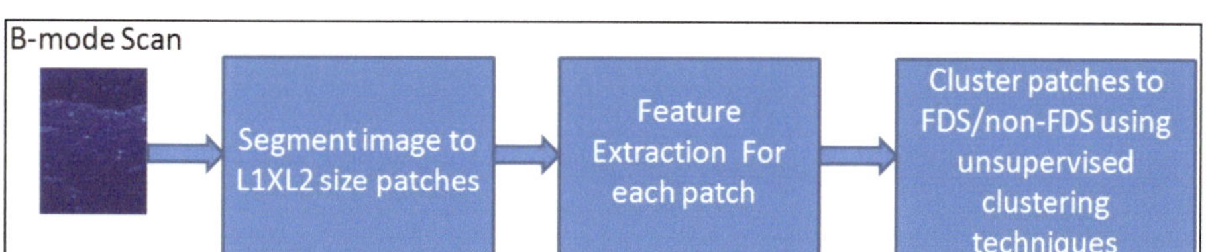

Fig. 2. Pipeline for Speckle detection.

2.3 Unsupervised clustering for speckle classification

Data clustering means partitioning data to fuzzy or crisp (hard) subsets. Hard clustering in a data set X means partitioning the data into a specified number of subsets of X with such a condition that an object either does or does not belong to a cluster. The number of subsets (clusters) is denoted by K. The hard partitioning is the simplest approach for data clustering, though its results are not always reliable and has numerical problems as well. However, fuzzy clustering allows objects to belong to multiple clusters in the same time, with different degrees of membership. In many real applications fuzzy clustering is more realistic than hard clustering, as objects on the boundaries between several classes are not forced to fully belong to one of the classes. In this study we used both hard (K-means and K-mediod) and fuzzy partitioning (Fuzzy C-Means, Gustafson-Kessel and Gath-Geva techniques) for speckle detection in a competitive manner.

2.3.1 K-means and K-medoid

The hard partitioning methods are simple and popular, though its results are not always reliable and these algorithms have numerical problems as well. From an Nxn dimensional data set K-means and K-medoid allocates algorithms allocates each data point to one of K clusters (in our case 2 for FDS and non-FDS) to minimize the within-cluster sum of squares (distance norm):

$$\sum_{i=1}^{K} \sum_{i \in A_j} \left\| X_i - V_j \right\| \tag{13}$$

where A_j is a set of objects (data points) in the j-th cluster. In k-means, V_j is the mean for that points over cluster j and is called the cluster prototypes or centers. While in K-medoid clustering the cluster centers are the nearest objects to the mean of data in one cluster. K-mediod is useful when there is no continuity in the data space.

2.3.2 Fuzzy C-means clustering

The Fuzzy C-means clustering algorithm is based on the minimization of an objective function called C-means functional. It is defined by Dunn as:

$$J = \sum_{j=1}^{C} \sum_{i=1}^{N} (\mu_{ji})^{m} \left\| X_i - V_j \right\|^2 \tag{14}$$

Where μ is membership degree, m is order, and V_j is center of the cluster j, which all of them have to be determined. The minimization of the c-means functional J (cost function) represents a nonlinear optimization problem that can be solved by using a variety of available methods, ranging from grouped coordinate minimization, over simulated annealing to genetic algorithms. The most popular method, however, is a simple Picard iteration through the first-order conditions for stationary points of J, known as the fuzzy c-means (FCM) algorithm.

The stationary points of the objective function J can be found by adjoining the following constraint for the fuzzy partitions $U=[\mu_{ji}]$:

$$\sum_{j=1}^{C} \mu_{ji} = 1, \quad 1 \le i \le N \tag{15}$$

If $||X_i - V_j||^2 > 0$ and m>1, then (U,V) may minimize J only if

$$\mu_{ji} = \frac{1}{\sum_{k=1}^{C} \left(\frac{\|X_i - V_j\|}{\|X_i - V_k\|} \right)^{\frac{2}{m-1}}}, \quad 1 \le j \le c, \quad 1 \le i \le N$$
$$V_j = \frac{\sum_{i=1}^{N} \mu_{ji}^{m} X_i}{\sum_{i=1}^{N} \mu_{ji}^{m}}, \quad 1 \le i \le N, \tag{16}$$

This solution also satisfies the constraints on fuzzy partitions. Note that equation for cluster centers gives V_j as the weighted mean of the data items that belong to a cluster, where the weights are the membership degrees. That is why the algorithm is called "c-means". The FCM algorithm computes with the standard Euclidean distance norm, which induces hyperspherical clusters. Hence it can only detect clusters with the same shape and orientation, because the common choice of norm matrix is the identical matrix.

2.3.3 Gustafson-Kessel clustering algorithm

It is extended version of the standard fuzzy c-means algorithm by employing an adaptive distance norm, in order to detect clusters of different geometrical shapes in one data set. Each cluster has its own norm-inducing matrix Ai:

$$D_{ikA}^{2} = (x_k - v_i)^T A_i (x_k - v_i), \qquad 1 \le i \le c, \quad 1 \le k \le N \tag{17}$$

The matrices Ai are used as optimization variables in the c-means functional, thus allowing each cluster to adapt the distance norm to the local topological structure of the data. Cost function for Gustafson-Kessel clustering algorithm (GK) algorithm is defined as following:

$$J = \sum_{i=1}^{C} \sum_{k=1}^{N} \mu_{ik}^{m} . D_{ikA_i}^{2} \tag{18}$$

where the N x C matrix $U=[\mu_{ik}]$ represents the fuzzy partitions. D means distance as defined in (17). To optimize the cluster's shape, it is proven that A_i should be as following:

$$A_i = [\rho_i \det(F_i)]^{1/n} . F_i^{-1} \tag{19}$$

where ρ_i is a fixed value for each cluster and det() means determinant of a matrix and F means fuzzy covariance matrix defined by:

$$F_i = \frac{\sum_{k=1}^{N} \mu_{ik}^{m} (X_k - V_i)(X_k - V_i)^T}{\sum_{k=1}^{N} \mu_{ik}^{m}} \tag{20}$$

Indeed A_i is a generalized squared Mahalanobis distance norm between point X_k and the cluster mean Vi, where the covariance is weighted by the membership degrees in $U=[\mu_{ik}]$. Mahalanobis distance is a distance based on correlations between variables by which different patterns can be identified and analyzed. It is a useful way of determining similarity of an unknown sample set to a known one. It differs from Euclidean distance in that it takes into account the correlations of the data set and is scale-invariant, i.e. not dependent on the scale of measurements.

2.3.4 Gath-Geva fuzzy classifier

The Gath-Geva fuzzy clustering algorithm employs a distance norm based on the fuzzy maximum likelihood estimates (FMLE), proposed by Bezdek and Dunn :

$$D_{ik}(X_k, V_i) = \frac{\sqrt{\det(F_{wi})}}{\alpha_i} \exp(0.5(X_k - V_i)^T F_{wi}^{-1}(X_k - V_i)) \tag{21}$$

Note that, contrary to the GK algorithm, this distance norm involves an exponential term and thus decreases faster. F_{wi} denotes the fuzzy covariance matrix of the i-the cluster, given by:

$$F_{wi} = \frac{\sum_{k=1}^{N} \mu_{ik}^{w}(X_k - V_i)(X_k - V_i)^T}{\sum_{k=1}^{N} \mu_{ik}^{w}}, \quad 1 \le i \le c \tag{22}$$

If w = 1, F_{wi} is identical to the original FMLE algorithm, but if w = 2, so that the partition becomes more fuzzy to compensate the exponential term of the distance norm. The difference between the matrix F_i in GK algoritm and the Fwi in (22) is that the latter does not involve the weighting exponent m, instead of this it consists of w = 1. This is because the two weighted covariance matrices arise as generalizations of the classical covariance from two different concepts. The α_i is the prior probability of selecting cluster is given by:

$$\alpha_i = \frac{1}{N} \sum_{k=1}^{N} \mu_{ik} \tag{23}$$

The membership degrees μ_{ik} are interpreted as the posterior probabilities of selecting the i-th cluster given the data point xk. Gath and Geva reported that the fuzzy maximum likelihood estimates clustering algorithm is able to detect clusters of varying shapes, sizes and densities. The cluster covariance matrix is used in conjunction with an "exponential" distance, and the clusters are not constrained in volume. However, this algorithm is less robust in the sense that it needs a good initialization, since due to the exponential distance norm, it converges to a near local optimum.

2.4 Echocardiographic images simulation

In order to quantitatively compare statistical features and classification methods, as ground truth, we used two different types of ultrasound simulation programs. To simulate short-axis echocardiographic images Field II simulator were used and to simulate left-ventricle

(LV) cardiac images the convolutional approach that ignores the geometry of the transducer were used. As opposed to the Field II simulator ignoring geometry allows to speed up simulations but at the cost of realism of the simulated images. For the simulation it is assumed that the imaging system has a linear, space-invariant point spread function (PSF) and the transducer is linear. We also applied our speckle classification scheme on other phantoms: fetus and cyst phantoms generated Field II simulator.

3. Results

To evaluate our proposed speckle classification scheme and calculate performance of each unsupervised classification technique, as the ground truth, we used B-mode images simulated by ultrasound simulation programs with 100,000 scatterers and 128 RF lines (see Figure 3). After resizing of reconstructed images to the size of 1200x800 pixels, they were segmented to 12x8 image patches, where each image patch had size of 100x100 pixels. We then calculated following statistical features for image patch: R, Skewness and Kurtosis features for the k-distribution and Maximum Likelihood (ML) for the Rayleigh distribution. After calculating statistical features for each image patch, we will have 4 dimensional features for each image patch and we can classify them to FDS and non-FDS using unsupervised clustering techniques. For this purpose in this study we applied five pattern classification techniques: K-means, K-medoid, Fuzzy C-means, Gustafson-Kessel fuzzy classifier and Gath-Geva fuzzy classifier. Figures 4,5,6 and 7 show performance of the classification methods for speckle detection, respectively for cyst, fetus, LV and short axes heart phantoms. Figure 8 show the specke detection performance for a real ultrasound image of a beating heart using 3D Ultrasound.

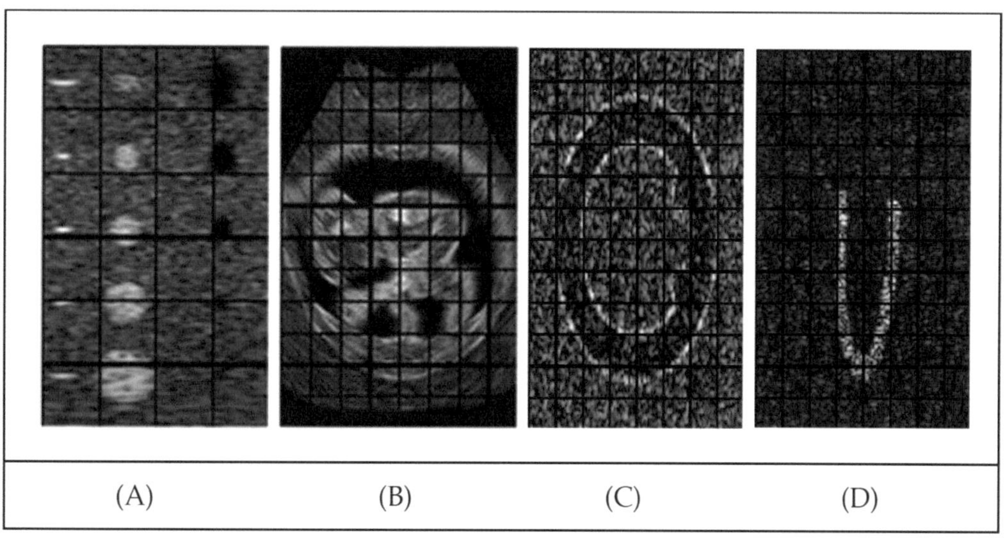

Fig. 3. Simulation Examples: A) short-axis, B) left ventricle, C) cyst and D) fetus phantoms and patches. Images were segmented to 12x8 image patches, where each image patch had size of 100x100 pixels.

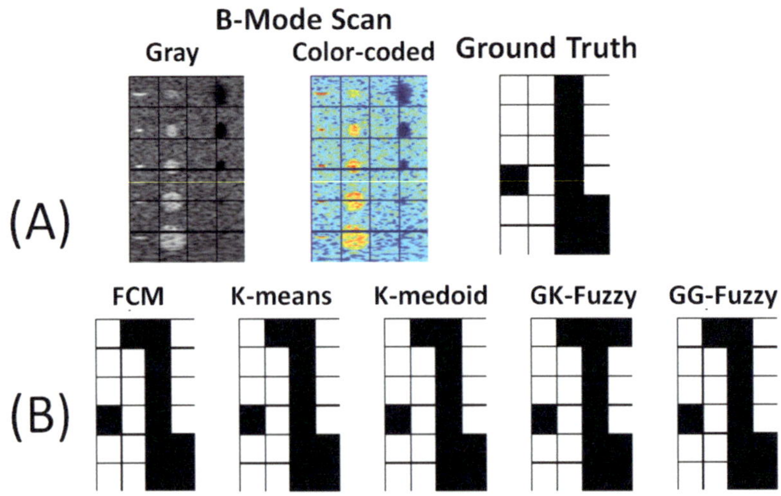

Dice Similarity	**0.97**	**0.97**	**0.97**	**0.93**	**0.97**

Fig. 4. Simulated ultrasound image of a cyst phantom (A) and speckle detection results for five different unsupervised classifiers. Total number of 100x100 patches for the phantom image was 24. Patches classified as fully developed speckles (FDS) are shown as black. All methods except GK-fuzzy classifier performed the same. Orders for statistical features respectively were 1,1 and 0.5.

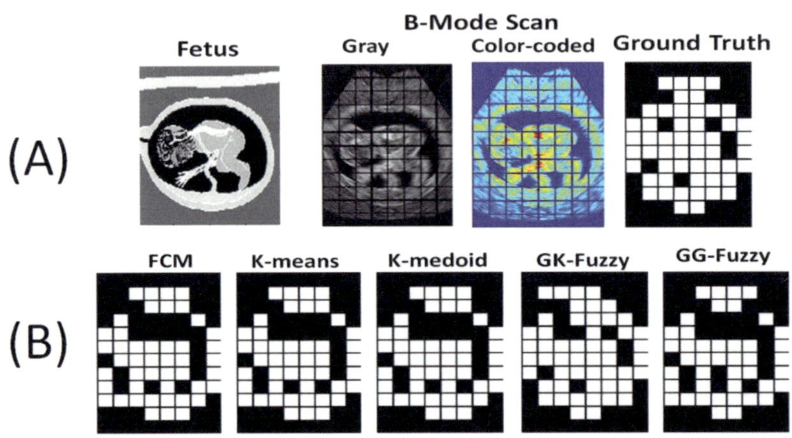

Dice Similarity	**0.85**	**0.85**	**0.85**	**0.96**	**0.85**

Fig. 5. Simulated ultrasound image of a fetus in 12th week (A) and speckle detection results for five different unsupervised classifiers. Patches classified as fully developed speckles (FDS) are shown as black. As can be seen, FCM,K-means and K-mediod performed the same. GK and GG fuzzy classifiers were able to decrease false positives and improve accuracy of the speckle detection. Total number of patches (100x100 pixels) for the phantom image was 96. Orders for statistical features respectively was 1,1 and 0.5.

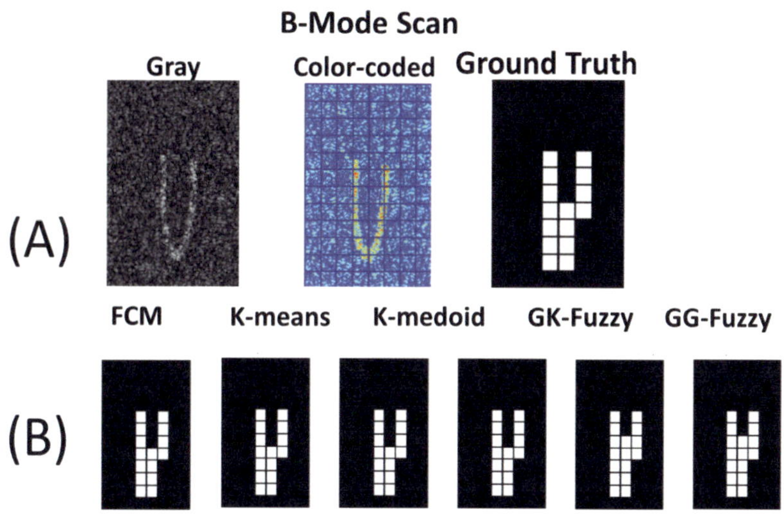

Dice Similarity	1	1	1	0.99	0.99

Fig. 6. Simulated ultrasound image of left ventricle (A) and speckle detection results for five different unsupervised classifiers. Patches classified as fully developed speckles (FDS) are shown as black. Total number of patches (100x100 pixels) for the phantom image was 96. Orders for statistical features respectively was 1,1 and 1.

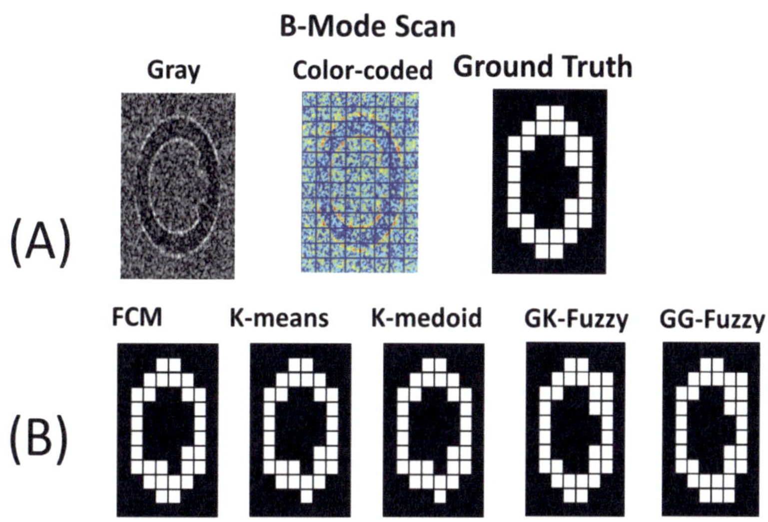

Dice Similarity	0.94	0.90	0.90	0.94	0.90

Fig. 7. Simulated ultrasound image of the heart in short axis (end diastolic) (A) and speckle detection results for five different unsupervised classifiers. Patches classified as fully developed speckles (FDS) are shown as black. Total number of patches (100x100 pixels) for the phantom image was 96. Orders for statistical features respectively was 1,1 and 1.

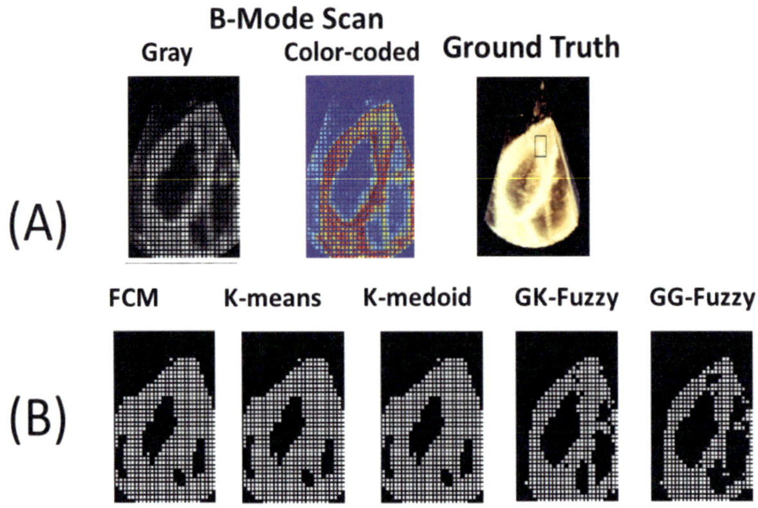

Dice Similarity	**0.86**	**0.86**	**0.86**	**0.97**	**0.91**

Fig. 8. Ultrasound image of the right ventricle (A) and speckle detection results for five different unsupervised classifiers. Patches classified as fully developed speckles (FDS) are shown as black. Total number of patches (30x30 pixels) for the ultrasound image was 96. Orders for statistical features respectively was 1,1 and 1.

4. Summary

In this study we reviewed the present statistical models to predict behaviour of the RF signal for different tissue types. In some ultrasonic imaging fields such as echocardiography Rayleigh distribution fits to reflect properties of reflections from blood but fails with complex structures such as myocardial tissue. However, another statistical model named K distribution have been proposed to model different kinds of tissue in ultrasound envelope imaging. To consider both statistical properties of the echocardiographic images we applied both Rayleigh and K-distributions and for each image patch A, we computed statistical features for K-distribution and Maximum Likelihood (ML) estimation of the image patch following the Rayleigh distribution. After extracting features for each image patch, we applied the unsupervised clustering techniques to classify each image patch to FDS and non-FDS. Based on our observation, we found when we use all statistical features (R-S-K- ML) together classifiers was able to separate classes in data space better than with other combinations out of R-S-K- ML features. Based on Table 1 ranking of the fuzzy classification methods performed better. To improve specificity and sensitivity of the proposed machine-learning speckle detection scheme, feature whitening and mapping techniques such as Sammon mapping can applied to increase distance between features before applying unsupervised classification techniques.

5. References

Abonyi, J., Babuska, R., Szeifert, F., 2002. Modified Gath-Geva fuzzy clustering for identification of Takagi-Sugeno fuzzy models. Systems, Man, and Cybernetics, Part B: Cybernetics, IEEE Transactions on. 32, 612-621.

Bamber, J.C., Dickinson, R.J., 1980. Ultrasonic B-scanning: a computer simulation. Phys Med Biol. 25, 463-79.

Bamber, J.C., Phelps, J.V., 1991. Real-time implementation of coherent speckle suppression in B-scan images. Ultrasonics. 29, 218-24.

Bankman, I.N., Nizialek, T., Simon, I., Gatewood, O.B., Weinberg, I.N., Brody, W.R., 1997. Segmentation algorithms for detecting microcalcifications in mammograms. IEEE Trans Inf Technol Biomed. 1, 141-9.

Bernard, O., D'Hooge, J., Friboulet, D., 2006. Statistics of the radio-frequency signal based on K distribution with application to echocardiography. Ultrasonics, Ferroelectrics and Frequency Control, IEEE Transactions on. 53, 1689-1694.

Bernard, O., Touil, B., Gelas, A., Prost, R., Friboulet, D., 2007. Segmentation of Myocardial Regions in Echocardiography Using the Statistics of the Radio-Frequency Signal. In: Functional Imaging and Modeling of the Heart. Lecture Notes in Computer Science, Vol. 4466, F. Sachse, G. Seemann, ed.^eds. Springer Berlin / Heidelberg, pp. 433-442.

Bezdek, J.C., 1975. Optimal Fuzzy Partitions: A Heuristic for Estimating the Parameters in a Mixture of Normal Distributions. IEEE Transactions on Computers. 24, 835-838.

Bezdek, J.C., Hall, L.O., Clarke, L.P., 1993. Review of MR image segmentation techniques using pattern recognition. Med Phys. 20, 1033-48.

Dutt, V., Greenleaf, J.F., 1994. Ultrasound echo envelope analysis using a homodyned K distribution signal model, Vol. 16, Dynamedia, Silver Spring, MD, ETATS-UNIS.

Gath, I., 1989. Unsupervised Optimal Fuzzy Clustering. IEEE Transactions on Pattern Analysis and Machine Intelligence. 11, 773-780.

Gullo, F., Ponti, G., Tagarelli, A., 2008. Clustering Uncertain Data Via K-Medoids. In: Proceedings of the 2nd international conference on Scalable Uncertainty Management. Vol., ed.^eds. Springer-Verlag, Naples, Italy, pp. 229-242.

Jensen, J.A., 2004. Simulation of advanced ultrasound systems using Field II. In: Biomedical Imaging: Nano to Macro, 2004. IEEE International Symposium on. Vol., ed.^eds., pp. 636-639 Vol. 1.

Kobayashi, T., Kida, Y., Tanaka, T., Kageyama, N., Kobayashi, H., Amemiya, Y., 1986. Magnetic induction hyperthermia for brain tumor using ferromagnetic implant with low Curie temperature. Journal of Neuro-Oncology. 4, 175-181.

Matsumoto, M., Yoshimura, N., Honda, Y., Hiraoka, M., Ohura, K., 1994. Ferromagnetic hyperthermia in rabbit eyes using a new glass-ceramic thermoseed. Graefe's Archive for Clinical and Experimental Ophthalmology. 232, 176-181.

Molthen, R.C., Shankar, P.M., Reid, J.M., 1995. Characterization of ultrasonic B-scans using non-rayleigh statistics. Ultrasound in medicine & biology. 21, 161-170.

Molthen, R.C., Shankar, P.M., Reid, J.M., Forsberg, F., Halpern, E.J., Piccoli, C.W., Goldberg, B.B., 1998. Comparisons of the Rayleigh and K-distribution models using in vivo breast and liver tissue. Ultrasound in medicine & biology. 24, 93-100.

Ordsmith, R.J., 1967. Abramowitz,M - Handbook Mathematical Functions with Formulas Graphs and Mathematical Tables. Computer Journal. 10, 45-&.

Ossant, F., Patat, F., Lebertre, M., Teriierooiterai, M.L., Pourcelot, L., 1998. Effective density estimators based on the K distribution: interest of low and fractional order moments. Ultrason Imaging. 20, 243-59.

Pham, D.L., Xu, C., Prince, J.L., 2000. Current methods in medical image segmentation. Annu Rev Biomed Eng. 2, 315-37.

Prager, R.W., Gee, A.H., Treece, G.M., Berman, L.H., 2003. Decompression and speckle detection for ultrasound images using the homodyned <i>K</i>-distribution. Pattern Recogn. Lett. 24, 705-713.

Rivaz, H., Boctor, E.M., Fichtinger, G., 2006. P3E-9 Ultrasound Speckle Detection Using Low Order Moments. In: Ultrasonics Symposium, 2006. IEEE. Vol., ed.^eds., pp. 2092-2095.

Sammon, J.W., Jr., 1969. A Nonlinear Mapping for Data Structure Analysis. Computers, IEEE Transactions on. C-18, 401-409.

Sanches, J.M., Marques, J.S., 2003. Compensation of log-compressed images for 3-D ultrasound. Ultrasound in medicine & biology. 29, 239-253.

Seabra, J., Sanches, J., 2008. Modeling log-compressed ultrasound images for radio frequency signal recovery. In: Engineering in Medicine and Biology Society, 2008. EMBS 2008. 30th Annual International Conference of the IEEE. Vol., ed.^eds., pp. 426-429.

Shankar, P.M., 1995. A model for ultrasonic scattering from tissues based on the K distribution. Physics in Medicine and Biology. 40, 1633.

Tatti, N., 2007. Distances between Data Sets Based on Summary Statistics. J. Mach. Learn. Res. 8, 131-154.

Thienphrapa, P., Elhawary, H., Ramachandran, B., D. Stanton, Popovic, A., 2011. Tracking and characterization of fragments in a beating heart using 3D ultrasound for interventional guidance. In: Medical Image Computing and Computer Assisted Intervention Conference (MICCAI). Vol., ed.^eds., Toronto, Canada.

Yih, J.-M., Huang, S.-F., 2010. Unsupervised clustering algorithm based on normalized Mahalanobis distances. In: Proceedings of the 9th WSEAS international conference on Applied computer and applied computational science. Vol., ed.^eds. World Scientific and Engineering Academy and Society (WSEAS), Hangzhou, China, pp. 180-184.

Part 2

New Techniques in Trans-Thoracic Echocardiography

Automated Segmentation of Real-Time 3D Echocardiography Using an Incompressibility Constraint

Yun Zhu, Xenophon Papademetris,
Albert Sinusas and James Duncan
Yale University
USA

1. Introduction

Coronary Heart Disease (CHD) is characterized by reduced blood flow and oxygen supply to the heart muscle, resulting from the occlusion of one or more major coronary arteries. CHD remains the most prevalent cause of mortality in developed countries and represents one of the major burdens on the healthcare systems today. Approximately every 25 seconds, an American will suffer from a coronary event, and about every minute, someone will die from one. According to the 2009 American Heart Association (AHS) report (Lloyd-Jones et al., 2009}, an estimated of 16.8 million American adults have CHD (extrapolated to US population in 2009 from National Health and Nutrition Examination Survey (NHANES) 2005-2006) and about 20% of total deaths in the United States are caused by CHD.

The advancements in noninvasive imaging techniques, such as real-time three-dimensional (RT3D) echocardiography, have enabled physicians to detect CHD in its earliest and most treatable stage. With cardiac imaging, physicians are able to evaluate essential global and local functional parameters, such as ejection fraction (EF), wall thickening, strain/strain rate, and etc. The rapid progress in cardiac imaging, however, has led to new challenges in handling of huge amount of image data involved in comprehensive functional patient studies. Manually analyzing these data sets becomes a formidable task for cardiologists, radiologists, and technicians in order to interpret the data and derive clinically useful information for diagnosis or decision support for surgical and pharmacological interventions. Also, manual analysis is subjective and therefore compromises the accuracy and reproducibility of quantitative measurements.

The abovementioned reasons have triggered a great demand for computerized techniques to automate the analysis of cardiac images. Various image-processing tasks need to be performed in order to recover diagnostically useful information, among which myocardial segmentation is one of the most important tasks. Myocardial segmentation aims to delineate the endocardial (ENDO) and epicardial (EPI) boundaries from cardiac images. Accurate segmentation of myocardial boundaries is essential for deriving cardiac global functional parameters such as ventricular mass/volume, ejection fraction, and wall thickening. It is also a prerequisite step for accurate myocardial deformation analysis.

However, myocardial segmentation is challenging, particularly for the EPI surface. This is due to the misleading, physically corrupted, and sometimes incomplete visual information of the EPI contours.

- Myocardium and liver are anatomically close to each other and often share similar intensity values. Thus, there is usually no clear and visible edge between them;
- The myocardium/lung air contrast is lower than the blood pool/myocardium contrast. This implies that myocardium and lung air have similar intensity properties, and might be misclassified as belonging in the same class;
- The right ventricle (RV) myocardium, which has similar intensity values as the left ventricular (LV) myocardium, often merges into the LV myocardium at the LV/RV juncture.

In this chapter, we present an automated coupled deformable model for the segmentation of LV myocardial borders from RT3D echocardiographic images. This approach was originally proposed in (Zhu et al., 2010). It incorporates the incompressibility property of myocardial, and therefore is able to handle fuzzy EPI borders. This model is formulated in a Bayesian framework, which maximizes the regional homogeneities of a cardiac image, while maintaining the myocardial volume during a cycle. By simultaneously evolving both ENDO and EPI surfaces, an automatic segmentation of the full myocardium is achieved from RT3D echocardiographic images.

The remaining sections are organized as follows. Section 2 presents background of echocardiographic image segmentation. Section 3 discusses the incompressibility property of the myocardium. Section 4 is the general framework and details of the method. Section 5 presents experimental results and finally section 6 is the conclusion.

2. Background

The heart is composed of four chambers: left atrium (LA), left ventricle, right atrium (RA), and right ventricle. Fig. 1(a) shows a long-axis cross-section of the heart. As shown in Fig. 1(a), the atria and ventricles are surrounded by muscle tissues called myocardium. Contraction and relaxation of the muscle fibers in the myocardium cause the pumping of the heart.

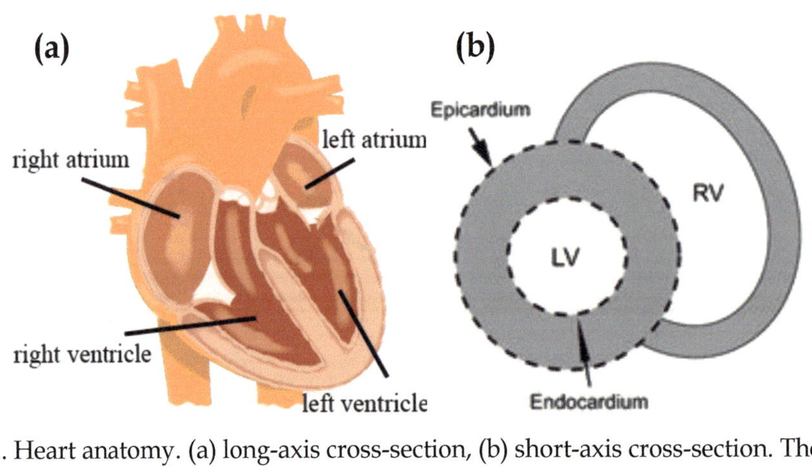

Fig. 1. Heart anatomy. (a) long-axis cross-section, (b) short-axis cross-section. The grey region represents the myocardium.

Fig. 1(b) shows a short-axis cross-section of the heart. The grey region represents the myocardium. The inner surface of the myocardium is called endocardium, and outer surface is called epicardium. As the LV is a powerful blood pump for the systemic circulation, the delineation of the LV endocardium and epicardium is often the object of interest for cardiologists, particularly because it is an important step for analyzing LV anatomical structure, quantifying cardiac function, and estimating LV motion.

Automatic LV segmentation algorithms can be broadly categorized into region-based and boundary-based methods. Region-based methods exploit the homogeneity of spatially dense information, e.g. pixel-wise grey level values, to produce segmented images. Examples of region-based segmentation methods include thresholding, region-growing, Markov random field-based approaches, and etc. In contrast to the region-based methods, boundary-based methods rely on the pixel-wise difference to guide the process of segmentation. They try to locate points of abrupt changes in the grey tone images. Examples of boundary-based methods include edge-detection, Hough transform, boundary-based snakes, and etc. However, in numerous medical imaging modalities, the LV boundaries cannot be reliably and accurately detected using the algorithms which rely only on boundary or edge information. Reasons for this include significant signal loss, noise, complicated geometric shapes. These problems are ever present for acquired in echocardiography, where the boundary detection problem is further complicated by the presence of attenuation, speckle, shadows, confusing anatomical structures.

In an effort to overcome these difficulties, various sources of image information have been used in the segmentation process. Most commonly used ones include grey level distribution, gradient, texture, and phase information. The choice of which information to use depends on imaging modality, image quality, and specific applications.

2.1 Grey level distribution

Incorporation of imaging physics as prior knowledge has been proven to be useful for cardiac segmentation (Paragios, 2002; Pluempitiwiriyawe et al., 2005, Chen et al., 2008). The random intensity distribution in ultrasound images, also known as speckle, is caused by the interference of energy from randomly distributed scatters, too small to be resolved by the imaging system. When an acoustic pulse travels through tissue or any medium, backscattering from the scatters in the range cell contributes to the returned echo. This contribution to the echo from the scatters in the range cell has been treated as a random walk because the locations of the scatters are considered to be random. The backscattered echo, therefore, is complex valued with a real part X and imagery part Y . By virtue of central limit theorem, X and Y have identical Gaussian distribution $N\left(0,\sigma^2\right)$, where σ^2 is its variance.

The envelop of the backscattered echo, I , is given by

$$I = \sqrt{X^2 + Y^2}$$

It has been shown that the envelop I has a Rayleigh distribution

$$P(I;\sigma) = \frac{I}{\sigma^2}\exp\left(-\frac{I^2}{2\sigma^2}\right)$$

The Rayleigh distribution has been proven to be one of the most popular models in ultrasound image analysis. For example, a Rayleigh distribution was incorporated into a region-based level-set approach for the segmentation of ultrasound images (Sarti et al., 2005). Also Cohen *et al.* proposed to use Rayleigh distribution as an image formation model in a maximum likelihood motion estimation scheme for noisy ultrasound images (Cohen and Dinstein 2002). Steen *et al.* proposed to use Rayleigh distribution for anisotropic diffusion-based edge detection (Steen and Olstad 1994).

While Rayleigh distribution is extensively used in ultrasound image processing, it is not always not norm because it is valid only in the special case of a large number of randomly distributed scatters. In this condition, the speckle is called fully developed. It has been shown that the echo envelop has a Rayleigh distribution when signal noise ratio (SNR)is approximately 1.91. Deviations from such special scattering conditions are called pre-Rayleigh condition when SNR <1.91, and post-Rayleigh condition when SNR>1.91 (Tuthill et al., 1988). The K-distribution has been proposed to model the pre-Rayleigh condition by accounting for low effective scatter density (Shankar et al., 1993; Shankar, 1995), and Rice distribution has been proposed to model the post-Rayleigh condition by accounting for a coherence component due to the presence of a regular structure of scatters within the tissue (Insana et al., 1986; Tuthill et al., 1988). However, the Rician family fails to model the pre-Rayleigh condition, and K-distribution model does not take into account the post-Rayleigh condition. Generalized K-distribution (Jakeman, 1999), homodyned K-distribution (Dutt and Greenleaf, 1994), and Rician Inverse of Gaussian distribution (Eltoft, 2003) have been proposed as general models to encompass pre-Rayleigh, Rayleigh, and post-Rayleigh conditions. Unfortunately, the complex nature of these models limited their practical applications.

Recently, Nakagami distribution has been proposed as a simple generalized model to collectively represent pre-Rayleigh, Rayleigh, and post-Rayleigh distributions (Shankar, 2000). It is a two-parameter distribution with analytical simplicity, which makes it relatively easy to estimate it parameters. The probability density function (pdf) of the Nakagami distribution is given by

$$P(I;\mu,\Omega) = \frac{2\mu^{\mu} I^{2\mu-1}}{\Gamma(\mu)\Omega^{\mu}}\exp\left(-\frac{\mu}{\Omega}I^2\right)$$

where $\Gamma(\bullet)$ is the Gamma function, μ is the shape parameter, and Ω is the scaling parameter. For $\mu = 1$ the pdf reduces to Rayleigh condition. For $\mu > 1$, the pdf can be described as post-Rayleigh, which is similar to Rician distribution, while for $\mu < 1$, the pdf can be described as pre-Rayleigh.

As shown in (Shankar, 2000), the shape parameter and scaling parameters can be obtained from the moments of the envelop as follows

$$\mu = \frac{\left[E\left(I^2\right)\right]^2}{E\left[I^2 - E\left(I^2\right)\right]^2}$$

and

$$\Omega = E\left(I^2\right)$$

where $E(\bullet)$ is the expectation.

Davignon *et al.* used a Nakagmi distribution to segment ultrasound images (Davignon et al., 2005).

Apart from the theoretical models mentioned above, empirical models have also been used in ultrasound image segmentation. For example, Tao *et al.* modeled the ultrasound speckle with a Gamma distribution and incorporated it into a tunneling descent optimization framework to overcome local minima (Tao and Tagare, 2007). Xiao *et al.* used a log-normal distribution for modeling speckle in breast images (Xiao et al., 2002). Qian *et al.* incorporated a log-normal distribution into a level-set framework to segment rat echocardiographic images with large dropout (Qian et al., 2006).

2.2 Gradient

Intensity gradient looks for intensity discontinuities between subregions corresponding to different tissue types. Intensity gradient can be computed from an image with standard differential operators (e.g. Sobel operator). A voxel is considered to be a boundary voxel if its intensity gradient is above a threshold. Gradient-based segmentation, such as such as gradient-based snake (Kass et al., 1987), Active Shape Model (ASM) (Cootes et al., 1995), and level-set approaches (Malladi et al., 1995), has been extensively used in cardiac applications (Lynch et al., 2006; Lynch et al., 2008; Assen et al., 2008; Chen et al., 2002; Corsi et al., 2002).

One limitation of intensity gradient is that it may suffer from spurious, missing, and discontinuous edges. This is especially evident in EPI segmentation because there are usually no clear and visible edges between the myocardium and background. In addition, intensity gradient is suboptimal for ultrasound images because a boundary response in ultrasound images is anisotropic and depends on the relative orientation of the transducer to the boundary. Therefore, intensity gradient information is often used in conjunction with other image features (Pluempitiwiriyawej et al., 2005; Chen et al, 2003).

2.3 Texture

Although no formal definition of texture exists, it can be loosely defined as one or more local patterns that are repeated in a periodic manner. Texture analysis has been attempted in numerous ways in medical image analysis, particularly for ultrasound images. The three principal approaches to describe texture are image pyramids, random fields, and statistical models.

The idea behind image pyramids is to generate a number of homogeneous parameters that represent the response of a bank of filters at different scales and possibly different orientations. Different filters have been proposed including Gabor filters (Xie et al., 2005; Zhan and Shen, 2006), Gaussian derivatives (Chen et al., 1998) and wavelet transforms (Mojsilovic et al., 1998; Yoshida et al., 2003). The idea behind random fields is that the value at each pixel/voxel is chosen by two-dimensional (2-D)/ three dimensional (3-D) stochastic process. Given a type of pdf of this stochastic process, one can estimate the value at a particular pixel/voxel given the values of other pixels/voxles in its neighborhood. The most commonly used random field is Markov Random Field (MRF) (Bouhlel et al., 2004). Statistical models analyze the spatial distribution of grey level values, by computing local features at each point in the image, and deriving a set of statistics from the distributions of the local features. Statistical approaches yield characterizations of textures as smooth, coarse, grainy, etc. Major statistical texture descriptors include co-occurrence matrix (Nicholas et al., 1986, Sahiner et al., 2004, Kuo et al., 2001), auto-correlation (Chen et al., 2000), edge frequency, run length, Law's texture energy, and fractal texture description. Several researchers have proposed to extract fractal texture features (Wu et al., 1992; Lee et al., 2003; Chen et al., 2005). In addition, several attempts have been made to combine multiple texture measures to improve discrimination abilities (Hao et al, 2001; Christodoulou et al., 2003; Stoitsis et al., 2006).

2.4 Phase

The local phase provides an alternative to intensity gradient to characterize structures in an image (Kovesi, 1996; Boukerroui et al., 2001; Mulet-Parada and Noble, 2000; Hacihaliloglu et al., 2008). Phase-based methods postulate that feature information is encoded at points where phase congruency is maximized, i.e. all the Fourier components are in phase. Generally, phase is estimated by quadrature filter bank. Thus, there is a link between phase-based methods and other wavelet methods. Phase-based methods are suggested to be more robust than intensity gradient for ultrasound images because intensity gradients in ultrasound images depend on the relative orientation of the transducer to the boundary. In addition, the presence of speckles and imaging artifacts might cause the variation of intensity gradient of equally significant features in the data. One limitation of phase-based methods, however, is that speckle also has its own phase signatures, and therefore an appropriate spatial scale has to be selected.

3. Incompressibility of myocardium

The heart is a remarkably efficient and during mechanical pump composed of complex biological materials. The main structural elements of the myocardium are inter-connected networks of muscle fibers and collagen fibers, as well as matrix that embeds them. The fibers are generally tangential to the ENDO and EPI surfaces, following a path of a right-handed helical geometry. The interstitial fluid carries only hydrostatic pressure, which in turn, is affected by the length and configuration changes of the fibers. These cause pressure gradients, which may result in the flow of the matrix. However, the fluid within the tissue is negligible for the duration of a cardiac cycle because the myocardium as low permeability. Consequently, the myocardium can be assumed to be nearly incompressible (Glass et al., 1990).

A few independent studies have been performed to quantitatively analyze the change of myocardial volume (MV) over an entire cardiac cycle. For example, Hamilton *et al.* performed experiments on frogs, turtles, and dogs, and discovered a relatively consistency of the MV during a cardiac cycle (Hamilton et al., 1932). Hoffman *et al.* used canine Dynamic Spatial Reconstructor data to study the changes in MV, obtaining a relatively constant volume that was consistent with Hamilton's findings (Hoffman and Ritman, 1987; Hoffman and Ritman, 1985). More recent work done by King *et al.*, who used freehand three dimensional (3-D) echocardiography to measure MV and mass, showed a 1.1% difference of volume between end-diastole(ED) and end-systole (ES) (King et al., 2002). Bowaman *et al.* found a variation of around 5% from ED to ES by using high-resolution magnetic resonance (MR) imaging (Bowman and Kovacs, 2003). O'Donnell also analyzed the myocardial volume using MR imaging, and found the difference of ED and ES to be around 2.5% (O'Donnell and Funka-Lea, 1998). The common conclusion of these studies is that the myocardial is nearly incompressible and the variation is less than 5% during a cardiac cycle. This incompressibility property of the myocardium is used an as important cardiac structure constraint which is taken into consideration in our approach, as will be detailed in Section 4.3.

4. Method

4.1 General framework

In this section, we formulate our segmentation problem in a maximum a posterior (MAP) framework combining image-derived information and the incompressibility property of the myocardium. Let I be a 3-D cardiac image, S_{in} be the ENDO surface, and S_{out} be the EPI surface. A MAP framework that combines image information and incompressibility constraint can be expressed as follows

$$\left(\hat{S}_{\text{in}}, \hat{S}_{\text{out}}\right) = \underset{S_{\text{in}}, S_{\text{out}}}{\arg\max}\, P(S_{\text{in}}, S_{\text{out}} \mid I) = \underset{S_{\text{in}}, S_{\text{out}}}{\arg\max}\, \underbrace{P(I \mid S_{\text{in}}, S_{\text{out}})}_{\text{data adherence}} \quad \underbrace{P(S_{\text{in}}, S_{\text{out}})}_{\text{incompressibility constraint}} \tag{1}$$

Equation (1) is a probability function which adheres to image data, modulated by the prior knowledge of incompressibility property of the myocardium. In particular, $P(I \mid S_{\text{in}}, S_{\text{out}})$ is the probability of producing an image I given S_{in} and S_{out} by assuming the piecewise homogeneities of each region enclosed by S_{in} and S_{out}. $P(S_{\text{in}}, S_{\text{out}})$ is the incompressibility constraint which keeps the MV enclosed by S_{in} and S_{out} nearly constant during a cardiac cycle. Since the myocardium is only nearly incompressible, it is more reasonable to define it within a probabilistic framework rather than imposing a deterministic constraint.

4.2 Data adherence

Region-based deformable models have been successfully applied in the segmentation of images with weak boundaries, due to their robustness (Chan and Vese, 2001). In this work, we evolve a three-phase region-based deformable model based on the statistical intensity distribution from RT3D echocardiographic images.

To evolve a region-based model, we first need to determine the intensity distribution of each region within a cardiac image. It is obvious that the entire cardiac image is partitioned by S_{in} and S_{out} into three regions, namely, LV blood pool, LV myocardium, and background, as shown in Fig. 2.

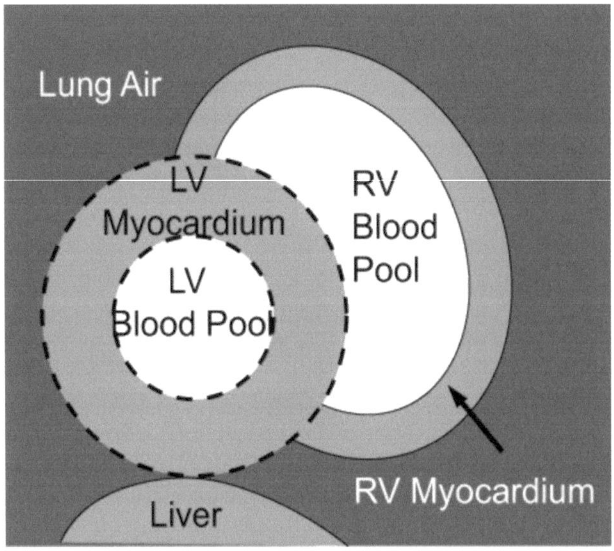

Fig. 2. The short-axis view of a heart. Two dotted circles are ENDO- and EPI contours, which partitioned the entire image into three regions: LV blood pool, LV myocardium, and background. The background is inhomogeneous because it contains more than one tissues, such as RV blood pool, RV myocardium, lung air, and liver.

The LV blood pool and myocardium are homogeneous, and therefore can modeled with a single pdf. In this work, we use Nakagami distribution (Shankar, 1995) (see Section 2.1) to model the intensity distributions of LV blood pool and myocardium as follows

$$P(I;\mu_l,\omega_l)=\frac{2\mu_l^{\mu_l}}{\Gamma(\mu_l)\omega_l^{\mu_l}}I^{2\mu_l-1}\exp\left(-\frac{\mu_l}{\omega_l}I^2\right) \tag{2}$$

where μ_l is the shape parameter of the Nakagami distribution, and ω_l is the scaling parameter. Equation (2) describes the intensity distribution for LV blood pool when l=1, and intensity distribution for LV myocardium when l=2.

Unlike LV blood pool and myocardium, the background (see Fig. 2) because it contains more than one tissues (RV blood pool, RV myocardium, and liver), and therefore modeling it with a single distribution function would be insufficient because it contains a wide range of intensities. To handle this problem, we use a mixture model (McLachlan and Peel, 2000) to describe the intensity distribution of the background.

$$P(I;\mu_3,\omega_3)=\sum_{k=1}^{M}\alpha_k P_{3,k}\left(I;\mu_{3,k},\omega_{3,k}\right)$$

where μ_3 and ω_3 are the shape and scaling parameters of the component distributions. For ultrasound images, we choose $M=2$ because the background histogram has two peaks, as shown in Fig. 3 (c). The first peak corresponds to RV blood pool and lung air, while the second peak corresponds to RV myocardium and liver.

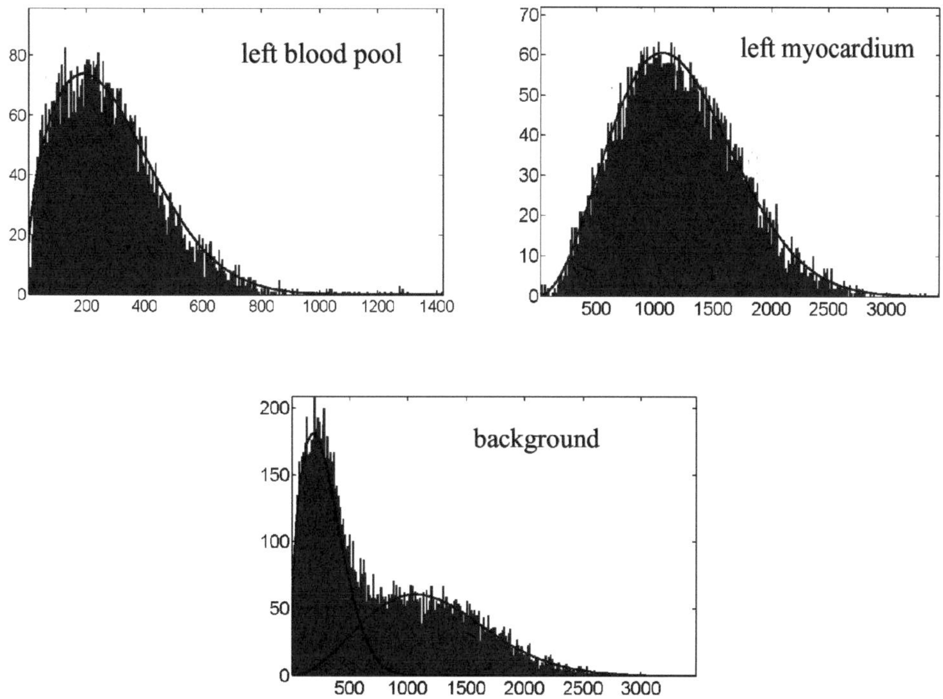

Fig. 3. The histograms of echocardiographic images with their fitted distributions.
(a) LV blood pool, (b) LV myocardium, (c) background.

Fig. 3 shows the histogram of each region for echocardiographic images.

Let Ω be a bounded open set of R^3, and be partitioned by S_{in} and S_{out} into three regions, namely, LV blood pool, LV myocardium, and background, which are denoted as Ω_1, Ω_2, and Ω_3 respectively. Thus, the data adherence term can be defined by a three-phase deformable model

$$\log P(I \mid S_{\text{in}}, S_{\text{out}}) = \sum_{l=1}^{3} \int_{\Omega_l} \log P(I; \mu_l, \omega_l) d\mathbf{x} \tag{3}$$

4.3 Incompressibility constraint

It is mentioned in Section 3 that the MV is nearly constant during cardiac cycle. Therefore, we assume that the MV has a Gaussian distribution $N(V_0, \sigma_V^2)$

$$P(S_{\text{in}}, S_{\text{out}}) = \frac{1}{\sqrt{2\pi}\sigma_V} \exp\left(-\frac{(V - V_0)^2}{2\sigma_V^2} \right) \tag{4}$$

where $V = \int_{\Omega_2} d\mathbf{x}$ is the MV enclosed by the deforming ENDO and EPI surfaces. Parameter V_0 is the average volume, which can be calculated from the manual segmentation of the first frame. As mentioned in Section 3, the MV changes by less than 5% during a cardiac cycle.

Assuming that $0.025V_0$ is the maximum deviation and using the three σ rule, we have the following relationship:

$$3\sigma_V = 0.025V_0$$

$$\sigma_V = \frac{1}{120}V_0$$

Therefore, the incompressibility constraint is encoded into a probability function which favors small variance of the MV while penalizing large deviations.

Combining Equations (1), (3), and (4), we arrive at the following optimization problem

$$\left(\hat{S}_{in},\hat{S}_{out}\right) = \underset{S_{in},S_{out}}{\arg\max}\, P\left(S_{in},S_{out} \mid I\right) = \underset{S_{in},S_{out}}{\arg\max}\left\{\sum_{l=1}^{3}\int_{\Omega_l} \log P\left(I;\mu_l,\omega_l\right)d\mathbf{x} - \frac{\left(V-V_0\right)^2}{2\sigma_V^2}\right\} \tag{5}$$

The maximization of Equation (5) can be identified by the coupled surface evolution equations

$$\frac{\partial S_{in}}{\partial \tau} = \left(\log\left(\frac{P\left(I;\mu_2,\omega_2\right)}{P\left(I;\mu_1,\omega_1\right)}\right) - \frac{V-V_0}{\sigma_V^2}\right)\mathbf{n}_{in} \tag{6}$$

$$\frac{\partial S_{out}}{\partial \tau} = \left(\log\left(\frac{P\left(I;\mu_3,\omega_3\right)}{P\left(I;\mu_2,\omega_2\right)}\right) + \frac{V-V_0}{\sigma_V^2}\right)\mathbf{n}_{out} \tag{7}$$

where $\mathbf{n}_{in}$ and $\mathbf{n}_{out}$ are the normals of S_{in} and S_{out} respectively, and τ is the propagation time step.

To implement the evolution of Equations (6) and (7), we embed the surface S_{in} and S_{out} in two higher dimensional functions $\varphi_{in}(\mathbf{x})$ and $\varphi_{out}(\mathbf{x})$, which implicitly represents S_{in} and S_{out} as zero level sets, i.e. $S_{in} = \{\mathbf{x} : \varphi_{in}(\mathbf{x}) = 0\}$ and $S_{out} = \{\mathbf{x} : \varphi_{out}(\mathbf{x}) = 0\}$.

To establish the relationship between surface evolution and level set function, we use the relation $\mathbf{n} = \frac{\nabla\varphi}{|\nabla\varphi|}$. Given the curve/surface evolution form

$$\frac{\partial S}{\partial \tau} = F\mathbf{n}$$

the correspondent level set evolution equation reads (Osher and Paragios, 2003)

$$\frac{\partial \varphi}{\partial \tau} = F|\nabla\varphi|$$

where ∇ is the gradient operator. Hence, the level set evolution equation for Equations (8) and (9) are

$$\frac{\partial \varphi_{\text{in}}}{\partial \tau} = \left(\log\left(\frac{P(I;\mu_2,\omega_2)}{P(I;\mu_1,\omega_1)} \right) - \frac{V - V_0}{\sigma_V^2} \right) |\nabla \varphi_{\text{in}}| \tag{8}$$

$$\frac{\partial \varphi_{\text{out}}}{\partial \tau} = \left(\log\left(\frac{P(I;\mu_3,\omega_3)}{P(I;\mu_2,\omega_2)} \right) + \frac{V - V_0}{\sigma_V^2} \right) |\nabla \varphi_{\text{out}}| \tag{9}$$

5. Experiments

5.1 Experimental setup

The ultrasound data were acquired using Philips echocardiographic system with a 4 MHz X4 xMatrix transducer. The transducer consists of 3000 miniaturized piezoelectric elements and offers steering in both azimuth and elevation of the beam, permitting real-time volumetric image acquisition and rendering (Philips, 2005). In this work, we acquired 11 sequences of canine images, and each sequence consists of 20-30 frames per cardiac cycle depending on the cardiac rate. Hence, we ran our program with a total of 286 sets of volumetric data.

5.2 Quantitative measures

To quantify the segmentation results, we used two distance error metrics and two area error metrics, namely, mean absolute distance (MAD), Hausdorff distance (HD), percentage of true positives (PTP), and percentage of false positives (PFP).

Let A and B be two surfaces from automatic and manual segmentation, respectively. Suppose they are represented by point sets, i.e. $A = \{\mathbf{a}_1, \mathbf{a}_2, \ldots, \mathbf{a}_N\}$ and $B = \{\mathbf{b}_1, \mathbf{b}_2, \ldots, \mathbf{b}_M\}$, we define

$$\text{MAD}(A,B) = \frac{1}{2}\left\{ \frac{1}{N}\sum_{i=1}^{N} d(\mathbf{a}_i, B) + \frac{1}{M}\sum_{j=1}^{M} d(\mathbf{b}_j, A) \right\}$$

$$\text{HD}(A,B) = \max\left\{ \max_i d(\mathbf{a}_i, B), \max_j d(\mathbf{b}_j, A) \right\}$$

where $d(\mathbf{a}_i, B) = \min_j \|\mathbf{a}_i - \mathbf{b}_j\|$ is the distance from point $\mathbf{a}_i$ to the closest point on surface B. While MAD represents the global agreement between two contours, HD compares their local similarities.

Let Ω_A and Ω_B be the region enclosed by surface A and B, we define

$$\text{PTP} = \frac{\text{Volume}(\Omega_A \cap \Omega_B)}{\text{Volume}(\Omega_A)}$$

$$\text{PFP} = \frac{\text{Volume}(\Omega_A) - \text{Volume}(\Omega_A \cap \Omega_B)}{\text{Volume}(\Omega_B)}$$

5.3 Experimental results

In Fig. 4, we show the long axis view of the automatically segmented ENDO- and EPI surfaces at frames 2, 4, 6, and 8 during ventricular systole.

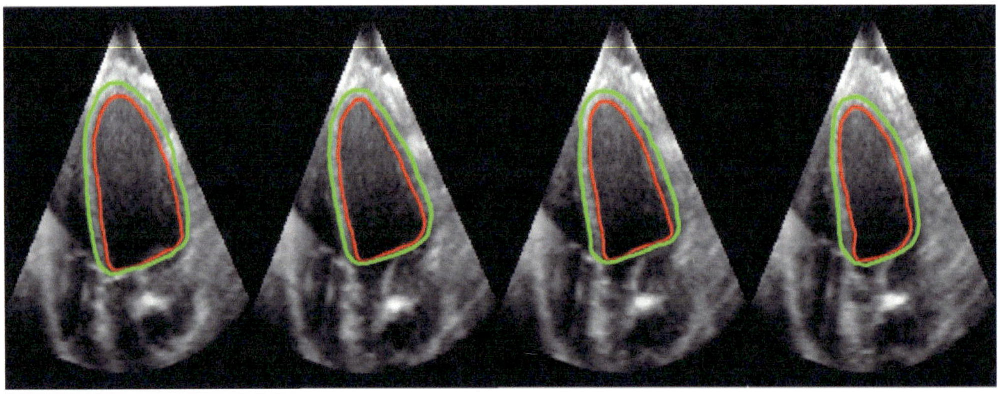

Fig. 4. Long axis view of segmented ENDO- and EPI contours at frames 2, 4, 6, and 8 during cardiac systole.

In Fig. 5, we compare the segmentation results of the EPI surface with and without incompressibility constraint. For a fair comparison, we used the same data adherence term for both cases. We observed that while the ENDO border was correctly detected even without the incompressibility constraint, the EPI contour leaked into other tissues, such as liver, that look like myocardium. This is because the LV myocardium/background contrast is lower than the LV blood pool/myocardium contrast, especially for the lateral and inferior sectors of myocardium. This low contrast obscures the exact location of the EPI boundary, making EPI segmentation more challenging than ENDO segmentation. When the incompressibility constraint was applied, however, the coupling of ENDO and EPI contours forced the evolution of the EPI contour to be consistent with that of the ENDO contour, thus preventing the leakage of the EPI contour.

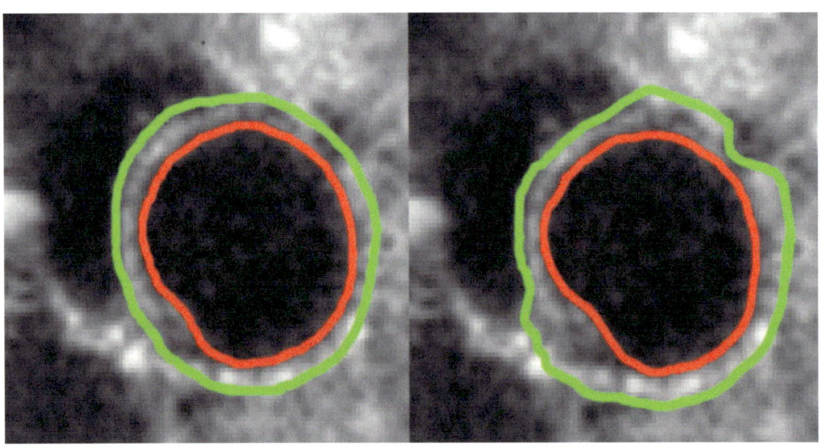

Fig. 5. Comparison of EPI segmentation with and without incompressibility constraint. (a) with incompressibility constraint; (b) without incompressibility constraint. Arrow: myocardium juncture.

As explained in Section 1, another challenge in the segmentation of the EPI boundary is the presence of the LV/RV myocardium junctures. The intensity similarity between the LV and RV myocardium makes the EPI boundary ambiguous at the juncture. When the incompressibility constraint was not applied, the EPI contour leaked out to segment RV myocardium. When the incompressibility constraint was applied, however, the LV myocardium was successfully separated from the RV myocardium at the juncture.

Fig. 6 compares the MV for an entire sequence from manual segmentation, automatic segmentation with incompressibility constraint, and automatic segmentation without incompressibility constraint. We took the mean value from three experts as the MV from manual segmentation. We observed that the variation of MV for manual segmentation is $\frac{92.1-88.2}{88.2}=4.42\%$, the variation of MV for automatic segmentation with incompressibility constraint is $\frac{92.2-88.1}{88.1}=4.65\%$. The variation of MV obtained without incompressibility constraint, however, is $\frac{143.2-106.1}{106.1}=34.97\%$. Also, we noticed that the MV obtained without incompressibility constraint is much larger than that from manual segmentation. This is because the EPI contour leaked into the background, leading to the over-estimation of the MV.

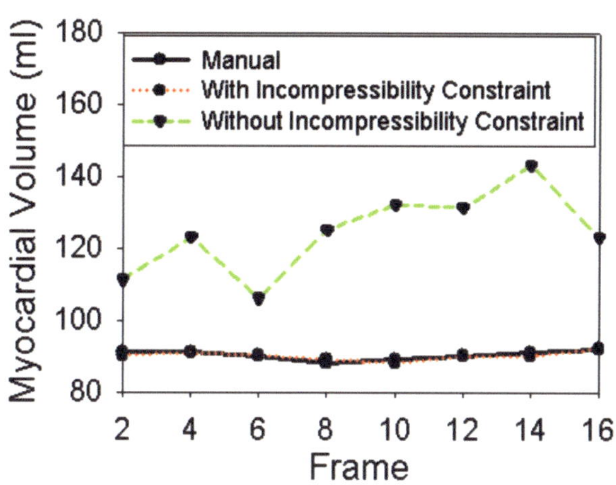

Fig. 6. Comparison of MV for an example sequence from manual segmentation, automatic segmentation with incompressibility constraint, and automatic segmentation without incompressibility constraint.

In addition, we performed Bland-Altman analysis (Bland and Altman, 1986) to assess the agreement of the MV measurements from manual segmentation and automatic segmentation. The Bland-Altman analysis revealed small bias and good coherence between the MV measurements from manual segmentation and automatic segmentation with incompressibility constraint. As shown in Fig. 7, the bias is -0.2%, and 95% of the computer measurements of MV can be expected to differ from expert measurements by less than 6.4% below and 5.9% above the mean. In comparison, when the incompressibility constraint was not applied, the MV largely deviated from the MV from manual segmentation (bias = 18.8%, 95% confidence interval = [2.4%,35.2%]).

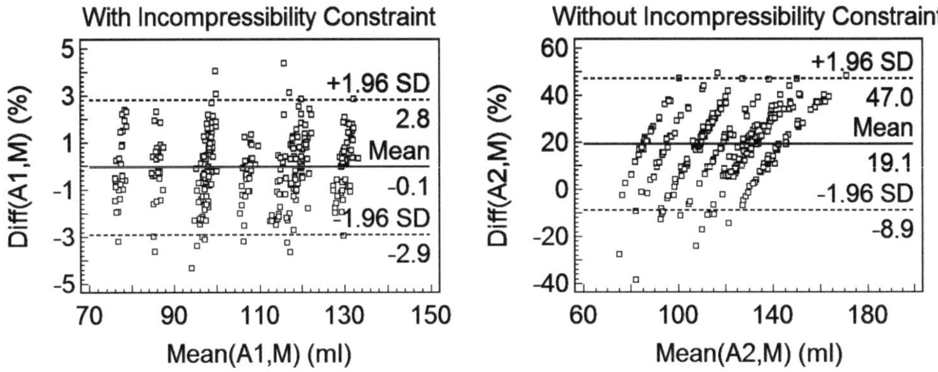

Fig. 7. Bland-Altman analysis showing the agreement between the MV measurements from manual segmentation and automatic segmentation.

Table 1 shows that the ENDO boundaries were detected with sufficient accuracy even if the incompressibility constraint was not applied. This is because that the ENDO boundaries are relatively clear compared to the EPI boundaries. However, we observed from Table 2 that for EPI boundaries, when the incompressibility constraint was not applied, the automatic-manual MAD was 2.78mm larger than the manual-manual MAD, the automatic-manual HD was 3.82mm larger than the manual-manual HD, and the automatic-manual PTP&PFP were 18%-20% worse than the manual-manual PTP&PFP. This is because of the leakage problem of EPI boundaries without incompressibility constraint. When the incompressibility constraint was applied, however, the automatic-manual MAD decreased by 3.38mm, the automatic-manual HD decreased by 4.11mm, and the automatic-manual PTP&PFP decreased by 16%-19%. We can see from Tables 1 and 2 that the automatic algorithm produced results with comparable accuracy to a manual segmentation. Furthermore, we observed from Tables 1 and 2 that the variability of manual-manual segmentation was smaller for the ENDO surface than for the EPI surface. This is probably because the EPI boundaries are more ambiguous for observers to detect, which was also the reason why we have multiple observers instead of a single one.

	MAD (mm)	HD (mm)	PTP (%)	PFP (%)
Automatic-manual (with constraint)	1.43 ± 0.29	2.40 ± 0.48	96.22 ± 1.97	3.99 ± 1.99
Automatic-manual (without constraint)	1.50 ± 0.29	2.42 ± 0.60	95.70 ± 1.76	4.29 ± 1.80
Manual-manual	1.31 ± 0.27	2.12 ± 0.50	96.21 ± 1.90	3.79 ± 1.84

Table 1. Comparison of automatic outline to three observers' outline of ENDO boundaries.

	MAD (mm)	HD (mm)	PTP (%)	PFP (%)
Automatic-manual (with constraint)	1.74 ± 0.49	2.91 ± 0.80	94.34 ± 1.21	5.66 ± 1.20
Automatic-manual (without constraint)	5.12 ± 2.12	7.02 ± 2.42	75.23 ± 7.17	22.45 ± 7.99
Manual-manual	2.34 ± 0.89	3.20 ± 0.99	95.90 ± 2.31	4.10 ± 2.30

Table 2. Comparison of automatic outline to three observers' outline of EPI boundaries.

6. Conclusion

In this chapter, we have presented a novel approach to segmenting the full myocardial volume from cardiac MR and ultrasound images. Motivated by the incompressibility property of myocardium during a cardiac cycle, we coupled the propagation of the ENDO and EPI surfaces according to image-derived information that maximized the piecewise homogeneities of a cardiac image, as well as the incompressibility constraint which constrains the variation of myocardial volume within 5%.

To validate our approach, we computed the MAD, HD, PTP, and PFP between the contours from automatic algorithm and manual segmentation. We observed that when the incompressibility constraint was not applied, the EPI boundaries leaked into other tissues. When incompressibility constraint was applied, however, the MAD, HD, PTP, and PFP were significantly improved.

7. References

Assen, H; Danilouchkine, M.; Dirksen, M.; Reiber, J. & Lelieveldt, B. (2008). A 3-D Active Shape Model Driven by Fuzzy Inference: Application to Cardiac CT and MR. *IEEE Trans. on Information Technology in Biomedicine*, vol.12, no.5 (2008), pp.595-605

Bland, J. & Altman, D. (1986). Statistical Methods for Assessing Agreement Betweeen Two Methods of Clinical Measurement. *Lancet*, vol.1 (1986)

Bouhlel, N.; Sevestre-Ghalila, S. & Rajhi, H. & Hamza, R. (2004). New Markov Random Field Model Based on K-Distribution for Textured Ultrasound Image. In *Proceedings of Medical Imaging: Ultrasonic Imaging and Signal Processing, ser. SPIE*, W.F. Walker and S.Y. Emelianov, pp.363-372

Boukerroui, D.; Noble, A.; Robini, M. & Brady, M. (2001). Enhancement of Contrast Region in Suboptimal Ultrasound Images with Application to Echocardiography. *Ultrasound in Medicine & Biology*, vol.27, no.12 (2001), pp.1583-1594

Bowman, A. & Kovacs, S. (2003). Assessment and Consequences of the Constant-Volume Attribute of the Four-Chamber Heart. *American Journal of Physiology - Heart Circulation Physiology*, vol.285 (2003), pp.H2027-2033

Chan, T. & Vese, L. (2001). Active Contours Without Edges. *IEEE Transactions on Image Processing*, vol.10, no.2 (2001), pp.266-277

Chen, C.; Pau, L. & Wang, P. (1998). Handbook of Pattern Recognition and Computer Vision (2nd edition). World Scientific

Chen, D.; Chang, R. & Huang, Y. (2000). Breast cancer diagnosis using self organizing map for sonography. *Ultrasound in Medicine and Biology*, vol.26, no.3 (2000), pp.405-411

Chen, D.; Chang, R.; Chen, C.; Ho, M.; Kuo, S.; Chen, S.; Hung, S. & Moon, W. (2005). Classification of breast ultrasound images using fractal feature. *Clinical Imaging*, vol.29 (2005), pp.235-245

Chen, T.; Babb, J.; Kellman, P.; Axel, L. & Kim, D. (2008). Semiautomated Segmentation of Myocardial Contours for Fast Strain Analysis in Cine Displacement-Encoded MRI. *IEEE Transactions on Medical Imaging*, vol.27, no.8 (2008), pp.1084-1094

Chen, Y.; Tagare, H.; Thiruvenkadam, S; Huang, F; Wilson, D; Gopinath, K; Briggs, R & Geiser, E (2002). Using Prior Shapes in Geometric Active Contours in a Variational Framework. *International Journal of Computer Vision*, vol.50, no.3 (2002), pp.315-328

Christodoulou, C.; Pattichis, C.; Pantziaris, M. & Nicolaides, A. (2003). Texture-Based Classification of Atherosclerotic Carotid Plaques. *IEEE Transactions on Medical Imaging* vol.22, no.7 (2003), pp.902-912

Chen, Y.; Huang, F.; Tagare, H.; Rao, M.; Wilson, D. & Geiser, E. (2003). Using Prior Shape and Intensity Prior Profile in Medical Image Segmentation. In *Proceedings of International Conference on Computer Vision and Pattern Recognition*, vol.2 (2003), pp.1117-1125

Cohen, B. & Dinstein, I. (2002). New Maximum Likelihood Motion Estimation Schemes for Noisy Ultraound Images. *Pattern Recognition*, vol.48, no.2 (2002), pp.455-463

Cootes, T. & Taylor, C.; Cooper, D. & Graham, J. (1995). Active Shape Models - Their Training and Application. *Computer Vision and Image Understanding*, vol.61, no.1 (1995), pp.38-59

Corsi, C; Saracino, G.; Sarti, A. & Lamberti, C. (2002). Left Ventricular Volume Estimation for Real-Time Three-Dimensional Echocardiography. *IEEE Transactions on Medical Imaging*, vol.21, no.9 (2002), pp.1202-1208

Davignon, F.; Deprez, J. & Basset, O. (2005). A Parametric Imaging Approach for the Segmentation of Ultrasound Data. *Ultrasonics*, vol.43 (2005), pp.789-801

Dutt, V. & Greenleaf, J. (1994). Ultrasound Echo Envelop Analysis Using A Homodyned K-distribution Signal Model. *Ultrasonic Imaging*, vol.16, no.4 (1994), pp.265-287

Eltoft, T. (2003). Speckle: Modeling and Filtering. In *Norwegian Signal Processing Symoposium* (2003)

Glass, L.; Hunter, P. & McCulloch, A. (1990). Theory of Heart: Biomechanics, Biophysics, and Nonlinear Dynamics of Cardiac Function. Springer-Verlag

Hacihaliloglu, I.; Abugharbieh, R.; Hodgson, A. & Rohling, R. (2008). Bone Segmentation and Fracture Detection in Ultrasound Using 3D Local Phase Features. In *Proceedings of International Conference on Medical Imaging and Computer Assisted Intervention* (2008), pp.287-295

Hamilton, W. & Rompf, J. (1932). Movement of the Base of the Ventricle and the Relative Constancy of the Cardiac Volume. *American Journal of Physiology*, vol.132 (1932), pp.559-565

Hao, X.; Bruce, C.; Pislaru, C. & Greenleaf, J. (2001). Segmenting High-Frequency Intracardiac Ultrasound Images of Myocardium Into Infarcted, Ischemic, and Normal Regions. *IEEE Transactions on Medical Imaging*, vol.20, no.12 (2001), pp.1373-1383

Hoffman, E. & Ritman, E. (1985). Invariant Total Heart Volume in the Intact Thorax. *American Journal of Physiology - Heart Circulation Physiology*, vol.249 (1985), pp.H883-890

Hoffman, E. & Ritman, E. (1987). Heart-Lung Interaction: Effect of Regional Lung Air Content and Total Heart Volume. *Annual Biomedical Engineering*, vol.15 (1987), pp.241-257

Insana, M.; Wagner, R.; Garra, B.; Brown D. & Shawker, T. (1986). Analysis of Ultrasound Image Texture via Generalized Rician Statistics. *Optical Engineering*, vol.25, no.6 (1986), pp.743-748

Jakeman, E. (1999). K-distributed Noise. *Journal of Optics A: Pure and Applied Optics*, vol.1 (1999), pp.784-789

Kass, M.; Witkin, A. & Terzopoulos, D. (1987). Snakes: Active Contour Models. *International Journal of Computer Vision*, vol.1 (1987), pp.321-331

King, D.; Coffin, L. & Maurer, M. (2002). Noncompressibility of Myocardium During Systole With Freehand Three-Dimensional Echocardiography. *Journal of the American Society of Echocardiogrpahy*, vol.15, no.12 (2002), pp.1503-1506

Kovesi, P. (1996). Invariant Measures of Image Features from Phase Information. PhD Thesis, University of Western Australia

Kuo, W.; Chang, R.; Chen, D. & Lee, C. (2001). Data mining with decision trees for diagnosis of breast tumor in medical ultrasonic images. *Breast Cancer Research and Treatment*, vol.66, no.1 (2001), pp.51-57

Lee, W.; Chen, Y. & Hsieh, K. (2003). Ultrasonic liver tissues classification by fractal feature vector based on M-band wavelet transform. *IEEE Transactions on Medical Imaging*, vol.22, no.3 (2003), pp.382-392

Lloyd-Jones, D.; et al. (2009). Heart Disease and Stroke Statistics 2009 Update: A Report From the American Heart Association Statistics Committee and Stroke Statistics Subcommittee. *Circulation*, vol.119, (2009), pp.e21-e181

Lynch, M.; Ghita, O. & Whelan, P. (2006). Left-Ventricle Myocardium Segmentation Using a Coupled Level-Set With a Prior Knowledge. *Computerized Medical Imaging and Graphics*, vol.30, no.4 (2006), pp.255-262

Lynch, M; Ghita, H & Whelan, P (2008). Segmentation of the Left Ventricle of the Heart in 3-D+t MRI Data Using an Optimized Nonrigid Temporal Model. *IEEE Transactions on Medical Imaging*, vol.27, no.2 (2008), pp.195-203

Malladi, R.; Sethian, J. & Vemuri, B. (1995). Shape Modeling with Front Propagation: A Level Set Approach. *IEEE Transactions on Pattern Analysis and Machine Intelligence*, vol.17, no.2 (1995), pp.158-175

Mojsilovic, A.; Popovic, M.; Markovic, S. & Krstic, M. (1998). Characterization of visually similar diffuse diseases from B-scan liver images using nonseparable wavelet transform. *IEEE Transactions on Medical Imaging*, vol.17, no.4 (1998), pp.541-549

Mulet-Parada, M. & Noble, A. (2000). 2D+T Acoustic Boundary Detection in Echocardiography. *Medical Image Analysis*, vol.4 (2000), pp.21-30

Nicholas, D.; Nassiri, D.; Garbutt, P.; Hill, C. (1986). Tissue characterization from ultrasound B-scan data. *Ultrasound in Medicine & Biology*, vol.12, no.2 (1986), pp.135-145

O'Donnell, T. & Funka-Lea, G. (1998). 3-D Cardiac Volume Analysis Using Magnetic Resonance Imaging. In *Proceedings of the Fourth IEEE Workshop on Applications of Computer Vision (WACV)* (1998), pp.240-241

Osher, S. & Paragios, N. (2003). Geometric Level Set Methods in Imaging, Vision, and Graphics. Springer

Paragios, N (2002). A VariationalApproach for the Segmentation of the Left Ventricle in Cardiac Image Analysis. *International Journal of Computer Vision*, vol.50, no.3 (2002), pp.345-362

Philips (2005). http://www.medical.philips.com/main/products/ultrasound/cardiology/. Philips Medical Systems Corporate Website

Pluempitiwiriyawej, C.; Moura, J.; Wu, Y. & Ho, C. (2005). STACS: New Active Contour Scheme for Cardiac MR Image Segmentation. *IEEE Transactions on Medical Imaging*, vol.24, no.5 (2005), pp.593-603

Qian, X.; Tagare H. & Tao, Z. (2006). Segmentation of Rat Cardiac Ultrasound Images with Large Dropout Regions. In *Proceedings of Mathematical Methods in Biomedical Image Analysis* (2006)

Sahiner, B.; Chan, H; Roubidoux, M.; Helvie, M; Hadjiiski, L.; Ramachandran, A.; Paramagul, C; LeCarpentier, G.; Nees, A. & Blane, C. (2004). Computerized characterization of breast masses on three dimensional ultrasound volumes. *Medical Physics*, vol.31, no.4 (2004), pp.744-754

Sarti, A.; Corsi, C; Mazzini, E. & Lamberti C. (2005). Maximum Likelihood Segmentation of Ultrasound Images with Rayleigh Distribution. *IEEE Tranactions on Ultrasonics, Ferroelectrics, and Frequency Control*, vol.52, no.6 (2005), pp.947-960

Shankar, P.; Reid, J.; Ortega H.; Piccoli C. & Goldberg, B. (1993). Use of Non-Rayleigh Statistics for the Identificiation of Tumors in Ultrasonic B-Scans of the Breast. *IEEE Transactions on Medical Imaging*, vol.12, no.4 (1993), pp.687-692

Shankar, P. (1995). A Model for Ultrasonic Scattering from Tissues Based on the K Distribution. *Physics in Medicine&Biology*, vol.40 (1995), pp.1633-1649

Shankar, P. (2000). A General Statistical Model for Ultrasonic Backscattering from Tissues. *IEEE Transactions on Ultrasonics, Ferroelectrics, and Frequency Control*, vol.47, no.3 (2000), pp.727-736

Steen, E. & Olstad, B. (1994). Scale-Space and Boundary Detection in Ultrasound Imaging, Using Signal-Adaptive Anisotropic Diffusion. In *Proceedings of SPIE Medical Imaging: Image Processing*

Stoitsis, J.; Golemati, S. & Nikita, K. (2006). A Modular Software System to Assist Interpretation of Medical Images—Application to Vascular Ultrasound Images. *IEEE Transactions on Instrumentation and Measurement*, vol.55, no.6 (2006), pp.1944-1952

Tao, Z. & Tagare, H. (2007). Tunneling Descent for M.A.P. Active Contours in Ultrasound Segmentation. *Medical Image Analysis*, vol.11, no.3 (2007), pp.266-281

Tuthill, T.; Sperry, R. & Parker, K. (1988). Deviations From Rayleigh Statistics in Ultrasonic Speckle. *Ultrasonic Imaging*, vol.10 (1988), pp.81-89

Wu, C.; Chen, Y. & Hsieh, K. (1992). Texture features for classification of ultrasonic liver images. *IEEE Transactions on Medical Imaging*, vol.11, no.2 (1992), pp.141-152

Xiao, G.; Brady, M.; Noble J. & Zhang, Y. (2002). Segmentation of Ultrasound B-mode Images with Intensity inhomogeneity Correction. *IEEE Transactions on Medical Imaging*, vol.21, no.1 (2002), pp.48-57

Xie, J.; Jiang, Y & Tsui, H. (2005). Segmentation of Kidney from Ultrasound Images Based on Texture and Shape Priors. *IEEE Transactions on Medical Imaging*, vol.24, no.1 (2005), pp.45-57

Yoshida, H.; Casalino, D.; Keserci, B.; Coskun, A.; Ozturk, O. & Savranlar, A. (2003). Wavelet-packet-based texture analysis for differentiation between benign and malignant liver tumours in ultrasound images. *Physics in Medicine and Biology*, vol.48 (2003), pp.3735-3753

Zhan, Y. & Shen, D. (2006). Deformable Segmentation of 3-D Ultrasound Prostate Images Using Statistical Texture Matching Method. *IEEE Transactions on Medical Imaging*, vol.25, no.3 (2006), pp.256-27

Zhu, Y.; Papademetris, X.; Sinusas, A. & Duncan, J. (2010). A Coupled Deformable Model for Tracking Myocardial Borders from Real-time Echocardiography Using an Incompressibility Constraint. *Medical Image Analysis*, vol.14, no.3 (2010), pp.428-449

6

Evaluation of Subvalvular Apparatus by 2-D Transthoracic Echocardiography

Yasushige Shingu, Suguru Kubota and Yoshiro Matsui
Hokkaido University Graduate School of Medicine,
Department of Cardiovascular Surgery
Japan

1. Introduction

Functional mitral regurgitation (MR) is one of the major contributing factors for heart failure and hospitalization in both nonischemic and ischemic dilated cardiomyopathy. The limitation of undersized mitral annuloplasty has been recognized. Recurrent late MR is associated with continued left ventricular (LV) remodeling and enhanced papillary muscle displacement outside posterior ring after mitral annuloplasty. Understanding of the tethering mechanism provided both annular and subvalvular targets for therapy and several procedures have been reported.

Kron et al. reported a novel approach to reduce tethering length and improve coaptation by approximating displaced posterior papillary muscle toward the annulus. Hvass et al. evolved a papillary muscle sling procedure using an ePTFE tube graft around the muscles and reported improved mitral tethering. Messas et al. proposed a chordal cutting procedure. Langer et al. reported transaortic repositioning of posterior papillary muscle to the midseptal fibrous annulus in a procedure named "RING plus STRING". Our group has reported papillary muscle approximation and its suspension to the mitral artificial ring.

However, there exists no standard method to determine the indication and effects of those various procedures and it makes the comparison between the procedures difficult. Although it would be ideal to determine 3-dimensional anatomy of submitral apparatus, we discuss here the usefulness and importance of 2-D transthoracic echocardiography in this area.

2. Methods

We developed our own submitral procedure, i.e., papillary muscle approximation and its suspension to the mitral ring. According to the method reported by Matsunaga et al., we measure the pre and postoperative values of those parameters relating to the submitral apparatus using 2-D transthoracic echocardiography in patients who need this submitral procedure for functional MR.

2.1 Submitral procedure

Fig. 1 shows our own surgical submitral procedure. Our recent surgical strategy for functional MR is to reconstruct the annulus and subvalvular apparatus of the mitral valve.

It consists of mitral annuloplasty with a semi-rigid total ring, papillary muscle approximation (PMA), and papillary muscle suspension (PMS). PMA is a surgical method to join the entire papillary muscle side-by-side from the bases to the heads by three pledgeted mattress sutures of 3-0 prolene. Shortening the distance between the papillary muscles reduces the lateral and backward tethering of the mitral valve. PMA is usually performed when the papillary muscle distance in the end-diastole is greater than 30 mm in the short axis view of the transthoracic echocardiography. We recently developed a PMS that fixes the distance between the approximated papillary muscle heads and the mitral annulus. This adjunctive method places a subvalvular CV-4 ePTFE suture between the site of the chordal attachment of the approximated papillary muscles and the mitral annulus. This suture is passed through the annuloplasty ring. We adjusted the length of artificial chordae to accomplish enough mitral coaptation length by saline infusion test. We believe that PMS maintains the mitral complex geometry and prevents future mitral tethering deterioration. PMA and PMS are usually performed by left ventriculotomy. The subjects were retrospectively divided into two groups: posterior-directional PMS (pPMS: ~ 2007, n=8) and anterior-directional PMS (aPMS: 2008 ~, n=12). The ePTFE suture was sewn to the middle of the posterior annuloplasty ring in the pPMS group and the anterior annuloplasty ring in the aPMS group. Nine (45%) patients had ischemic and 11 (55%) patients had non-ischemic etiology. Most of the patients had NYHA class over III. Mean age was 62±9 years and MR grade was 3.4±0.8.

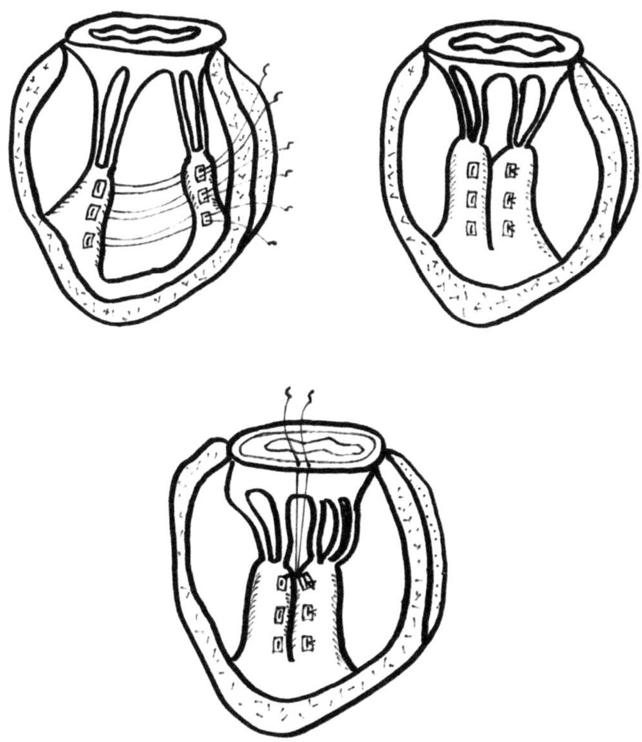

Fig. 1. Submitral procedure named papillary muscle approximation and suspension.

Mitral complex reconstruction consists of mitral annuloplasty with a semi-rigid total ring, papillary muscle approximation (PMA), and papillary muscle suspension (PMS). The entire papillary muscles are joined side-by-side from the bases to the heads by three pledgeted mattress sutures of 3-0 prolene.

Figure 2 shows a surgical method of LV volume reduction surgery named "Overlapping left ventriculoplasty". To reshape the severely remodeled LV, we perform Overlapping left ventriculoplasty, as previously reported. This procedure is based on volume reduction without a patch or ventriculectomy. Basically, it is adopted to cases with LV end-diastolic dimension greater than 65 mm.

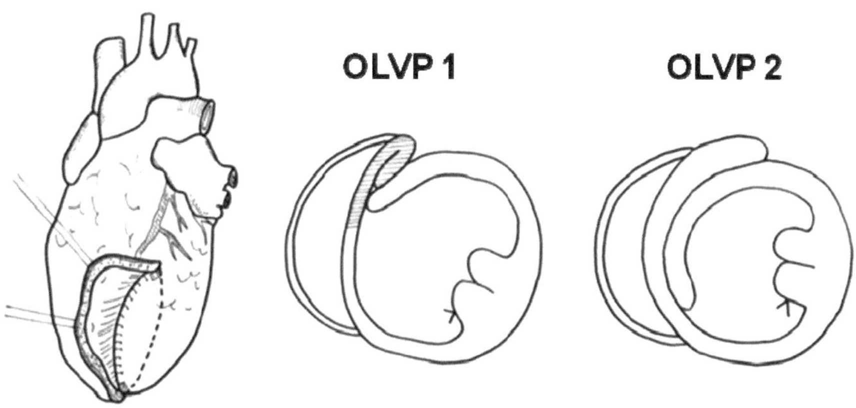

Fig. 2. LV volume reduction surgery named "Overlapping left ventriculoplasty (OLVP)".

LV anterior free wall incision is made parallel to the left anterior descending artery. Left incision margin is sutured to the septal wall, and part of excluded myocardium is sutured to just above the first suture line when the septal wall is scar (OLVP 1). When the septal wall is viable mostly in the idiopathic dilated cardiomyopathy, the excluded myocardium is largely overlapped on the lateral LV wall (OLVP 2).

2.2 Measurement of cardiac function and anatomy of submitral apparatus by 2-D transthoracic echocardiography

Preoperative and postoperative echocardiographic studies were performed a few days before and about four weeks after the operations, respectively. We used a Sonos 5500 ultrasound system (Philips Medical Systems, Andover, Massachusetts, USA) with a 3S transducer (3-5 MHz), a Vivid Seven system (GE/Vingmed, Milwaukee, Wis, USA) with an M3S (2.5-3.5 MHz) transducer, or an Aplio system (Toshiba Medical Systems, Tokyo, Japan) with a 2.5 MHz transducer. These were performed by experienced examiners who were blinded about the study population. The following basic variables were measured from the parasternal long axis view: LV end-diastolic and end-systolic dimensions (mm), LV percent fractional shortening (%), left atrial dimension (mm), interventricular septal thickness and left ventricular posterior wall thickness (mm). Left ventricular ejection fraction (%) was measured by biplane method of discs. On an apical long-axis color Doppler flow image, a sample volume of pulsed Doppler was located at the tip of the mitral valve leaflets to obtain the transmitral flow velocity. Peak early and late transmitral flow velocities (E and A, respectively, cm/s), the ratio of early to late peak velocities (E/A), and the deceleration time (ms) of the early transmitral flow velocity were measured. MR grade was categorized from +1 to +4 by color Doppler images.

Fig. 2 shows the parameters of the submitral apparatus reported by Matsunaga et al. Based on this, we measured the following parameters of mitral systolic tethering on the apical 2 chamber view for the posterior papillary muscle and the apical 4 chamber view for the anterior papillary muscle: mitral valve coaptation height (mm), tenting area (cm^2), papillary muscle tethering distance (mm), papillary muscle depth (mm), and papillary muscle angle(°). We averaged these values measured by 2 and 4 chamber view. The papillary muscle distance was measured on the short axis view of the papillary muscle level in end-diastole. In the apical 2 chamber view, to determine diastolic mitral tethering, the mitral inflow direction was measured using Doppler color flow mapping at the time of maximal early diastolic rapid filling, as the line connecting the center of the filling flow signal at the mitral annulus and chordal levels between the leaflets and papillary muscles. The angle between this line and the annulus was measured as the mitral inflow angle. The echocardiographic study and the use of the clinical records for research were approved by the institutional ethics review board.

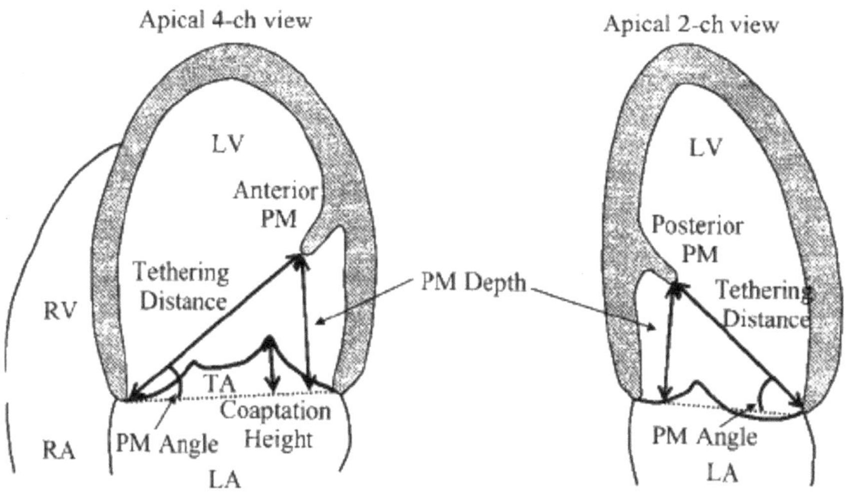

Fig. 2. Measurement of the parameters of the submitral apparatus.

The parameters for the anterior papillary muscle were measured on the apical 4-chamber view and those for the posterior papillary muscle were measured on the apical 2-chamber view. These values were averaged. LA, left atrium; LV, left ventricle; PM, papillary muscle; RA, right atrium; RV, right ventricle; TA, tenting area.

2.3 Statistical analysis

All the descriptive data are given as mean ± standard deviation. Statistical analysis was performed with SPSS version 17.0 software (SPSS Inc. Chicago, Ill). The *t* test was used for comparing the continuous variables between independent groups. The paired *t* test was used for comparing the continuous variables before and after the operation. A p value <0.05 was considered statistically significant.

3. Results

Table 1 shows preoperative patients' characteristics and operative data. Most of the cases had NYHA class over III. All patients underwent PMA and PMS procedures. Overlapping left ventriculoplasty was performed in 11 (55%) patients.

	all cases (n=20)
age (years)	62±9
male/female	17/3
ischemic/idiopathic etiology	9/11
NYHA class III/IV	13/5
beta blocker (%)	16 (80%)
chronic atrial fibrillation (%)	4 (20)
operative data	
cardiopulmonary bypass time (min)	258±54
aortic cross clamp time (min)	144±40
CABG (%)	8 (40)
tricuspid valve annuloplasty (%)	17 (85)
MAZE (%)	5 (25)
intraoperative IABP	5 (25)
left ventricular volume reduction (overlapping) (%)	11 (55)
posterior directional PMS (%)	8 (40)
anterior directional PMS (%)	12 (60)

Values±standard deviation. CABG, coronary artery bypass grafting; IABP, intra aortic balloon pumping; PMS, papillary muscle suspension.

Table 1. Preoperative patients' characteristics and operative data

Table 2 shows pre and postoperative functional parameters of all patients. LV end-diastolic and systolic diameters significantly decreased after operation. While transmitral E and A waves increased, E/A did not change. MR grade significantly decreased after operation (3.4±0.8 vs 0.2±0.4, p<0.001). Deceleration time significantly increased after operation.

Deceleration time was below 150 ms in only 3 cases (15%) after operation, although it was below 150 ms in 10 cases (50%) before operation.

	preOP (n=20)	postOP (n=20)	P value
LVDd (mm)	73±9	64±8	<0.001
LVDs (mm)	64±10	55±8	<0.001
FS (%)	12±5	14±7	0.38
LVEF (%)	27±6	30±7	0.077
IVST (mm)	9.5±1.9	10±2.0	0.11
PWT (mm)	9.0±1.6	9.4±1.6	0.068
E (m/s)	1.1±0.3	1.3±0.3	0.006
A (m/s)	0.5±0.3	0.8±0.5	0.024
E/A	2.9±1.9	2.4±1.5	0.33
DcT (ms)	167±66	223±71	0.008
MR grade	3.4±0.8	0.2±0.4	<0.001

Values±standard deviation. A, late diastolic wave; DcT, deceleration time; E, early diastolic wave; FS, fractional shortening; IVST, interventricular septal thickness; LVDd, left ventricular end-diastolic dimension; LVDs, left ventricular end-systolic dimension; LVEF, left ventricular ejection fraction; MR, mitral regurgitation; PWT, posterior wall thickness. P values were derived from paired t test.

Table 2. Pre and postoperative functional parameters of all patients

Table 3 shows pre and postoperative values of parameters for the submitral apparatus. Our data are the average of the parameters for the anterior and posterior papillary muscles and the normal values are those of the posterior papillary muscle. Mitral valve coaptation height and tenting area significantly decreased after operation. While tethering distance and papillary muscle angle significantly improved to normal values for reference, papillary muscle distance, which indicates the distance between papillary muscle heads to the mitral annular plain, did not change. By PMA, papillary muscle distance significantly decreased below the normal value after operation.

	preOP (n=20)	postOP (n=20)	normal values
coaptation height (mm)	11±3	5±3*	-
tenting area (cm^2)	2.3±0.7	0.6±0.3*	-
tethering distance (mm)	44±6	37±6*	33±5
papillary muscle depth (mm)	29±4	29±6	27±6
papillary muscle angle (°)	42±7	52±10*	51±7
papillary muscle distance (mm)	35±7	13±6*	25±1

Values±standard deviation. The normal values were derived from the reports by Nordblom P et al. and Vergnat M et al. *P<0.001.

Table 3. Pre and postoperative values of parameters for the submitral apparatus

Table 4 shows the postoperative values of parameters for the submitral apparatus, transmitral flow, and stroke volume index in the posterior directional PMS group and the anterior directional PMS group. Papillary muscle angle was significantly larger in the anterior PMS group than posterior PMS group, which suggests more anterior repositioning of the papillary muscles in the anterior PMS group. Peak mitral pressure gradient, which derives from mitral E wave, was smaller in the anterior PMS group than the posterior PMS group. There was no deference in stroke volume index between the groups. LV inflow angle was significantly larger in the anterior PMS group, which may be also an evidence of more anterior repositioning of the papillary muscles in the anterior PMS group.

	posterior PMS (n=8)	anterior PMS (n=12)	P value
coaptation height (mm)	3.3±1.2	5.9±3.3	0.055
tenting area (cm^2)	0.41±0.32	0.69±0.29	0.056
tethering distance (mm)	37±5	37±6	0.92
papillary muscle depth (mm)	26±6	30±5	0.11
papillary muscle angle (°)	46±9	56±9	0.025
papillary muscle distance (mm)	13±4	12±8	0.71
E (m/s)	1.6±0.2	1.1±0.2	0.001
DcT (ms)	186±45	247±80	0.073
peak pressure gradient (mmHg)	10±3	5±2	0.001
left ventricular inflow angle	60±6	78±9	<0.001
stroke volume index (ml/m^2)	28±5	33±11	0.23

Values±standard deviation. DcT, deceleration time; E, early diastolic wave; PMS, papillary muscle suspension. P values were derived from t test.

Table 4. Postoperative values of parameters for the submitral apparatus, transmitral flow, and stroke volume index in the posterior directional PMS group and the anterior directional PMS group.

4. Discussion

We demonstrate that we can precisely assess the change of geometry of the submitral apparatus after operation by using 2-D transthoracic echocardiography. The geometry of the submitral apparatus dramatically changed after operation and most of the parameters normalized in the anterior PMS group. Furthermore, we could detect the postoperative geometric deference between the two methods of papillary muscle suspension i.e. anterior and posterior direction. The papillary muscles positioned more anterior in the anterior PMS group compared to the posterior PMS group. This effect corresponded to the optimal diastolic LV filling i.e. lower transmitral gradient in the anterior PMS group.

There exists no standard method to determine the indication and effects of the surgical submitral procedures. Most of the clinical data after other submitral procedures are only basic echocardiographic values and MR grade. We performed PMA and PMS based on the criteria of preoperative papillary muscle distance > 30mm in short axis view and assessed the geometry of the submitral apparatus both before and after surgery. Therefore, this chapter would be the first step for establishing a guideline for proper comparison between the deferent submitral procedures by using 2-D transthoracic echocardiography.

4.1 Modalities for assessment of subvalvular apparatus

In order to clarify the mechanism of functional MR, there have been amounts of experimental studies in which 3-dimentional anatomy of submitral apparatus has been documented in several large animal models. In those models, they needed to place tantalum myocardial makers to detect the motion by videofluoroscopy and it cannot be used in clinic. Three-dimentional echocardiography has recently emerged and it enabled comprehensive preoperative evaluation of prolapsed mitral valve. Furthermore, mitral tenting volume has been studied in normal and patients with functional MR by using this modality. However, the analysis of submitral apparatus including papillary muscles is still controversial. The quality of the transthoracic echocardiography would be one problem especially in the early postoperative period. In our recent study using 2-D transthoracic echocardiography, all the measurements were completed without difficulty even in the postoperative state.

Vergnat et al recently reported the anatomy of the submitral apparatus using 3-D echocardiography. In their study, the normal tethering distance was 37 mm for the anterior and 39 mm for the posterior papillary muscles, respectively. These values well corresponds to the postoperative values in our population. Normal inter-papillary distance was reported 25 mm. By our PMA procedure, the distance is over-corrected from 35 mm to 13 mm on average after surgery. Although we need 3-D echocardiography to assess specific volume like mitral tenting volume, 2-D echocardiography would be enough to assess the length between the anatomical points of mitral valve complex.

4.2 Submitral procedures for functional MR

Our surgical strategy consists of mitral annuloplasty with semi-rigid total ring, PMA and PMS. Although we first performed posterior-directional PMS (pPMS) because it was easy, even through the mitral annulus from left atrial approach, we considered more physiological geometry of mitral complex and recently changed the PMS direction from the posterior to the anterior. Anterior-directional PMS (aPMS) is sometimes difficult due to submitral apparatus, but it becomes easier with a large needle even through mitral annulus. We recently preferred a true-sized ring to an undersized one because adequate coaptation length is accomplished with subvalvular reconstruction. Although this is a short-term study, we found no recurrence of significant mitral regurgitation during two years of follow-up (data are not shown).

Kron et al. reported a novel approach to reduce tethering length and improve coaptation by approximating displaced posterior papillary muscle toward the annulus. The efficacy of this procedure was confirmed in an acute experimental model of posterior myocardial infarction. Hvass et al evolved a papillary muscle sling procedure using an ePTFE tube graft around the muscles and reported improved mitral tethering. Messas et al. proposed a chordal cutting procedure. Basal chordal cutting eliminates the anterior leaflet bend and can make the leaflets less taut and improve coaptation. Although several surgeons have performed this procedure and argued for its efficacy without left ventricular dysfunction, we still do not know the long-term clinical effect. Furthermore, adverse effects of chordal cutting have also been reported. Borger et al. reported that the late recurrence of a grade 2 MR was 15% two years after chordal cutting. Langer et al. reported transaortic repositioning of posterior papillary muscle to the midseptal fibrous annulus in a procedure named "RING plus STRING". They first determined in an experimental model of sheep the geometric and functional effects of this procedure. STRING alone did not significantly shift the posterior papillary muscle to the septum and did not improve MR. The major deference between "RING plus STRING" and our PMA and PMS is the direction of the papillary muscle suspension. While the direction of suspension by "STRING" is lateral side of the anterior mitral annulus, we place the suspension in the middle of the anterior mitral annulus in the PMA and PMS procedure. As determined by trasthoracic echocardiography in this chapter, the approximated papillary muscles shift to antero-septal side of the ventricle, papillary muscle angle normalizes, and MR disappears by our anterior directional PMS procedure.

As mentioned above, thus far various kinds of surgical methods have emerged to correct the geometry of the submitral apparatus and to prevent late recurrence of MR. However, there exists no standard method to determine the indication and effects of those various procedures and it makes the comparison between the procedures difficult. In this chapter, we suggested the usefulness and importance of 2-D transthoracic echocardiography in this controversial issue. By the routine assessment of submitral apparatus pre and postoperatively, we may compare the results of different procedures and it would be also important information for the mechanism of late recurrence of functional MR.

4.3 Beneficial effects of antero-septal directional papillary muscle suspension – prevention of functional mitral stenosis after surgery

Left ventricular inflow angle was significantly larger in the anterior PMS group and mitral peak pressure gradient was significantly smaller in the anterior PMS group than the posterior PMS group. We consider that mitral valve tethering during diastole could be ameliorated by anterior PMS which can relocate the papillary muscles toward antero-septal side of the ventricle but not posterior side. Furthermore, because stroke volume index was relatively larger even with lower transmitral gradient, mitral valve opening area during diastole may be larger in the anterior PMS group

In the recent report by Kubota et al, they have given a new insight in the mechanism of "functional mitral stenosis (MS)" after mitral annuloplasty (MAP) for ischemic MR. Persistent subvalvular leaflet tethering in the presence of down-sized MAP causes functional MS, which is related to heart failure symptom after surgery. Down-sized MAP has been a standard procedure for ischemic MR and believed to be safe and effective over ten years. In 2008 Magne et al. first reported functional MS after MAP. However its mechanism was not clarified in this study. On the other hand, Kubota et al. examined subvalvular apparatus during exertion and indicated that not only MAP but also further mitral tethering causes functional MS. This study has a considerable impact on the surgical strategy for ischemic MR in the future. It would be necessary to consider not only the elimination of MR but also functional effects of various submitral procedures.

5. Conclusion

We can precisely assess the change of geometry of the submitral apparatus after operation by using 2-D transthoracic echocardiography. It would be useful for the comparison between different surgical procedures.

6. References

Borger MA, Murphy PM, Alam A, et al. (2007) J Thorac Cardiovasc Surg. *Initial results of the chordal-cutting operation for ischemic mitral regurgitation.* 133:1483-1492.

Goetz WA, Lim HS, Pekar F, et al. (2003) Circulation. *Anterior mitral leaflet mobility is limited by the basal stay chords.* 107:2969 –2974.

Hvass U, Tapia M, Baron F, et al. (2003) Ann Thorac Surg. *Papillary muscle sling: a new functional approach to mitral repair in patients with ischemic left ventricular dysfunction and functional mitral regurgitation.* 75:809-811.

Kron IL, Green GR & Cope JT. (2002) Ann Thorac Surg. *Surgical relocation of the posterior papillary muscle in chronic ischemic mitral regurgitation.* 74:600-601.

Kubota K, Otsuji Y, Ueno T, et al. (2010) J Thorac Cardiovasc Surg. *Functional mitral stenosis after surgical annuloplasty for ischemic mitral regurgitation: Importance of subvalvular tethering in the mechanism and dynamic deterioration during exertion.* 140:617-623.

Langer F, Rodriguez F, Ortiz S, et al. (2005) Circulation. *Subvalvular repair: the key to repairing ischemic mitral regurgitation?* 112:383-389.

Langer F, Schäfers HJ. (2007) J Thorac Cardiovasc Surg. *RING plus STRING: papillary muscle repositioning as an adjunctive repair technique for ischemic mitral regurgitation.* 133:247-249.

Magne J, Sénéchal M, Mathieu P, et al. (2008) J Am Coll Cardiol. *Restrictive annuloplasty for ischemic mitral regurgitation may induce functional mitral stenosis.* 51:1692-1701.

Matsui Y, Suto Y, Shimura S, et al. (2005) Ann Thorac Cardiovasc Surg. *Impact of papillary muscles approximation on the adequacy of mitral coaptation in functional mitral regurgitation due to dilated cardiomyopathy.* 11:164-171.

Matsunaga A, Tahta SA & Duran CM. (2004) J Heart Valve Dis. *Failure of reduction annuloplasty for functional ischemic mitral regurgitation.*13:390-397.

Messas E, Guerrero JL, Handschumacher MD, et al. (2001) Circulation. *Chordal cutting: a new therapeutic approach for ischemic mitral regurgitation.* 104:1958-1963.

Messas E, Pouzet B, Touchot B, et al. (2003) Circulation. *Efficacy of chordal cutting to relieve chronic persistent ischemic mitral regurgitation.* 108:111-115.

Nordblom P, Bech-Hanssen O. (2007) Echocardiography. *Reference values describing the normal mitral valve and the position of the papillary muscles.*24:665-672.

Rodriguez F, Langer F, Harrington KB, et al. (2004) Circulation. *Cutting second-order chords does not prevent acute ischemic mitral regurgitation.* 110:91-97.

Shingu Y, Yamada S, Ooka T, et al. (2009) Circ J. *Papillary muscle suspension concomitant with approximation for functional mitral regurgitation.*73:2061-2067.

Vergnat M, Jassar AS, Jackson BM, et al. (2011) Ann Thorac Surg. *Ischemic mitral regurgitation: a quantitative three-dimensional echocardiographic analysis.* 91:157-164.

7

Role of Transthoracic Echocardiography in Visualization of the Coronary Arteries and Assessment of Coronary Flow Reserve

Yasser Baghdady, Hussein Hishmat and Heba Farook
Cairo University
Egypt

1. Introduction

Visualization of the epicardial coronary arteries by echocardiography is technically challenging. The physical nature of ultrasound waves prevents them from delineating the coronary tree because of multiple factors. The resolution of tansthoracic echo using a 2.5-3.5MHz probe is only 2mm while the diameter of the epicardial coronary arteries ranges from 1.5 to 4mm. The epicardial coronaries are relatively superficial in the chest, so the lie in near field of the ultrasound waves. The translational and rotational motion of the coronary arteries in the AV grooves poses a challenge in obtaining stable Doppler signals. The relatively low velocity of coronary flow compared to the flow velocity in the ventricles makes color signals hard to discern. Finally, the tomographic nature of the echocardiographic study makes differentiation between adjacent vessels e.g. the LAD and the diagonal branches extremely difficult. Despite these difficulties, the need for a non-invasive bedside tool that could allow inference of the coronary arteries pushed towards more efforts in using echo for that aspect. Using dedicated high-frequency probes made assessment of the left main coronary, the LAD and even the posterior descending branch of the RCA feasible in a large proportion of patients (Hozumi et al., 1998). Transthoracic and transesophageal echo can provide data regarding coronary patency, the presence of coronary stenosis or coronary ectasia (Iliceto S, et al., 1991, Kozakova M, et al., 1997, Lambertz et al., 2000).

2. Coronary flow and Doppler analysis

Normal antegrade coronary flow is predominant diastolic with a small systolic component (Heinz Lambertz et al., 2004). Systolic flow is less important and is a less stable measure as it can be eve retrograde. It may be difficult to record both diastolic and systolic flow in the same cardiac cycle in all patients, because of cardiac motion that displaces the coronary artery from the ultrasound beam in systole. Diastolic flow is antegrade in both epicardial and intramural vessels, whereas systolic flow is antegrade in epicardial but retrograde in intramural vessels, because blood is squeezed backwards by myocardial contraction (Vernon Anderson H et al., 2000). As a result of the two opposite forces, the magnitude of systolic flow velocity may change along the coronary tree and close to the origin of a perforator there might be a watershed area with stagnation of systolic flow. Therefore, the epicardial anterograde systolic flow is mainly a capacitance, rather than a nutrient flow, and may not reflect myocardial perfusion.

2.1 The parameters that can be assessed by coronary Doppler imaging include

- Diastolic flow velocity
- Systolic flow velocity
- Diastolic Deceleration time
- Coronary flow reserve

The baseline coronary flow velocity may change from one beat to the other of even 5–10 cm/s. Elevated resting flow velocities may occur in tachycardia, anaemia, hyperthyroidism, severe left ventricular hypertrophy etc (Czernin J er al, 1993, Voci P et al., 2004). Coronary vasodilators increase the diameter of the epicardial artery and reduce baseline flow velocity. Analysis of the coronary Doppler waveform can provide useful information about vessel patency and the presence of severe stenosis or moderate stenosis. Noninvasive Doppler has some alleged advantages over IVUS/FFR. Echocardiography avoids contact with the coronary artery, which may be reactive during myocardial infarction. Echo also measuring velocities in regions inaccessible to IVUS such as the septal perforators. The most important limitation of transthoracic Doppler measurement is the difficulty of obtaining accurate adjustment of the Doppler beam parallel to the coronary flow. If the angle between the Doppler beam and the coronary artery is >60°, diastolic flow velocity could be underestimated.

3. Visualization of different coronary artery segments by Echo-Doppler

3.1 Transthoracic echocardiography

In general, assessment of coronary blood flow differs in different coronary arteries. The LAD blood flow can be assessed by using high frequency transducers due to the proximity of this vessel to the chest wall. However, this technique is not suitable for imaging peripheral RCA flow because of the distance between the transducer and the basal inferior cardiac wall (7-10cm). Therefore a lower frequency transducer is required to overcome the problem of inadequate penetration depth of a high frequency transducer. Individual coronary anatomy shows considerable patient to patient variability. Therefore it is not possible to visualize a segment of the right coronary artery in the posterior interventricular grove in every patient (Lethen H et al., 2003, Meimoun P et al., 2004, 2005, Tokai K et al., 2003, Ueno Y et al., 2002, 2003). Recording an accurate systolic-diastolic pulsed wave Doppler signal is often hampered by respiratory movements and lateral as well as vertical motion of the basal inferior cardiac wall during the cardiac cycle. This problem can partially be resolved by obtaining Doppler signals in apnea.

3.2 LMT and proximal segments of the left and right coronary arteries

The proximal portion of the left coronary artery can be visualized from a modified high parasternal short axis view. First obtain the classic parasternal short axis view at the level of the aortic valve. Then make slight clockwise rotation and anterior tilt of the transducer to visualize the left main trunk as seen in the figure below.

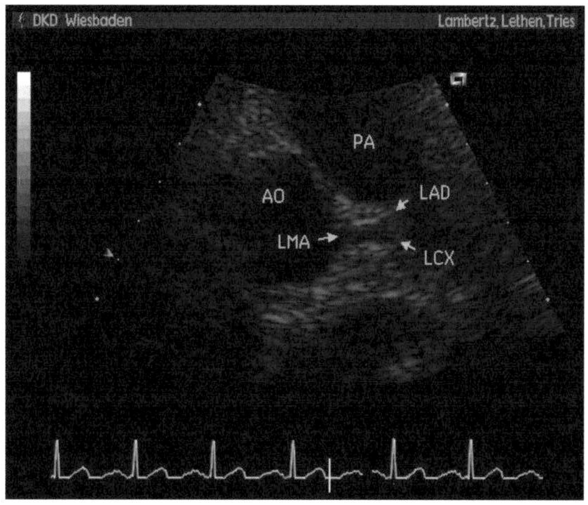

Fig. 1. Parasternal short axis view showing left main stem and its bifurcation into LAD and LCX branches (Heinz Lambertz et al., 2004).

Color Doppler imaging of the coronary flow in the proximal portion of the left coronary artery is technically difficult for two reasons: First, the almost orthogonal alignment of coronary flow to the ultrasound beam and second, the interposition of the right ventricular outflow tract and pulmonary artery. The left main coronary artery can also be imaged from an apical transducer position. From the classical five chamber view, the transducer is carefully angled more anteriorly until the ascending aorta is visualized. With slight tilting and rotation of the transducer, the left and the right coronary arteries can be recorded in one imaging plane: The orifice of the left coronary artery is located approximately three O'clock. The orifice of the RCA can be detected at approximately ten O'clock.

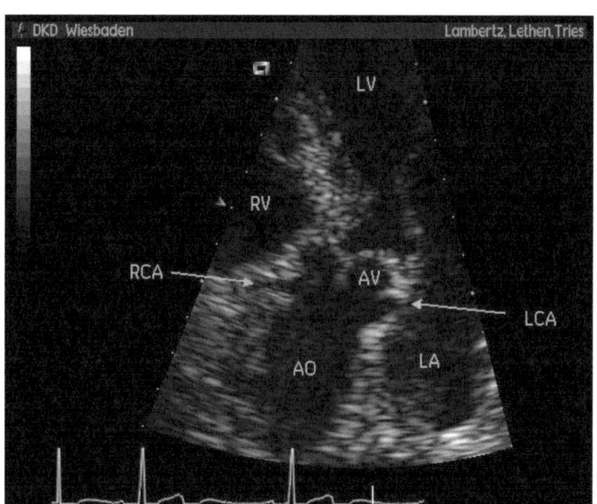

Fig. 2. Modified apical five-chamber view illustrating the origin of the left and right coronary artery from the aortic bulbus (Heinz Lambertz et al., 2004).

3.3 Visualization of the middle segment of the LAD

The middle and distal portion of the left anterior descending artery lies in the anterior ventricular groove close to the anterior chest wall. Due to the proximity of the middle and distal left anterior descending artery to a precordially located transducer, these coronary segments are ideal for transthoracic echocardiographic examination. From the classic parasternal short axis view at the level of the papillary muscles, a lateral displacement of the transducer by 2-3cm allows the visualization of the anterior interventricular groove. With caudal displacement of the transducer of 1-2 intercostal spaces, Color Doppler is used to identify the coronary flow in the anterior groove. Once a predominant diastolic flow signal is detected from a vessel within the anterior interventricular groove, activate the zoom mode while keeping the Doppler box small with adjustment of the velocity range at 12-24cm/s. From the previous view, the transducer is rotated 70 to 90° to obtain the best LAD long axis view. For measurement of the coronary flow velocity, pulsed wave Doppler is used with a sample size of 3mm and care should be taken to avoid an angle exceeding 35 to 45°.

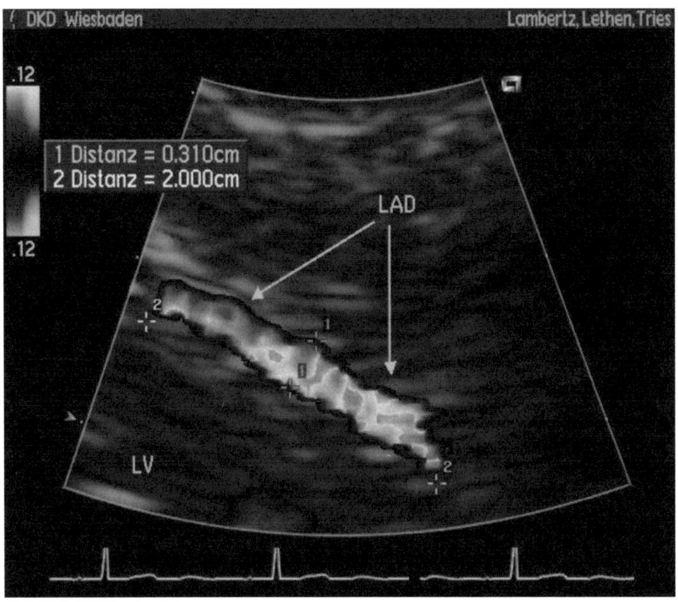

Fig. 3. Modified PLAX view allowing color Doppler assessment of coronary blood flow in the mid segment of the LAD (Heinz Lambertz et al., 2004).

3.4 Visualization of the distal segment of the LAD

The distal part of the left anterior descending artery can be recorded in a modified foreshortened three-chamber view from an apical window. From the conventional apical 2 chamber view the transducer is rotated anti-clockwise to obtain an apical long axis view, showing the left ventricle and left ventricular outflow tract. Using the color Doppler, the distal segment of the LAD, located in the apical part of the interventricular groove can be detected close to the apex of the left ventricle. From this view, the transducer is shifted 1 to 2 intercostal spaces cranially with anterior tilt to visualize the peripheral epicardial segments of the LAD.

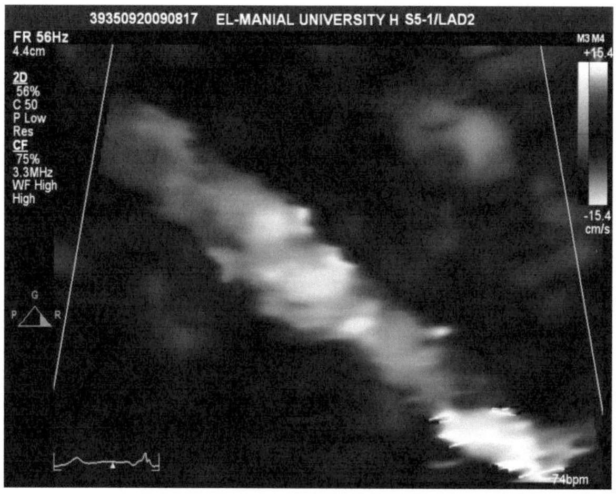

Fig. 4. Modified apical view showing the distal segment of the LAD (H. Farouk, et al., 2010).

3.5 Visualization of the RCA

To visualize the posterior descending branch of the RCA, the left ventricle is first imaged in a conventional apical two-chamber view. From this position, the transducer is slightly rotated anti-clockwise and carefully tilted anteriorly. Using color Doppler, coronary blood flow in the posterior interventricular groove can be identified.

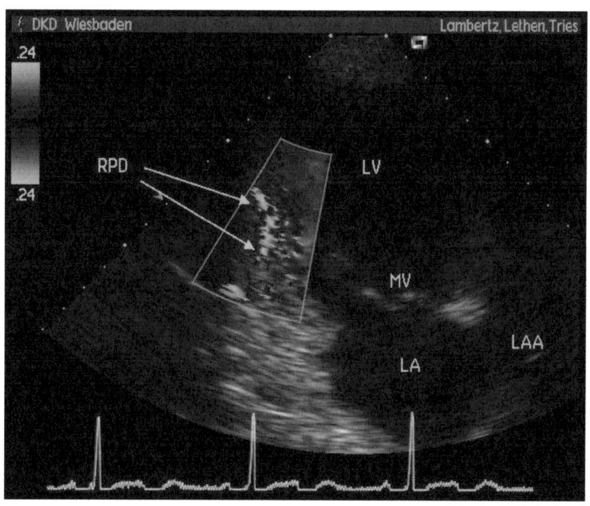

Fig. 5. Modified apical two-chamber view. Color Doppler flow map showing the proximal part of the posterior interventricular branch in the posterior interventricular groove (Heinz Lambertz et al., 2004).

After detection of the characteristic predominant diastolic blood flow in the basal part of the posterior interventricular groove, the sample volume (2.0-3.5mm) is positioned for spectral Doppler analysis of coronary blood flow.

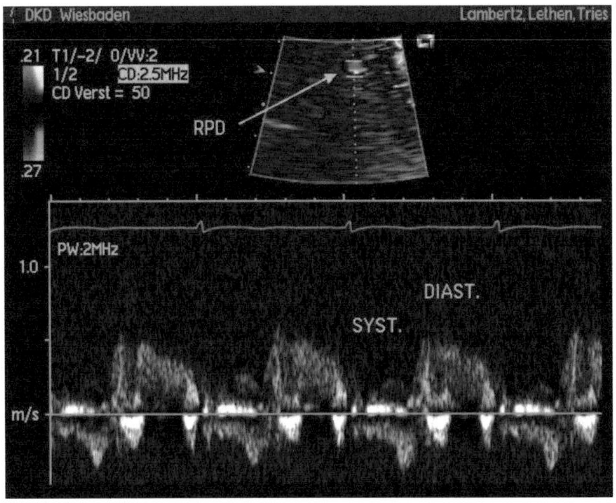

Fig. 6. Characteristic biphasic spectral Doppler recording of coronary blood flow velocity in the distal RCA (Heinz Lambertz et al., 2004).

The modified apical two-chamber view used for assessment of the right coronary artery blood flow allows alignment of the ultrasound beam roughly parallel to the course of the posterior descending artery, thus, unlike assessment of the flow of the left anterior descending artery, provide an adequate registration of the coronary flow velocity.

3.6 Detection of the left circumflex artery by TTE

The proximal third of the LCX can be examined using an apical or parasternal short axis view approach. To assess the distal left circumflex artery, we use the apical 5 chamber view with the transducer is rotated clockwise to direct the imaging plane posteriorly and inferiorly. The direction of the CBF of the circumflex artery is not parallel to the ultrasound beam. Because the success rate in visualizing the flow in the mid and distal circumflex is limited, assessment of the coronary flow reserve is of limited clinical significance in cases of suspected left circumflex artery disease (Heinz Lambertz et al., 2004)

3.7 Detection of the left internal mammary artery

The proximal mammary artery is best visualized from a supraclavicular view using high frequency transducer (8 MHz linear transducer). A patent mammary artery graft is recognized by its typical baseline spectral Doppler flow profile, showing considerably higher diastolic blood flow velocity compared to the other vessels originating in close proximity to the subclavian artery.

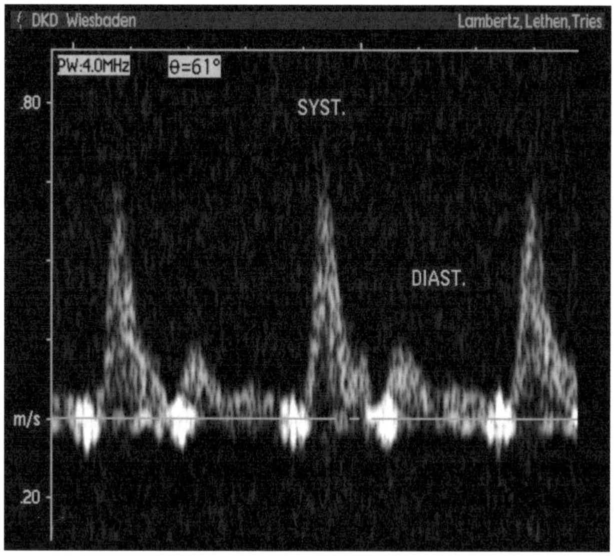

Fig. 7. Pulsed wave Doppler profile of mammary artery. The systolic flow velocity is typically higher than the diastolic (Heinz Lambertz et al., 2004).

3.8 Detection of the septal branches of the LAD by TTE

In immediate proximity of the mid and distal portion of the left anterior descending artery, septal side branches with varying caliber can be seen by color Doppler analysis. Frequently, the vessel course can be followed over a longer distance within the ventricular septum. Diagonal branches or a dominant intermediate branch can't always be clearly differentiated from the left anterior descending artery, as they may have approximately the same diameter and an almost parallel course.

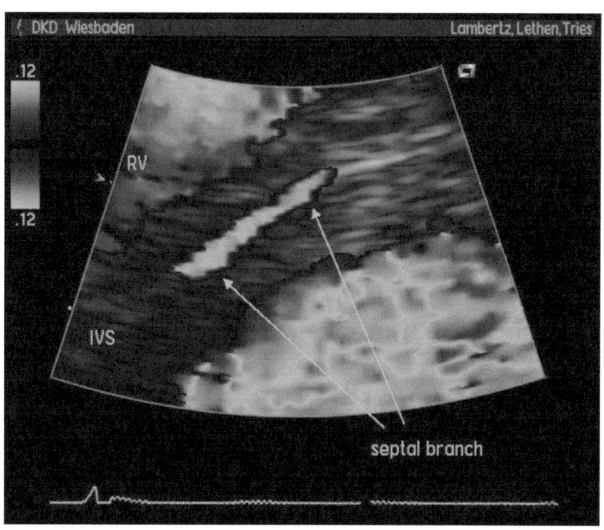

Fig. 8. Parasternal short axis view illustrating a perforator branch in the mid septum (Heinz Lambertz et al., 2004).

3.9 Transesophageal echocardiography

The best way to image the proximal segment of the coronary artery is a transesophageal short axis view at the level of the aortic bulb with a slight anteflexion of the probe. From this view the left main stem and the proximal LAD can be visualized in about 70 to 90% of patients. The success rate in imaging the proximal segment of the left circumflex is even higher (75 to 90%). The best way to visualize the ostuim of the right coronary artery is a sagittal scanning plane showing the ascending aorta in a long axis (Lambertz H et al., 2000). With a slight clockwise rotation of the probe, a short segment of the right coronary artery originating from the aortic bulb can be imaged from the majority of patients.

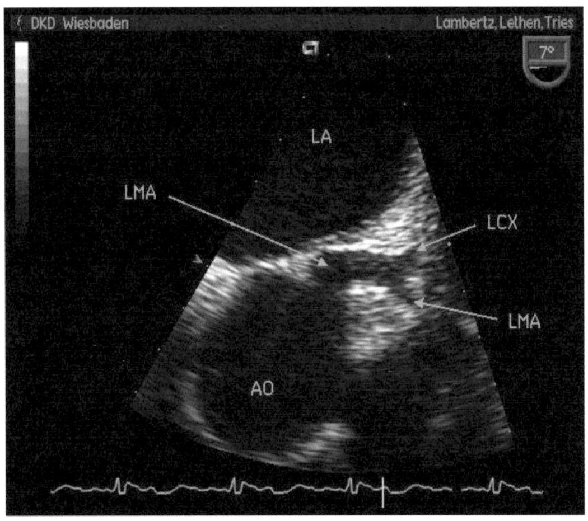

Fig. 9. Transesophageal echocardiography illustrating the left main stem and its bifurcation into LAD and LCX ((Heinz Lambertz et al., 2004).

With a pulsed wave Doppler, sample volume positioned in the proximal portion of the left anterior descending coronary artery, systolic as well as diastolic flow can be recorded (Iliceto S, et al. , 1991)

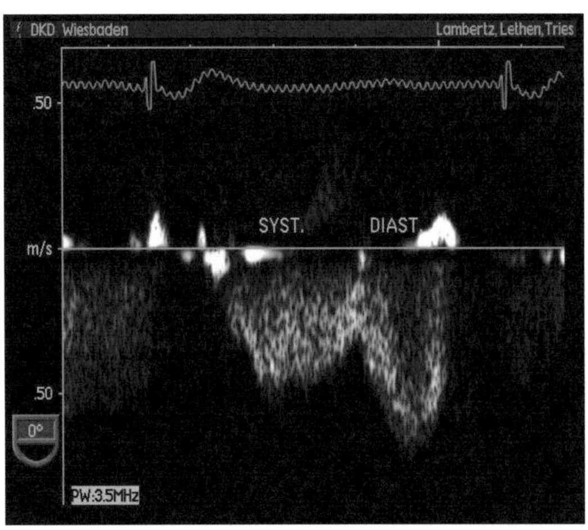

Fig. 10. TEE recording from a normal LAD.CBF occurs systolic-diastolic with the highest velocity during diastole (Heinz Lambertz et al., 2004).

In contrast to the transthoracic approach, TEE imaging allows a reliable Doppler flow analysis in the proximal left anterior descending artery, because the ultrasound beam can be aligned almost parallel to the anatomical course of the vessel. However, due to motion artifacts caused by respiratory excursions and ventricular contraction, adequate recording of the coronary blood flow can be obtained more easily during a short period of apnea.

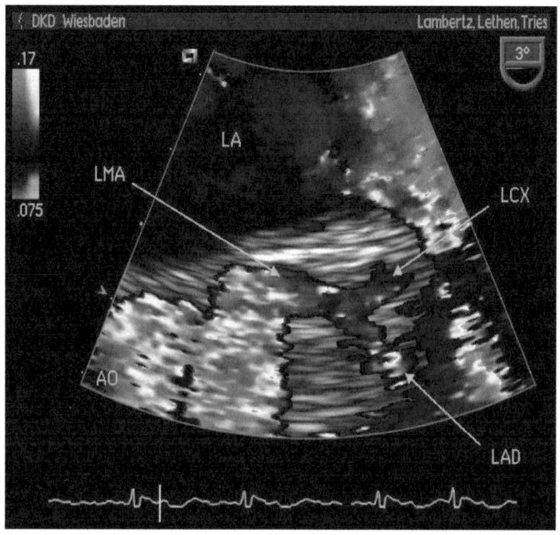

Fig. 11. Color Doppler illustrating normal coronary blood flow within the left main artery and its bifurcation into LAD and LCX (Heinz Lambertz et al., 2004).

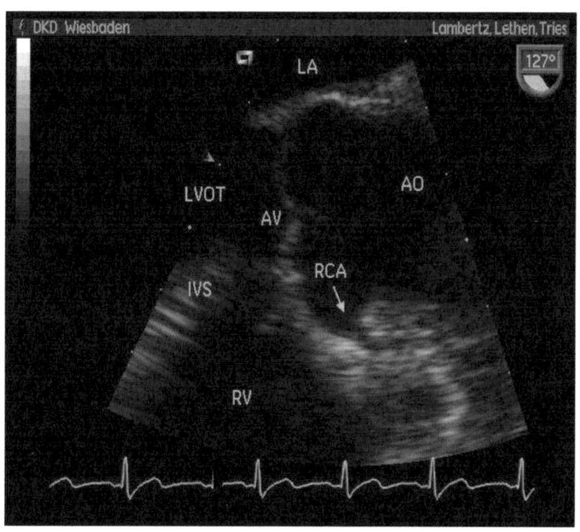

Fig. 12. Orifice of the right coronary artery. The TEE scanning plane is aligned roughly parallel to a long axis of the ascending aorta ((Heinz Lambertz et al., 2004)

Transesophageal echocardiography, with or without contrast, is a low cost method and easily repeatable, which can be used to evaluate coronary circulation in selected patients. However, this approach has less clinical importance in evaluating the hemodynamic relevance of a left anterior descending artery stenosis. This is based on the fact that most of the left anterior descending artery stenoses are located distal to those left anterior descending artery segments that can be visualized by Transesophageal echocardiography.

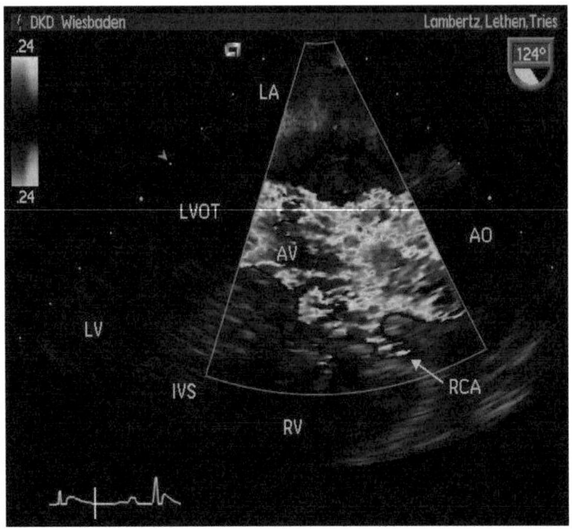

Fig. 13. Visualization of the coronary blood flow in the proximal right coronary artery (Heinz Lambertz et al., 2004).

It has to be taken also into consideration that approximately 20% to 30% of the patients cannot be investigated by Doppler because of respiration, obesity, chest deformity and emphysema, acute changes in cardiac volume, or inadequately stable position of the Doppler signal. Flow in the branches could be erroneously interpreted as the flow in the main trunk. In particular, this could happen for LAD in the two-chamber or in the short axis view, where a long diagonal branch or the first septal perforator might also be visualized.

4. Clinical utilization of echocardiographic coronary imaging

4.1 Coronary artery patency

In the particular situation of acute myocardial infarction, a non-invasive way to visualize the LAD should be of great help to diagnose the success of reperfusion. In this setting, the sensitivity, specificity, positive predictive value, negative predictive value and accuracy of the transthoracic echo Doppler in the noninvasive assessment of the LAD reperfusion with 2.5MHz transducer were 81.6%, 64%, 90.7%, 54% and 78% respectively (H. Farouk et al., 2010). Detection of the distal LAD flow by TTDE was significantly correlated with the reperfusion as assessed by coronary angiography.

Epicardial coronary flow is not always synonymous with cellular myocardial perfusion as seen in the no-reflow phenomenon. Visualization of septal perforator flow can be a more reliable marker of reperfusion. Voci et al (Voci P et al., 2004) considered a myocardial segment to be reperfused when at least two of the predicted four to five perforators could be visualized by transthoracic echo after acute MI. A recanalization score (RS) of 1 to 4 was used—where 1 = LAD closed, no perforators; 2 = LAD open, no perforators; 3 = LAD open, 1 to 2 segments with perforators; 4 = LAD open, 3 to 4 segments with perforators. RS discriminated recovery of ventricular function better than TIMI flow. The RS was the best single multivariate predictor ($p < 0.0001$) of percent changes in wall motion score index and the ejection fraction.

Antti Saraste et al, (Saraste M et al., 2005) found that diastolic deceleration time of the LAD flow velocity correlated with myocardial fluorodeoxyglucose uptake in the LAD territory.

Diastolic deceleration time was markedly longer in patients with viable myocardium than partially viable or non-viable myocardium. A DDT <190ms is always associated with non-viable myocardium. However, this finding was not consistent among different studies.

4.2 Coronary artery occlusion

Coronary flow can be measured by transthoracic coronary Doppler ultrasound in occluded coronary arteries receiving collateral flow. Reverse diastolic flow at rest, reflecting retrograde filling of the artery by collaterals, is a very specific marker of coronary occlusion but it unfortunately has a low sensitivity, since collaterals may perfuse the vessel either retrogradely or anterogradely.

4.3 Severe coronary stenosis

Coronary artery stenosis could be identified with color Doppler as local spot of turbulence. An abnormal maximal-to-prestenotic blood flow velocity ratio greater than 2.0 would signify a critical stenosis. These findings have an overall sensitivity of 82% and specificity of 92%. The sensitivity and specificity were, respectively, 73% and 92% for left anterior descending coronary artery, 63% and 96% for right coronary artery, and 38% and 99% for left circumflex coronary artery stenoses. For left main coronary stenosis, echo showed a 92% sensitivity and 62% specificity to identify IVUS significant (MLA < 6 mm2) left main stenosis if taking a peak diastolic velocity cut off of 112 cm/sec (Gerkens U, et al. , 1989, Samdarshi TE et al.,1990)

4.4 Moderate coronary stenosis

The assessment of moderate-severity coronary stenosis by angiography has limitations related to the "lumenographic "nature of angiography (Topol EJ, et al., 1995). The concept of coronary flow reserve performed by Doppler intracoronary wire during coronary angiography can be also performed by echocardiography. The major advantages of coronary flow assessment by TTDE are that it is completely non-invasive, relatively inexpensive, and gives objective and accurate information on the physiological significance both in epicardial native coronary stenosis as well as in detecting coronary restenosis following coronary percutaneous interventions (Caiati C et al., 1999, 1999, Hozumi T et al., 1998). Another important value of TTDE study of CFVR is the assessment of microvascular coronary circulation.

4.5 Coronary flow reserve

Coronary flow reserve is defined as the maximal increase in coronary blood flow (by using a strong coronary vasodilator) above its basal level for a given perfusion pressure. So, it is a ratio of maximal (stimulated) to baseline (resting) coronary blood flow. The best sampling site of the coronary flow, for assessing the functional significance of a stenosis, is the distal tract of the vessel which could be easily obtained with TDE. Proximal to the stenosis CFR may be normal as there are side branches between the sampling site and the stenosis, which reflects perfusion in normal territories (Voci P et al., 2004). The angle correction is redundant given that CFR is the ratio between hyperemic and baseline flow velocity, and it is not affected by the actual flow velocity. However, the angle has to be kept as small as possible. Blood flow velocity measurements are performed offline by contouring the spectral Doppler signals, using the integrated software package of the ultrasound system. Final values of flow velocity represent an average of three cardiac cycles. TDE-CFR is defined as hyperemic diastolic mean (or peak) flow velocity divided by baseline flow velocity. It is important to underscore that during administration of the vasodilating agent, the transducer probe is in the same position as baseline, and machine settings including size of sample volume and velocity scale are not changed. The mean time required to complete a CFR test is around 10–15 min.

Adenosine is the most commonly used vasodilator to assess TDE-CFR. It is a potent vasodilator producing maximal coronary vasodilatation within 40-50 seconds. Given its short half life (10s) and rapid onset of action, it allows CFR measurements more rapidly than other vasodilators. Furthermore, Adenosine acts mainly at the level of the microcirculation and does not alter significantly the diameter of the coronary artery. Adenosine is administered intravenously (0.140 mg/kg/min) for 5 minutes (Lapeyre AC III et al., 2004, Sudhir K et al., 1993, Verani MS, 1991, Wilson R et al., 1990). The normal range of CFVR for both men and women is ≥ 2.7. The cut-off value of 2 of CFR for detecting significant epicardial coronary stenosis or to predict ischemia in the underlying territory has been demonstrated in various studies (Kern MJ et al., 1996, Matsumara Y et al., 2003).

The feasibility of TDE-CFR for LAD artery is very high, with more than 90% in experienced hands, and nearly 100% with the use of intravenous contrast agents (Caiati C et al., 1999). The feasibility is less in the PDA artery, between 54 and 86% due to technical limitations (Hozumi T et al., 1998, Lethen H et al., 2003, Ueno Y et al., 2002). The measurements of TDE-CFR, in the LAD as in the PDA arteries, are closely correlated with invasive measurements using a Doppler flow wire. The feasibility of TDE-CFR in the circumflex artery is more challenging given the particular anatomy of this artery and the poor resolution of the lateral wall.

4.6 Kawasaki disease and congenital coronary anomalies

In the pediatric population, visualization of the proximal portions of the left and the right coronaries by transthoracic echo is achievable in almost all cases. Therefore, it is routine to comment on the origin and the course of the proximal left and right coronary arteries in all pediatric studies. The aneurysms of the proximal RCA and proximal LAD in Kawasaki disease provide the diagnosis in infants with febrile illness and the classic rash and can be useful in follow up of this condition (Satomi G et al., 1984, Yoshikawa J et al., 1979). Also, failure of visualization of one of the coronary arteries in children with cardiomyopathy should prompt excluding the diagnosis of anomalous origin of the coronary from the pulmonary artery. Also anomalous origin of the right coronary from the left sinus of valsalva which poses a threat of sudden cardiac death can be readily diagnosed in children by transthoracic echo.

5. Conclusion

Echocardiography can be used to visualize the epicardial coronary arteries directly in a large proportion of patients. The success is greatest in children, ostia of the left and right coronary arteries and in the LAD. However, it is unlikely, at least in the near future, that echo can provide complete anatomical assessment of the coronary tree. X-ray bases modalities, namely angiography and CT are still superior in providing anatomical details. Nevertheless, in some clinical situations, echo can provide very useful data regarding coronary patency, severe stenosis, moderate coronary lesions, the state of the microcirculation and congenital coronary anomalies.

6. References

Caiati C, Montaldo C, Zedda N, Bina A, Iliceto S. A new noninvasive method for coronary flow reserve assessment: contrast-enhanced transthoracic second harmonic echo Doppler. Circulation 1999; 99: 771–778.

Caiati C, Montaldo C, Zedda N, Montisci R, Ruscazio M, Lai G et al. Validation of a non-invasive method (contrast enhanced transthoracic second harmonic echo Doppler) for the evaluation of coronary flow reserve: comparison with intracoronary Doppler flow wire. J Am Coll Cardiol 1999;34:1193 - 200.

Caiati C, Zedda N, Montaldo C, Montisci R, Iliceto S. Contrast-enhanced transthroacic second harmonic echoDoppler with adenosine. A noninvasive, rapid and effective method for coronary flow reserve assessment. JACC 1999; 34:122–130

Czernin J, Muller P, Chan S, Brunken RC, Porenta G, Krivokapitch J et al. Influence of age and hemodynamics on myocardial blood flow and flow reserve. Circulation 1993;88:62 - 9.

Gerkens U, et al. detection of proximal coronary artery stenosis by transesophageal echocardiography. Eur Heart J. 1989; 10:121

Heba F. Saleh, Hussien Heshmat, Y.Baghdady, K. Sorour. Faculty of medicine, Cairo University.

Heinz Lambertz, Hans-Peter Tries, Harald Lethen. Coronary flow reserve: a practical echocardiographic approach. Second edition. 2004.

Hozumi T, Yoshida K, Akasaka T et al. Noninvasive assessment of coronary flow velocity and coronary flow velocity reserve in the left anterior descending coronary artery by Doppler echocardiography: comparison with invasive technique. J Am Coll Cardiol 1998; 32: 1251–1259.

Hozumi T, Yoshida K, Akasaka T et al. Noninvasive assessment of coronary flow velocity and coronary flow velocity reserve in the left anterior descending coronary artery by Doppler echocardiography: comparison with invasive technique. J Am Coll Cardiol 1998; 32: 1251–1259.

Iliceto S. Transesophageal Doppler echocardiography evaluation of coronary flow velocity in baseline conditions and during dipyridamole-induced coronary vasodilation. Circulation 83:61-69, 1991.

Kern MJ, Bach RG, Mechem CJ, et al. Variations in normal coronary vasodilatory reserve stratified by artery, gender, heart transplantation and coronary artery disease. J Am Coll Cardiol. 1996;28:1154-1160.

Kozakova M. Mechanisms of coronary flow impairments in human hypertension. Hypertension 29:551-559, 1997.

Lambertz H, Lethen H. Lehratlas der transősophagealen Echokardiographie, 2000; Thieme Verlag Stuttgart, New York 1-273.

Lapeyre AC III, Goraya TY, Johnston DL, Gibbons RJ. The impact of caffeine on vasodilator stress perfusion studies. J Nucl Cardiol. 2004;11:506–511.

Lethen H, Tries HP, Kersting S, Lambertz H. Validation of noninvasive assessment of coronary flow velocity reserve in the right coronary artery: a comparison of transthoracic echocardiographic results with intracoronary Doppler flow wire measurements. Eur Heart J 2003;24:1567 - 75.

Matsumara Y, Hozumi T, Watanabe H, Fujimoto K, Sugioka K, Takemoto Y et al. Cut-off value of coronary flow velocity reserve by transthoracic Doppler echocardiography for diagnosis of significant left anterior descending artery stenosis in patients with coronary risk factors. Am J Cardiol 2003;92:1389 - 93.

Meimoun P, Benali T, Sayah S, Luycx-Bore A, Boulanger J, Zemir H et al. Evaluation of left anterior descending coronary artery stenosis of intermediate severity using transthoracic coronary flow reserve and dobutamine stress echocardiography. J Am Soc Echocardiogr 2005;12:1233 - 40.

Meimoun P, Sayah S, Maitre B, Luycx-Bore A, Benali T, Beausoleil M et al. Measurement of coronary flow reserve with transthoracic echocardiography: an old concept, a new tool, a lot of applications. Ann Cardiol Angiol 2004;53:325 - 34.

Samdarshi TE et al. Transesophageal color Doppler echocardiography in assessing proximal coronary artery stenosis. J Am Coll Cardiol. 1990; 15:93

Saraste M, Vesalainen RK, Ylitalo A, Saraste A, Koskenvuo JW, Toikka JO, Vaittinen MA, Hartiala JJ, Airaksinen KE: Transthoracic Doppler echocardiography as a noninvasive tool to assess coronary artery stenoses-a comparison with quantitative coronary angiography. J Am Soc Echocardiogr 2005, 18:679-85.

Satomi G, Nakamura K, Narai S, et al. Systematic visualization of coronary arteries by two-dimensional echocardiography in children and infants: evaluation in Kawasaki's disease and coronary arteriovenous fistulas. Am Heart J 107:497-505, 1984.

Sudhir K, MacGregor JS, Barbant SD, Foster E, Fitzgerald PJ, Chaterjee Ket al. Assessment of coronary conductance and resistance vessel reactivity in response to nitroglycerin, ergonovine, and adenosine: in vivo studies with simultaneous intravascular two-dimensional and Doppler ultrasound. J Am Coll Cardiol 1993;21:1261 - 8.

Tokai K, Watanabe H, Hirata K, Otsuka R, Muro T, Yamagishi H et al. Noninvasive assessment of myocardial ischemia in the left ventricular inferior regions by coronary flow reserve measurement using transthoracic Doppler echocardiography. J Am Soc Echocardiogr 2003;16:1252 - 7.

Topol EJ, Nissen SE. Our preoccupation with coronary luminology. The dissociation between clinical and angiographic findings in ischemic heart disease. Circulation 1995; 92: 2333–2342.

Ueno Y, Nakamura Y, Kinoshita M, Fujita T, Sakamoto T, Okamura H. Noninvasive assessment of significant right coronary artery stenosis based on coronary flow velocity reserve in the right coronary artery by transthoracic Doppler echocardiography. Echocardiography 2003;20:495 - 501.

Ueno Y, Nakamura Y, Takashima H, Kinoshita M, Soma A. Noninvasive assessment of coronary flow velocity and coronary flow velocity reserve in the right coronary artery by transthoracic Doppler echocardiography: comparison with intracoronary Doppler guidewire. J Am Soc Echocardiogr 2002;15:1074 - 9.

Verani MS. Adenosine thallium-201 myocardial perfusion scintigraphy. Am Heart J. 1991;122:269–278.

Vernon Anderson H, Stockes MJ, Leon M, Abu-Hawala SA, Stuart Y, Kireeide RL. Coronary artery flow velocity is related to lumen area and regional left ventricular mass. Circulation 2000;102:48 - 54.89.

Voci P, Pizzuto F, Romeo F. Coronary flow: a new asset for the echo lab? Eur Heart J 2004;25:1867–79.

Wilson R, Wyche K, Christensen BV, Zimmer S, Laxson DD. Effects of adenosine on human coronary arterial circulation. Circulation 1990;82: 1595 - 606.

Yoshikawa J, Yanagihara K, Owaki T, et al. Cross-sectional echocardiographic diagnosis of coronary artery aneurysms in patients with mucoucutaneous lymph node syndrome. Circulation 59:133-9, 1979.

8

3D Myocardial Contrast Echocardiography

Katsuomi Iwakura
Division of Cardiology, Sakurabashi Watanabe Hospital
Japan

1. Introduction

Early restoration of coronary perfusion is the most important objective in the management of ST-segment elevation myocardial infarction (STEMI), and primary percutaneous coronary intervention (PCI) is established as the most effective strategy for it. Advances in interventional techniques and pharmacological therapy have made it possible to achieve Thrombolysis in Myocardial Infarction (TIMI) grade 3 flow in as many as 95% of patients undergoing primary PCI. Nevertheless, optimal myocardial perfusion is not achieved in approximately 15% of patients despite of successful opening of infarct-related artery. The inadequate myocardial perfusion, or "no-reflow" phenomenon, may be caused by microvascular damage after myocardial ischemia, distal coronary emboli resulting from thrombus, platelets and atheroma, in situ thrombosis, vasospasm, or cell necrosis and regional inflammatory responses induced by reperfusion. The no-reflow phenomenon is associated with worse functional and clinical outcomes after STEMI. It was linked to larger infarction size, lower ejection fraction, ventricular arrhythmias(Aiello *et al.*,1995), early congestive heart failure(Ito *et al.*,1996), and even cardiac rupture(Morishima *et al.*,1995). It may have an adverse effect on left ventricular (LV) remodeling(Gerber *et al.*,2000). Therefore, detection of no-reflow early after primary `PCI is important for the risk stratification of patients with STEMI. Several invasive and non-invasive imaging modalities have been developed to detect no-reflow. We had focused on one of these modalities, myocardial contrast echocardiography (MCE), and used it in several clinical studies to investigate the pathogenesis of the no-reflow. In this article, we investigated the ability of newly developed, real-time 3D MCE to assess the microvascular dysfunction in patients with AMI.

2. Imaging modalities for assessment of the no-reflow phenomenon

No-reflow can be assessed during PCI with Thrombolysis In Myocardial Infarction (TIMI) flow grade(TIMI Study Group,1985), with TIMI-myocardial perfusion grade(van 't Hof *et al.*,1998) (TMPG), or with coronary flow velocity pattern assessed by Doppler guidewire(Iwakura *et al.*,1996). It can be better quantified by noninvasive imaging techniques, such as myocardial contrast echocardiography (MCE), cardiac CT, and contrast-enhanced cardiac magnetic resonance (CMR).

2.1 CMR and contrast-enhanced CT

CMR using gadolinium can diagnose the no-reflow as: 1) lack of gadolinium enhancement during first pass (microvascular obstruction); and 2) lack of gadolinium enhancement within a necrotic region, identified by late gadolinium hyperenhancement (Albert *et al.*,2006) (Ingkanisorn *et al.*,2004). There is a good correlation between gadolinium enhancement during first pass and TMPG, thus suggesting that these two parameters might reflect the microvascular integrity within the infarct zone (Porto *et al.*,2007). There is a significant correlation between area of microvascular obstruction and that of hyperenhancement on CMR (Lund *et al.*,2004). Presence of substantial microvascular obstruction on CMR also predicts LV remodeling (Gerber *et al.*,2000) (Hombach *et al.*,2005) and major adverse cardiac events (Hombach *et al.*,2005). Contrast enhanced multi-detector CT also delineates infarct zone as hyperenhancement area. Transmural hyperenhancement was observed immediately after successful PCI, and its area was correlated with non-viable area assessed by dobutamine stress echocardiography (Habis *et al.*,2007). Thus, hyperenhancement observed early after PCI on contrast enhanced CT could be associated with the no-reflow phenomenon.

2.2 Myocardial contrast echocardiography (MCE)

MCE uses ultrasonic contrast agent containing microbubbles which are strong scatters in an ultrasonic field and send compression and rarefaction waves back to the scanner. MCE has been proven useful in evaluating patients with AMI receiving reperfusion therapy. Ito et al. examined myocardial microvascular perfusion with MCE in patients with AMI, and found that some patients showed a lack of contrast enhancement (no-reflow) after successful PCI(Ito *et al.*,1992). Their finding is the first clinical report of the no-reflow phenomenon in patients with AMI. They demonstrated patients with substantial no-reflow have poor functional and clinical outcomes after AMI (Ito *et al.*,1996). They performed MCE using intracoronary injection of fragile microbubbles through catheter. The no-reflow phenomenon was also observed by MCE with intravenous administration of stable microbubbles, which is capable of passing through pulmonary circulation and into coronary microcirculation (Porter *et al.*,1998). These studies indicated that no-reflow phenomenon is observed in 25-40% of patients receiving successful primary PCI resulting into TIMI-3 flow grade. The substantial myocardial contrast defect on MCE predicts poor recovery of contractile function (Ito *et al.*,1992)(Balcells *et al.*,2003) and is associated with both death and recurrent infarction on the later stage (Dwivedi *et al.*,2007). Multicenter studies have recently demonstrated that the extent of microvascular damage, assessed on day 1 after reperfusion therapy in AMI, is the most powerful independent predictor of development of LV remodeling (Galiuto *et al.*,2008).

Accumulating study results proved the usefulness of MCE as a clinical tool for evaluating myocardial perfusion, though no contrast agent is approved for this indication currently. MCE has its pros and cons comparing to other imaging modalities such as CMR (Table 1).

	CMR	MCE
Contrast Agent	Gadomium	Microbubbles
Resolution	High Spatial Resolution	High Temporal Resolution
Image quality	Good in almost all cases	Sometimes inappropriate
Reproducibility	Excellent	Moderate
Acquisition	About 30 minutes	Real-time
Image mode	2D/3D	2D
Measurement	Area/Volume	Area
Operation	In MRI lab	Bedside / in cath-lab

Table 1. Characteritics of CMR and MCE

MCE is a very easy method not requiring a large apparatus, and it can be performed not only in the echo-lab but also in bed side or in the cath-lab. MCE is a suitable imaging modality for assessing myocardial perfusion soon after PCI. On the other hand, interpretation of MCE depends on the quality of obtained images and it could be difficult to obtain reliable images in some cases. Quantification of contrast enhancement on MCE is possible but is still difficult and requires complicated techniques. Even the subjective evaluation of myocardial perfusion is difficult in some cases because of attenuation, lung and rib shadowing, apical bubble distraction by ultrasound.

2.3 Potential of real-time 3D-MCE

3D-image reconstruction is the other advantage of CMR over MCE. Precise assessment of myocardial perfusion in a whole LV can be achieved by 3D-imaging. 2D-MCE observes myocardial opacification only on very limited slices, and assessment of contrast defect could be insufficient. Most of myocardial wall thickening is determined by contractile function of the subendocardial layer (Hashimoto *et al.*,2003), and recovery of contractility after AMI mostly depends on the viability of the subendocardial layer (Garot *et al.*,2000). Ischemic myocardial injury progress from endocardial- to epicardial layers (wavefront phenomenon), and subendocardium is the most vulnerable layer to ischemic insults (Grattan *et al.*,1986). Assessment of subendocardial perfusion is important for prediction of contratile function after AMI. 2D-MCE has only limited ability to visualize subendocardial perfusion.

3D- echocardiography visualizes the whole LV, and it is superior to 2D-echocardiography in assessment of regional wall motion abnormalities (Corsi *et al.*,2005). It also visualizes endocardial surface structure within a beating heart (Inoue *et al.*,2006). In the next chapter, we investigated whether real-time 3D-MCE could assess subendocardial perfusion in patients with AMI undergoing primary PCI , and compared its perfusion patterns to those obtained with 2D-MCE (Iwakura *et al.*,2007). We also compared the ability of these two modalities to assess infarct size and to predict functional recovery.

3. Assessment of subendocardial perfusion by real-time 3D-MCE

3.1 Study population and protocol

Between October 2004 and December 2005, consecutive 68 patients with AMI underwent primary PCI within 24 hours after symptom onset, and subsequently underwent intracoronary 2D- and 3D-MCE study. The diagnosis of AMI was based on the chest pain prolonged ≥ 30 minutes, ST segment elevation of ≥ 2 mm in at least two contiguous electrocardiograph leads, and greater than 3 fold increase in serum creatine kinase (CK) levels. Seven patients were excluded because of poor echocardiograph images, including 2 patients in whom 2D-MCE was adequate but 3D-MCE was suboptimal. We excluded 14 patients who did not undergo follow-up left ventriculography (LVG) study. Therefore, the final study population consisted of 47 patients.

After the admission, we performed echocardiography examination with SONOS 7500 (Philips Medical Systems), and defined the risk area as myocardial segments showing dyskinesia, akinesia or severe hypokinesia. After aspirin (243 mg) and intravenous heparin

(100 U/kg) administration, we performed coronary angiography (CAG) using the right femoral approach. We determined the culprit lesion and performed primary PCI to achieve the residual diameter stenosis < 25 %. After the PCI procedure, we assessed TMPG on CAG from the view chosen to minimize superimposition of non-infarcted territories(Gibson *et al.*,2000).

A mean of 15 minutes after the last PCI procedure, we performed 2D-MCE with SONOS 7500 using a S4 transducer. We made microbubbles of a mean size of 12 μm by sonicating iodinated contrast medium, Ioxagate (Hexabrix-320, Tanabe), using an ultrasonic homogenizer with a sterilized tip (Figure 1). We injected 2 mL of sonicated medium into the right coronary artery in patients with inferior wall AMI and into the left coronary artery in those with anterior or posterior wall AMI. We recorded 2D-echocardiogram from the apical two- or four-chamber view. Then, we performed real time 3D-MCE using Live 3D system without ECG gating. We observed 3D images from apical 2- or 4-chamber view with an X4 matrix array transducer on second harmonic mode. We adjusted time-gain compensation and lateral gain control carefully to obtain clear view of endocardial surface. Then, we injected microbubbles into culprit coronary artery again, and recorded a 3D-MCE image for 20 heartbeats. All MCE images were digitally stored for the further analysis.

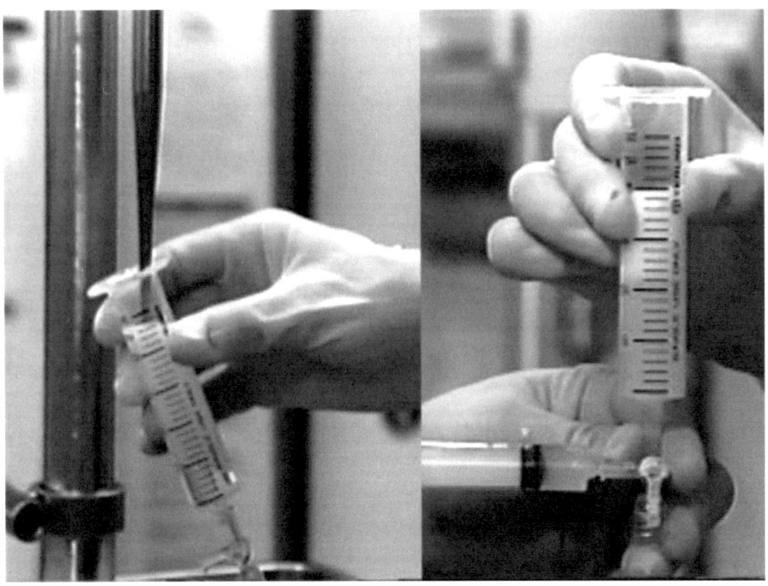

Fig. 1. Sonification of contrast medium to make microbubbles for MCE

We performed LVG in 42 patients (89.4%) following MCE study, and measured left ventricular end-diastolic and end-systolic volume index (LVEDVI and LVESVI, mL/m^2) and LV ejection fraction (LVEF, %) by the biapical Simpson's rule. Regional wall motion (RWM, SD/chord) within the culprit artery territory was analyzed using the centerline method. Follow-up coronary angiography and LVG were performed in all patients at a mean of 4.6±2.7 months later.

An experienced echocardiographer analyzed 2D-MCE images to determine myocardial perfusion within the risk area. We used the apical long-axis view or apical 4-chamber view for the patients with anterior wall AMI and posterior wall AMI and the apical 2-chamber view for the patients with inferior wall AMI. We divided LV wall into myocardial segments based on 16-segment model endorsed by American Society of Echocardiography(Cerqueira *et al.*,2002), and scored myocardial opacification in each segment as 1 (homogenous opacification), 0.5 (patchy opacification or opacification only in epicardium), or 0 (no opacification)(Ragosta *et al.*,1994). We calculated the averaged contrast score by dividing the sum of contrast scores in the segments within risk area by the number of these segments. We graded myocardial perfusion in each patient as good- (the averaged score = 1), poor- ($0.5 \leq$ score <1.0) and no-reflow (score <0.5).

A sonographer blinded to 2D-MCE data assessed subendocardial contrast opacification on end-systolic 3D-MCE images. For assessing the risk area and myocardial perfusion, we used the echo windows to include the whole risk area within 3D echocardiograph image. We observed myocardial opacification from LV cavity side. The "shade" mode was activated to reduce the effect of opacification from the epicardial layers. If necessary, some parts of the LV were cropped to obtain clear image of endocardial surface (Figure 2). Risk area was defined as myocardium showing no contraction of endocardial surface. We divided whole LV into myocardial segments corresponding to those of 16-segment model in 2D-echocardiogram(Kapetanakis *et al.*,2005), and scored endocardial opacification within each segment as 1 (enhancement as good as that within nearby normal segment), 0.5 (enhancement was observed but not as strong as that within the normal area), or 0 (no clear enhancement). We calculated the averaged endocardial contrast score in the segments within the risk area. We graded myocardial opacification in endocardium (MOE) into 3 groups; good- (the averaged score = 1), poor- ($0.5 \leq$ score <1.0) and no-MOE (score <0.5).

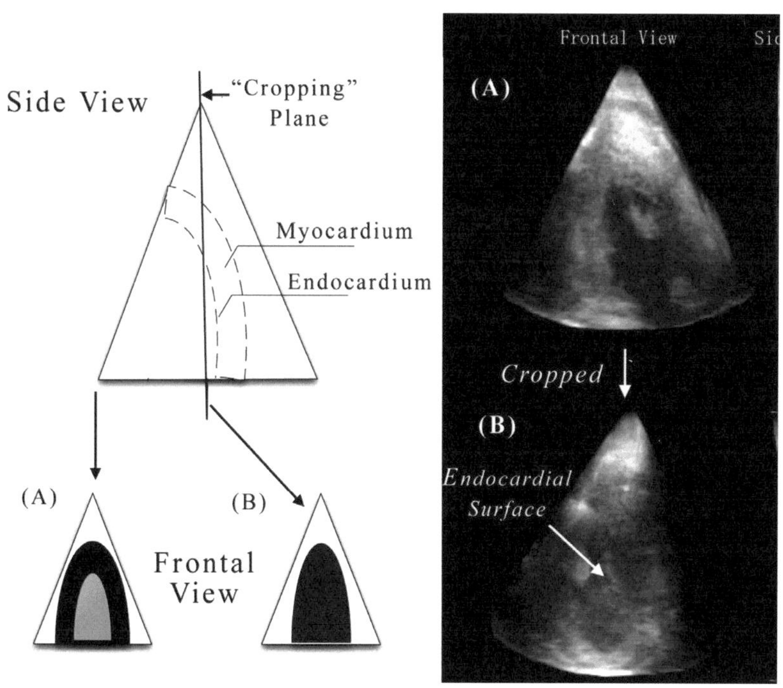

Fig. 2. Cropping of 3D-MCE images to reveal endocardial surface

All data are expressed as mean ± SD. We made comparisons by one-way ANOVA for continuous variables, and significance of difference was calculated with Tukey's HSD test for factor analysis. Categorical variables were compared with the Fisher's exact test. The differences in the changes of RWM from the initial- to the follow-up LVG study among the groups were analyzed with multivariate analysis of variance (MANOVA). Differences were considered significant at $P < 0.05$ (two-sided).

3.2 Patient characteristics

The mean age of the 47 study patients was 61±11 years (range 40 to 81 years), and 38 patients (80.9%) were male. The culprit artery was the left anterior descending artery in 28 patients, the left circumflex artery in 6 patients and the right coronary artery in 13 patients. Multivessel disease was observed in 12 patients. The mean time from the symptom onset to coronary reperfusion was 12.3 ± 14.2 hours. The peak CK and CK-MB level was 3069±2490 IU/L and 235±185 IU/L, respectively.

3.3 Representative cases of 3D-MCE

Figures 3 shows 2D- and 3D-MCE images in a patient with inferior wall AMI. 2D-MCE (upper left) showed good-reflow within the risk area (between arrows). On 3D-echocardiograph before injection, endocardial surface of area at risk was revealed through cropping (lower left). After microbubble injection, contrast enhancement was observed within the risk area, and we judged this case as good-MOE. Peak CK and CK-MB of this case were 1977 IU/L and 118 IU/L, respectively.

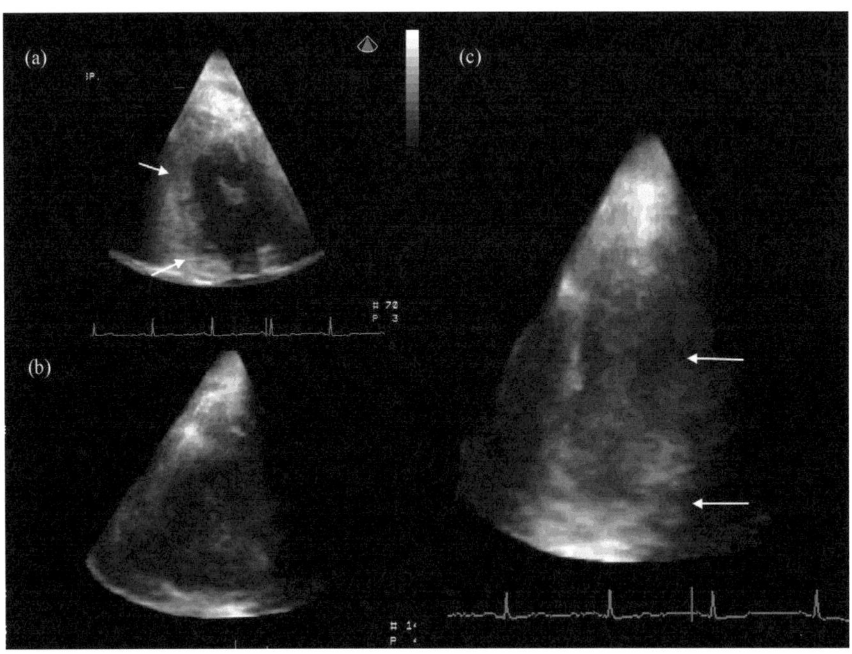

Fig. 3. A representative case showing good-reflow on 2D-MCE (a) and good-MOE on 3D-MCE (c).

Figure 4 showed MCE images in a patient with posterior wall AMI. 2D-MCE (upper left) showed good-reflow within the risk area (between arrows). 3D-MCE (right) showed almost no endocardial contrast enhancement (no-MOE) within the risk area (between arrows). A good contrast enhancement was observed in the normal myocardium around the risk are (Compare it to the 3D-image before contrast injection, on lower left). Peak CK and CK-MB of this case were 4758 IU/L and 414 IU/L, respectively.

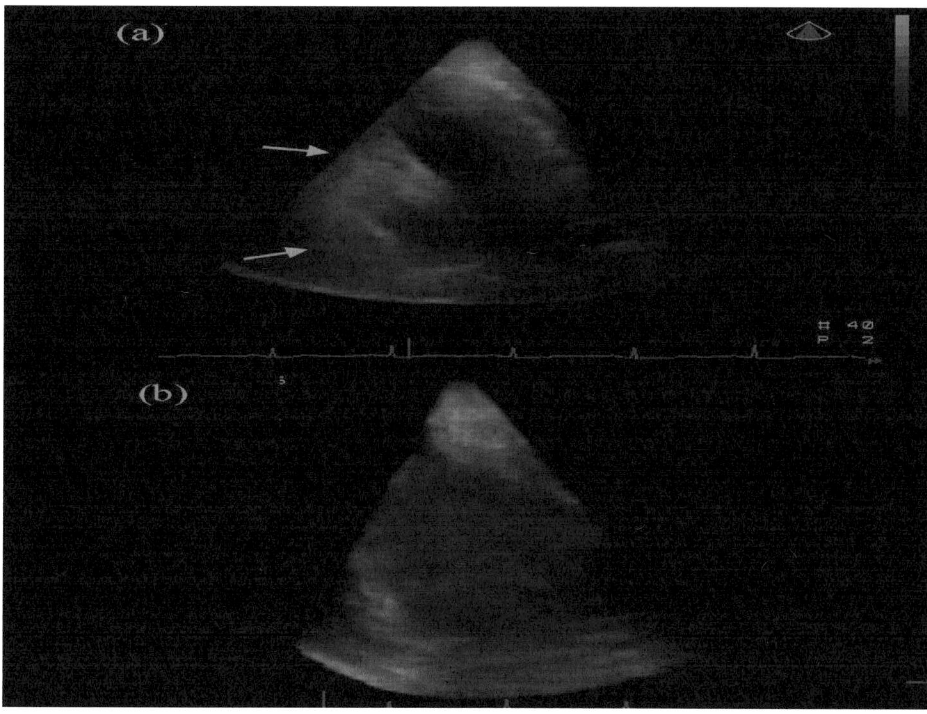

Fig. 4. A case with posterior AMI showing good-reflow on 2D-MCE (a) but no-MOE on 3D-MCE (c).

Figure 5 showed interesting images obtained in other case with anterior wall AMI. Good opacification was observed on endocardial surface of septum on 3D-MCE at 790msec after injection of microbubbles (b). Then, a jet of contrast medium was observed to flow out directly from the apical myocardium (arrow) at 2220 msec (c) and 2990 msec (d) after injection ((e) and (f) are zoomed images of (c) and (d)). These images demonstrated that endocardial hemorrhage occurred immediately after AMI. Possibly rupture of subendocardial hematoma occurred in this case (Iwakura, 2011).

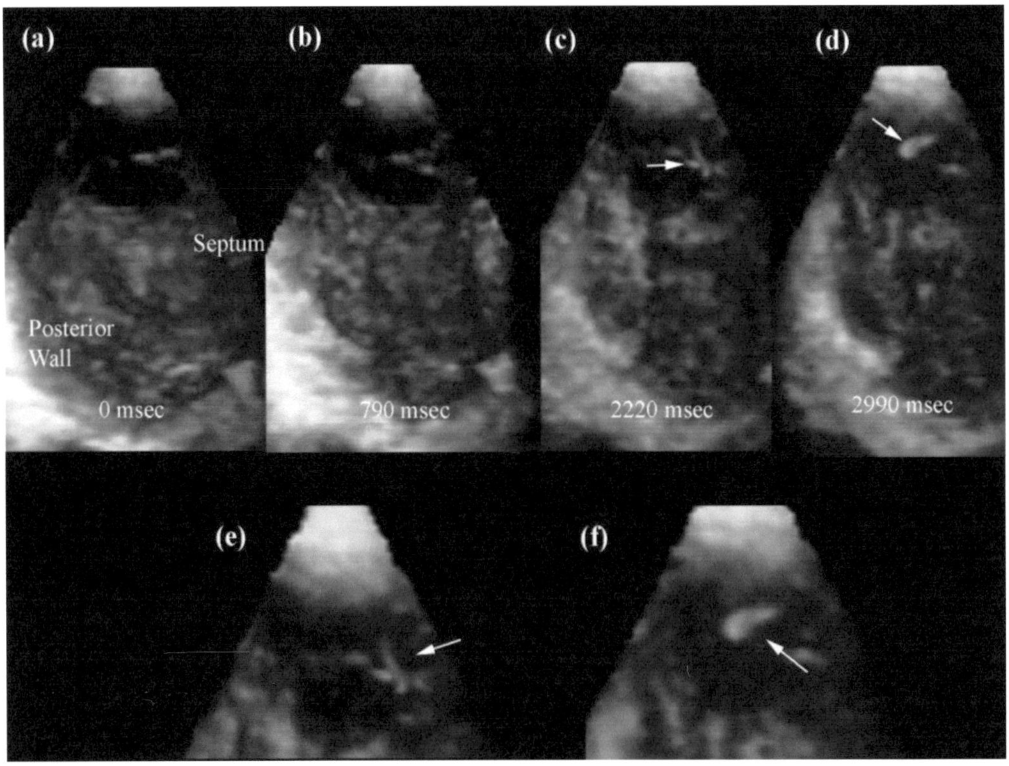

Fig. 5. Endocardial hemorrhage observed immediately after primary PCI.

3.4 Assessment of endocardial perfusion with 3D-MCE.

2D-MCE showed good-reflow in 31 out of 47 study patients (66.0%), poor-reflow in 9 patients (19.1%) and no-reflow in 7 patients (14.9%). Patient characteristics of each group were illustrated in Table 2. The incidence of anterior wall AMI was significantly higher in the no- and poor-reflow than the good-reflow (p=.01). The additional ST elevation after reperfusion was more frequently observed in the no-reflow (p=.04). There were significant differences in the incidence of the multivessel disease (p=.02) and the collateral grade (p=.03) among three subsets (Table 2).

	2D-MCE				3D-MCE			
	Good-reflow	Poor-reflow	No-reflow	P	Good-MO	Poor-MOE	No-MOE	P
Number of Patients	31	9	7		17	16	14	
Age, y	62±11	60±10	55±11	.30	63±12	63±9	55±10	.08
Gender, male/female	24/7	9/0	5/2	.25	15/2	13/3	10/4	.50
Peak CK, IU/L	2516±2186	3195±2209	5240±3040	.03	1166±1081	2796±1700	5583±2345	<.0001
Peak CK-MB, IU/L	204±185	259±166	349±177	.16	100±100	261±189	383±144	<.0001
Diabetes Mellitus, n (%)	12 (38.8)	4 (44.4)	3 (42.9)	.94	6 (35.3)	7 (43.8)	6 (42.9)	.86
Hypertension, n (%)	19 (61.3)	5 (55.6)	5 (71.4)	.81	10 (58.8)	11 (68.8)	8 (57.1)	.77
Hyperlipidemia, n (%)	16 (51.6)	6 (66.7)	2 (28.6)	.32	12 (70.6)	5 (31.3)	7 (50.0)	.08
Smoking, n (%)	22 (71.0)	8 (88.9)	6 (85.7)	.44	12 (70.6)	12 (75.0)	12 (85.7)	.60
Onset to reperfusion , h	13.0±13.1	15.1±20.9	5.9±4.9	.41	11.2±13.4	18.7±17.9	5.8±4.3	.04
Stent implantation, n (%)	29 (93.4)	9 (100)	5 (71.4)	.10	16 (94.1)	15 (93.8)	12 (85.7)	.65
Thrombectomy, n (%)	21 (67.7)	7 (77.8)	6 (85.7)	.58	12 (70.6)	11 (68.8)	11 (78.6)	.82
Anterior wall MI, n (%)	17 (54.8)	6 (66.7)	5 (71.4)	.64	11 (64.7)	7 (43.8)	10 (71.4)	.26
Multivessel disease, n	8 (25.8)	3 (33.3)	1 (14.3)	.68	4 (23.5)	5 (31.2)	3 (21.4)	.80
ST re-elevation, n (%)	11 (35.5)	1 (11.1)	5 (71.4)	.04	2 (11.8)	7 (43.8)	8 (57.1)	.02

Table 2. Clinical parameters of the study patients.

Good-MOE was observed on 3D-MCE only in 17 patients (36.2%). Poor-MOE was observed in 16 patients (34.0%) and no-MOE in 14 patients (29.8%). Among the 31 patients with good-reflow on 2D-MCE, only 14 patients (45.2 %) showed good-MOE, and 4 patients (12.9%) showed no-MOE. In contrast, all 7 patients with no-reflow on 2D-MCE showed no-MOE on 3D-MCE (Table 3).

	3D-MCE			
2D-MCE	Good-MOE, n	Poor-MOE, n	No-MOE, n	Total, n
Good-reflow, n	14	13	3	31
Poor-reflow, n	3	3	3	9
No-reflow, n	0	0	7	7
Total, n	17	16	14	47

Table 3. Distribution of myocardial perfusion grade on 2D- and 3D-MCE

Among the 31 patients with good-reflow, only 19 patients (61.3%) showed TMPG-3, and 6 patients showed TMPG-0/1 on CAG after PCI. On the other hand, 16 out of 17 patients (94.1%) with good-MOE showed TMPG-3.

3.5 Prediction of infarct size with 2D- and 3D-MCE

Among the 3 groups classified with 2D-MCE, the no-reflow had the highest peak-CK value (5240±3040 IU/L), followed by the poor-reflow (3195±2209 IU/L) and the good-reflow (2516±2186 IU/L). The differences in peak CK among three subsets were significant (p=.03), and the no-reflow had significantly higher peak CK than the good-reflow. However, the differences in peak CK between the poor-reflow and the good- or the no-reflow did not reach statistical significance (Figure 6). There were no significant differences in CK-MB values among the three subsets (p=0.16).

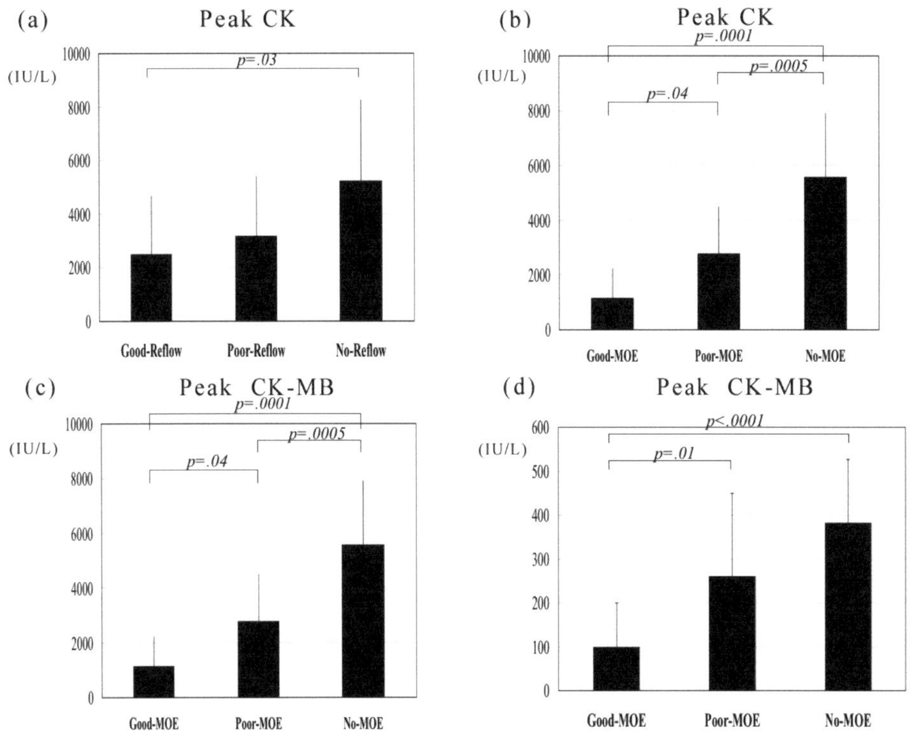

Fig. 6. Peak CK/CK-MB and myocardial perfusion grade on 2D/3D-MCE

The no-MOE on 3D-MCE also had the highest peak CK value (5583±2345 IU/L), followed by the poor-MOE (2796±1700 IU/L) and by the good –MOE (1166±1080 IU/L). The differences in peak CK were significant not only among 3 groups (p<.0001) but also in each pair of groups (Figure 6). Moreover, there were significant differences in CK-MB among 3 groups (p<.0001). The good-MOE had significantly lower CK-MB then the poor- (p=.01) or the no-MOE (p<.0001) (Figure 6). These results indicated that myocardial perfusion grade by 3D-MCE predicted infarct size more distinctively than that by 2D-MCE does.

3.6 Prediction of LV functional and morphological outcomes with 2D- and 3D-MCE

At baseline study, there was no significant difference in RWM among 3 groups based on 2D-MCE. The good-MOE had the highest RWM among 3 groups based on 3D-MCE at baseline study (good-/poor-/no-MOE = -2.28±0.91/-3.03±0.67/-2.99±0.71, p=0.02). A mean of 4.6±2.7 months later, RWM of the no-reflow (-2.84±0.83) was lower than that of the good-reflow (-1.37±1.11, p=.004). However, RWM was not statistically different between the poor-reflow (-1.73±0.71) and the good-reflow or the no-reflow (Figure 7). On the other hand, there were significant differences in RWM in each pair of the 3 groups defined by 3D-MCE (Figure 7).

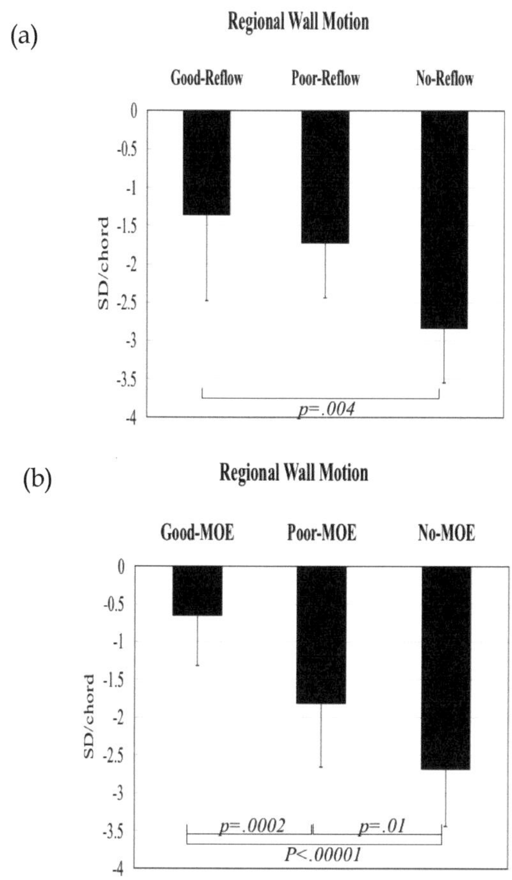

Fig. 7. RWM on the chronic stage and myocardial perfusion grade on 2D/3D-MCE

Among the 42 patients in whom initial ventriculography study was performed, the improvement of RWM from baseline to follow-up study was the highest in the good-MOE, followed by the poor-MOE and the no-MOE (1.59±0.98 vs. 1.19±0.71 vs. 0.31±0.84, p=.001). Although RWM improvement was also the highest in the good-reflow, but it showed significant overlap among 3 groups, and no significant differences were observed among them (p=0.10). These results implied that myocardial perfusion pattern assessed with 3D-MCE predicts the functional recovery more definitively than that with 2D-MCE.

There were no differences in LVEDVI and LVESVI at baseline study among 3 groups based on 2D-MCE, and there were no significant differences in LVEDVI and LVESVI among 3 groups at follow-up study. The no-reflow had significantly lower ejection fraction than the good-reflow at baseline study. At the follow-up study, the good-reflow showed higher LVEF than the no-reflow, but LVEF of the poor-reflow showed significant overlap with those of other two subsets (Figure 8). At baseline, LVEDVI was comparable among 3 groups defined by 3D-MCE. The good-MOE had smaller LVESVI than the no-MOE and better LVEF than other two groups on initial LVG. At the follow-up study, the no-MOE had larger LVEDVI than the good-MOE, and larger LVESVI and LVEF fraction than two other groups (Figure 8).

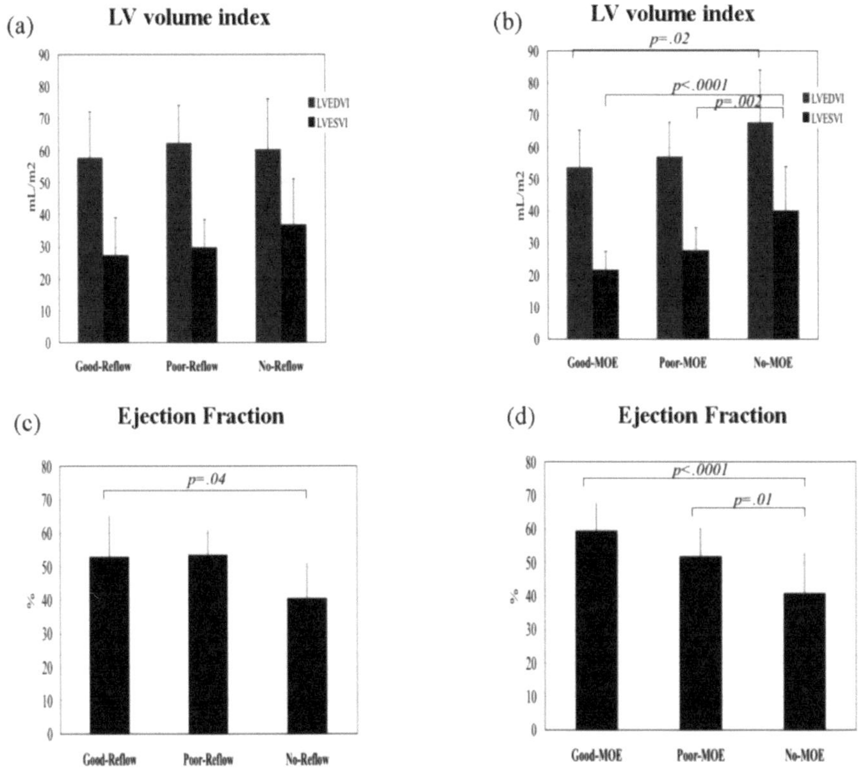

Fig. 8. LV volume index and LVEF on the chronic stage

4. 3D-MCE as a novel method for assessment of subendocardial perfusion

The present study demonstrated that subendocardial perfusion after coronary recanalization was well visualized with 3D-MCE in patients with AMI. Assessment of subendocardial perfusion with 3D-MCE predicted infarct size and discriminated patients with poor functional outcome more precisely than 2D-MCE. We used intracoronary injection of microbubbles for 3D-MCE rather than intravenous injection because intravenous injection of contrast agent would make LV filled with microbubbles, which make endocardial surface invisible.

4.1 Comparison between 2D- and 3D-MCE for detection of the no-reflow

While the no-reflow assessed by 2D-MCE is associated with poor functional recovery after AMI, the microvascular integrity does not always go along with functional recovery on the chronic stage(Galiuto *et al.*,1998). TMPG-3 on coronary angiogram is generally achieved only in less than 30% of the patients with AMI after primary PCI(Gibson *et al.*,2000)(Costantini *et al.*,2004), while good reflow is observed on 2D-MCE in about 70% of the patients(Ito *et al.*,1992)(Galiuto *et al.*,1998)(Porter *et al.*,1998). TMPG grade was far better correlated with MOE on 3D-MCE than with perfusion pattern on 2D-MCE in the present study. Thus, 2D-MCE might overestimate myocardial reperfusion and predict functional recovery excessively(Bolognese *et al.*,1996).

Myocardial perfusion patterns assessed by 3D-MCE were not necessarily coincident with those with 2D-MCE. The frequency of good-MOE on 3D-MCE was significantly lower than that of good reflow on 2D-MCE (36.2% vs. 66.0%) in the present study. Although 2D-MCE might detect subendocardial perfusion defect in some cases(Ragosta *et al.*,1994), it basically could not well assess transmural differences in myocardial perfusion(Kaul *et al.*,1992). 3D-MCE observes contrast opacification on the endocardial surface directly from the view point of LV cavity, and could assess subendocardial perfusion more precisely than 2D-MCE. Nevertheless, direct observation of subendocardial opacification has some limitations for precise subendocardial perfusion. Contrast signal from the mid-layers might contaminate the subendocardial opacification, even with adjustment of recording conditions to reduce such interference. We used sonicated contrast medium for intracoronary MCE, which contains various sized microbubbles(Ito *et al.*,1992). Large bubbles work as scatters rather than reflectors of ultrasound, and ultrasound scatter would produce false ultrasound signals in the neighboring myocardium. This interference has the potential for inhibiting the discrimination between endocardium and epicardium on 3D-MCE(Kaul *et al.*,1992).

While 2D-MCE observed myocardial perfusion only in a slice of the risk area, 3D-MCE observed spatial distribution of perfusion more widely. If the echo-plane on 2D-MCE is not placed at the center area of the infarct zone, we would observe myocardial perfusion at the marginal zone. Microvascular injury in the peripheral zone is not as severe as in the center area, and myocardial perfusion could be overestimated. The 3D-MCE image in Figure 4 showed high contrast enhancement area around the central risk area. This could be hyperemic response occurring at the marginal area. Presence of hyperemia might make 2D-MCE overestimate myocardial perfusion.

4.2 Limitation of the study

In the present study, we used real-time 3D echocardiography (Live-3D) instead of full-volume imaging. Real-time 3D acquisition is limited to an angle of about 30° - 50° degrees, and provides only a partial view of LV. To cover the complete LV, acquisition of wide-angle ('full-volume') volumetric data sets using ECG gating is required. 3D-contrast echocardiography, using intravenous contrast agents, assesses LV volumes more precisely than 2D-contrast echocardiography or 3D-echocardiography in patients with a history of myocardial infarction(Jenkins *et al.*,2009). LV volumes measured with 3D-contrast echocardiography is compatible with those measured on CMR. However, 3D-contrast echocardiography was used to delineate endocardial border clearly (LV opacification), and myocardial perfusion was not assessed in these studies. Full-volume 3D-MCE will not only assess myocardial perfusion within a complete LV, but will be able to measure myocardial volume showing microvascular dysfunction. At the time of the present study, the image-analysis software for SONOS 7500 was not suitable for observation of contrast enhancement in a full-volume image, let alone measurement of the volume of microvascular dysfunction. New software should be developed to analyze a full-volume 3D-MCE image quantitatively.

Despite of the limitation described above, real-time 3D-MCE has some advantages over full-volume imaging, including direct and easy observation of changes in endocardial structures. In one of the present study patients, we observed eruption of contrast medium from endocardial surface immediately after intracoronary injection of microbubbles. We considered this phenomenon as indicating rupture of subendocardial hematoma. In an experimental model, intramural hemorrhage is not observed early after coronary reperfusion on intracoronary 2D-MCE (Shishido *et al.*,1997). The contrast defect spread significantly with time after reperfusion in the cases developing intramural hemorrhage, but enhancement immediately after reperfusion was compatible between those with and without hemorrhage (Shishido *et al.*,1997). 2D-MCE might fail to detect small hemorrhage limited to the subendocardial layer, while 3D-MCE could detect it by direct observation of endocardial surface. Thus, real time 3D-MCE is a promising method not only to observe on endocardial perfusion but also to observe pathological events occurring endocardial surface.

The present real time 3D-MCE technique has other limitations. The spatial resolution of 3D-echocardiograhy is still inferior to that of 2D-echocardiography, which might lead to the poorer 3D-MCE image quality. We evaluated perfusion pattern and MOE only visually, because the present system does not have the objective method to measure myocardial opacification on 3D-images. The quantitative measures using replenishment curves which is available in 2D-MCE (Wei *et al.*,1998) still could not be performed in 3D-MCE. We hope that the technical progress would soon resolve these technical issues.

5. Conclusion

Newly developed, real time 3D-MCE was a feasible method to assess endocardial perfusion in patients with AMI. 3D-MCE assessed infarct size and predicted functional outcomes after AMI better than 2D-MCE did. It also observed endocardial hemorrhage occurred after PCI in one of the study patients. Thus, 3D-MCE is a promising method for assessment of microvascular function and of endocardial structural changes immediately after primary PCI for AMI.

6. References

Aiello, E.A., Jabr, R.I. & Cole, W.C. (1995) Arrhythmia and delayed recovery of cardiac action potential during reperfusion after ischemia. role of oxygen radical-induced no-reflow phenomenon. *Circ. Res.*, Vol.77, No.1, (Jul, 1995), pp. 153-162, ISBN0009-7330

Ito, H., Maruyama, A., Iwakura, K., Takiuchi, S., Masuyama, T., Hori, M., Higashino, Y., Fujii, K. & Minamino, T. (1996) Clinical implications of the 'no reflow' phenomenon. a predictor of complications and left ventricular remodeling in reperfused anterior wall myocardial infarction. *Circulation*, Vol.93, No.2, (Jan, 1996), pp. 223-228, ISBN0009-7322

Morishima, I., Sone, T., Mokuno, S., Taga, S., Shimauchi, A., Oki, Y., Kondo, J., Tsuboi, H. & Sassa, H. (1995) Clinical significance of no-reflow phenomenon observed on angiography after successful treatment of acute myocardial infarction with percutaneous transluminal coronary angioplasty. *Am. Heart J.*, Vol.130, No.2, (Aug, 1995), pp. 239-243, ISBN0002-8703

Gerber, B.L., Rochitte, C.E., Melin, J.A., McVeigh, E.R., Bluemke, D.A., Wu, K.C., Becker, L.C. & Lima, J.A. (2000) Microvascular obstruction and left ventricular remodeling early after acute myocardial infarction. *Circulation*, Vol.101, No.23, (Jun, 2000), pp. 2734-2741, ISBN1524-4539

TIMI Study Group (1985) The thrombolysis in myocardial infarction (TIMI) trial. phase i findings.. *N. Engl. J. Med.*, Vol.312, No.14, (Apr, 1985), pp. 932-936, ISBN0028-4793

van 't Hof, A.W., Liem, A., Suryapranata, H., Hoorntje, J.C., de Boer, M.J. & Zijlstra, F. (1998) Angiographic assessment of myocardial reperfusion in patients treated with primary angioplasty for acute myocardial infarction: myocardial blush grade. zwolle myocardial infarction study group. *Circulation*, Vol.97, No.23, (Jun, 1998), pp. 2302-2306, ISBN0009-7322

Iwakura, K., Ito, H., Takiuchi, S., Taniyama, Y., Nakatsuchi, Y., Negoro, S., Higashino, Y., Okamura, A., Masuyama, T., Hori, M., Fujii, K. & Minamino, T. (1996) Alternation in the coronary blood flow velocity pattern in patients with no reflow and reperfused acute myocardial infarction. *Circulation*, Vol.94, No.6, (Sep, 1996), pp. 1269-1275, ISBN0009-7322

Albert, T.S.E., Kim, R.J. & Judd, R.M. (2006) Assessment of no-reflow regions using cardiac mri. *Basic Res. Cardiol.*, Vol.101, No.5, (Sep, 2006), pp. 383-390, ISBN0300-8428

Ingkanisorn, W.P., Rhoads, K.L., Aletras, A.H., Kellman, P. & Arai, A.E. (2004) Gadolinium delayed enhancement cardiovascular magnetic resonance correlates with clinical measures of myocardial infarction. *J. Am. Coll. Cardiol.*, Vol.43, No.12, (Jun, 2004), pp. 2253-2259, ISBN0735-1097

Porto, I., Burzotta, F., Brancati, M., Trani, C., Lombardo, A., Romagnoli, E., Niccoli, G., Natale, L., Bonomo, L. & Crea, F. (2007) Relation of myocardial blush grade to microvascular perfusion and myocardial infarct size after primary or rescue percutaneous coronary intervention. *Am. J. Cardiol.*, Vol.99, No.12, (Jun, 2007), pp. 1671-1673, ISBN0002-9149

Lund, G.K., Stork, A., Saeed, M., Bansmann, M.P., Gerken, J.H., Müller, V., Mester, J., Higgins, C.B., Adam, G. & Meinertz, T. (2004) Acute myocardial infarction: evaluation with first-pass enhancement and delayed enhancement mr imaging compared with 201tl spect imaging. *Radiology*, Vol.232, No.1, (Jul, 2004), pp. 49-57, ISBN0033-8419

Hombach, V., Grebe, O., Merkle, N., Waldenmaier, S., Höher, M., Kochs, M., Wöhrle, J. & Kestler, H.A. (2005) Sequelae of acute myocardial infarction regarding cardiac structure and function and their prognostic significance as assessed by magnetic resonance imaging. *Eur. Heart J.*, Vol.26, No.6, (Mar, 2005), pp. 549-557, ISBN0195-668X

Habis, M., Capderou, A., Ghostine, S., Daoud, B., Caussin, C., Riou, J., Brenot, P., Angel, C.Y., Lancelin, B. & Paul, J. (2007) Acute myocardial infarction early viability assessment by 64-slice computed tomography immediately after coronary angiography: comparison with low-dose dobutamine echocardiography. *J. Am. Coll. Cardiol.*, Vol.49, No.11, (Mar, 2007), pp. 1178-1185, ISBN1558-3597

Ito, H., Tomooka, T., Sakai, N., Yu, H., Higashino, Y., Fujii, K., Masuyama, T., Kitabatake, A. & Minamino, T. (1992) Lack of myocardial perfusion immediately after successful thrombolysis. a predictor of poor recovery of left ventricular function in anterior myocardial infarction. *Circulation,* Vol.85, No.5, (May, 1992), pp. 1699-1705, ISBN0009-7322

Porter, T.R., Li, S., Oster, R. & Deligonul, U. (1998) The clinical implications of no reflow demonstrated with intravenous perfluorocarbon containing microbubbles following restoration of thrombolysis in myocardial infarction (TIMI) 3 flow in patients with acute myocardial infarction. *Am. J. Cardiol.,* Vol.82, No.10, (Nov, 1998), pp. 1173-1177, ISBN0002-9149

Balcells, E., Powers, E.R., Lepper, W., Belcik, T., Wei, K., Ragosta, M., Samady, H. & Lindner, J.R. (2003) Detection of myocardial viability by contrast echocardiography in acute infarction predicts recovery of resting function and contractile reserve. *J. Am. Coll. Cardiol.,* Vol.41, No.5, (Mar, 2003), pp. 827-833, ISBN0735-1097

Dwivedi, G., Janardhanan, R., Hayat, S.A., Swinburn, J.M. & Senior, R. (2007) Prognostic value of myocardial viability detected by myocardial contrast echocardiography early after acute myocardial infarction. *J. Am. Coll. Cardiol.,* Vol.50, No.4, (Jul, 2007), pp. 327-334, ISBN1558-3597

Galiuto, L., Garramone, B., Scarà, A., Rebuzzi, A.G., Crea, F., La Torre, G., Funaro, S., Madonna, M., Fedele, F., Agati, L. (2008) The extent of microvascular damage during myocardial contrast echocardiography is superior to other known indexes of post-infarct reperfusion in predicting left ventricular remodeling: results of the multicenter amici study. *J. Am. Coll. Cardiol.,* Vol.51, No.5, (Feb, 2008), pp. 552-559, ISBN1558-3597

Hashimoto, I., Li, X., Hejmadi Bhat, A., Jones, M., Zetts, A.D. & Sahn, D.J. (2003) Myocardial strain rate is a superior method for evaluation of left ventricular subendocardial function compared with tissue doppler imaging. *J. Am. Coll. Cardiol.,* Vol.42, No.9, (Nov, 2003), pp. 1574-1583, ISBN0735-1097

Garot, J., Bluemke, D.A., Osman, N.F., Rochitte, C.E., Zerhouni, E.A., Prince, J.L. & Lima, J.A. (2000) Transmural contractile reserve after reperfused myocardial infarction in dogs. *J. Am. Coll. Cardiol.,* Vol.36, No.7, (Dec, 2000), pp. 2339-2346, ISBN0735-1097

Grattan, M.T., Hanley, F.L., Stevens, M.B. & Hoffman, J.I. (1986) Transmural coronary flow reserve patterns in dogs. *Am. J. Physiol.,* Vol.250, No.2 Pt 2, (Feb, 1986), p. H276-83, ISBN0002-9513

Corsi, C., Lang, R.M., Veronesi, F., Weinert, L., Caiani, E.G., MacEneaney, P., Lamberti, C. & Mor-Avi, V. (2005) Volumetric quantification of global and regional left ventricular function from real-time three-dimensional echocardiographic images. *Circulation,* Vol.112, No.8, (Aug, 2005), pp. 1161-1170, ISBN1524-4539

Inoue, K., Ito, H., Iwakura, K., Kawano, S., Okamura, A., Kurotobi, T., Date, M., Otsu, K., Hori, M. & Fujii, K. (2006) Usefulness of high-resolution real-time three-dimensional echocardiography to visualize the left ventricular endocardial surface in myocardial infarction. *Am. J. Cardiol.,* Vol.97, No.11, (Jun, 2006), pp. 1578-1581, ISBN0002-9149

Iwakura, K., Ito, H., Okamura, A., Kurotobi, T., Koyama, Y., Date, M., Inoue, K., Nagai, H., Imai, M., Arita, Y., Toyoshima, Y., Ozawa, M. & Fujii, K. (2007) Comparison of two-versus three-dimensional myocardial contrast echocardiography for assessing subendocardial perfusion abnormality after percutaneous coronary intervention in patients with acute myocardial infarction. *Am. J. Cardiol.*, Vol.100, No.10, (Nov, 2007), pp. 1502-1510, ISBN0002-9149

Gibson, C.M., Cannon, C.P., Murphy, S.A., Ryan, K.A., Mesley, R., Marble, S.J., McCabe, C.H., Van De Werf, F. & Braunwald, E. (2000) Relationship of timi myocardial perfusion grade to mortality after administration of thrombolytic drugs. *Circulation*, Vol.101, No.2, (Jan, 2000), pp. 125-130, ISBN1524-4539

Iwakura, K (2011) . Visualization of Myocardial Hemorrhage with Real Time Three-Dimensional Myocardial Contrast Echocardiography in Patients with Acute Myocardial Infarction. *J Echocardiogr, in press*

[Cerqueira2002] Standardized myocardial segmentation and nomenclature for tomographic imaging of the heart: a statement for healthcare professionals from the cardiac imaging committee of the council on clinical cardiology of the american heart association. . 2002.

Ragosta, M., Camarano, G., Kaul, S., Powers, E.R., Sarembock, I.J. & Gimple, L.W. (1994) Microvascular integrity indicates myocellular viability in patients with recent myocardial infarction. new insights using myocardial contrast echocardiography. *Circulation*, Vol.89, No.6, (Jun, 1994), pp. 2562-2569, ISBN0009-7322

Kapetanakis, S., Kearney, M.T., Siva, A., Gall, N., Cooklin, M. & Monaghan, M.J. (2005) Real-time three-dimensional echocardiography: a novel technique to quantify global left ventricular mechanical dyssynchrony. *Circulation*, Vol.112, No.7, (Aug, 2005), pp. 992-1000, ISBN1524-4539

Galiuto, L. & Iliceto, S. (1998) Myocardial contrast echocardiography in the evaluation of viable myocardium after acute myocardial infarction. *Am. J. Cardiol.*, Vol.81, No.12A, (Jun, 1998), p. 29G-32G, ISBN0002-9149

Costantini, C.O., Stone, G.W., Mehran, R., Aymong, E., Grines, C.L., Cox, D.A., Stuckey, T., Turco, M., Gersh, B.J., Tcheng, J.E., Garcia, E., Griffin, J.J., Guagliumi, G., Leon, M.B. & Lansky, A.J. (2004) Frequency, correlates, and clinical implications of myocardial perfusion after primary angioplasty and stenting, with and without glycoprotein iib/iiia inhibition, in acute myocardial infarction. *J. Am. Coll. Cardiol.*, Vol.44, No.2, (Jul, 2004), pp. 305-312, ISBN0735-1097

Bolognese, L., Antoniucci, D., Rovai, D., Buonamici, P., Cerisano, G., Santoro, G.M., Marini, C., L'Abbate, A. & Fazzini, P.F. (1996) Myocardial contrast echocardiography versus dobutamine echocardiography for predicting functional recovery after acute myocardial infarction treated with primary coronary angioplasty. *J. Am. Coll. Cardiol.*, Vol.28, No.7, (Dec, 1996), pp. 1677-1683, ISBN0735-1097

Kaul, S., Jayaweera, A.R., Glasheen, W.P., Villanueva, F.S., Gutgesell, H.P. & Spotnitz, W.D. (1992) Myocardial contrast echocardiography and the transmural distribution of flow: a critical appraisal during myocardial ischemia not associated with infarction. *J. Am. Coll. Cardiol.*, Vol.20, No.4, (Oct, 1992), pp. 1005-1016, ISBN0735-1097

Jenkins, C., Moir, S., Chan, J., Rakhit, D., Haluska, B. & Marwick, T.H. (2009) Left ventricular volume measurement with echocardiography: a comparison of left ventricular opacification, three-dimensional echocardiography, or both with magnetic resonance imaging. *Eur. Heart J.*, Vol.30, No.1, (Jan, 2009), pp. 98-106, ISBN1522-9645

Shishido, T., Beppu, S., Matsuda, H., Yutani, C. & Miyatake, K. (1997) Extension of hemorrhage after reperfusion of occluded coronary artery: contrast echocardiographic assessment in dogs. *J. Am. Coll. Cardiol.*, Vol.30, No.2, (Aug, 1997), pp. 585-591, ISBN0735-1097

Wei, K., Jayaweera, A.R., Firoozan, S., Linka, A., Skyba, D.M. & Kaul, S. (1998) Quantification of myocardial blood flow with ultrasound-induced destruction of microbubbles administered as a constant venous infusion. *Circulation*, Vol.97, No.5, (Feb, 1998), pp. 473-483, ISBN0009-7322

Part 3

Fetal Imagine Techniques

9

Fetal Echocardiography

Ahmet Cantug Caliskan
Samsun Education and Training Hospital Department of Obstetrics and Gynecology Samsun Turkey

1. Introduction

This is a test using sound waves to show the structure of an unborn baby's heart. An obstetrician may get a limited view of a baby's heart during a routine pregnancy ultrasound. However, a specialist in fetal echocardiography can study a baby's heart in great detail using a fetal echocardiogram.Some pregnant women are at higher risk of giving birth to a baby with a heart defect. They should be considered for referral for a specialized fetal echocardiogram. The ultrasound scanning may be done through the vagina or through the abdomen. There are no known risks to the mother or fetus.

Congenital heart disease is the most common birth defect, occurring at a rate of 8/1,000 births.Because there are many different types of heart defects, ranging from minor to life-threatening problems, examination of the fetal heart before birth has been mandated as a requirement when examining a fetus between 15 and 40 weeks of pregnancy. This has been called the Standard ultrasound evaluation of the heart and has been defined by the American College of Obstetricians and Gynecologists, the American Institute of Ultrasound in Medicine, and the American College of Radiology.In Los Angeles it has been estimated that less than 10% of serious heart defects are detected before birth when the examination is performed by an obstetrician or radiologist who does not have special training evaluating the fetal heart. Fetal Echocardiography is a more comprehensive examination of the fetal heart than the standard examination and includes identification of additional cardiac structures not defined in the standard evaluation. The physician who performs Fetal Echocardiography often uses color Doppler ultrasound and may utilize pulsed Doppler, 3D, and 4D ultrasound; depending upon the circumstances of the examination. Fetal Echocardiography is an important part of Genetic Ultrasound, a new test that identifies over 95% of fetuses with Down syndrome when performed during the second-trimester of pregnancy.

Fetal echocardiography is the primary diagnostic tool used to assess fetal cardiac structure and function.This is a specialized sonogram that is a certainly indicated when there is an increased risk of fetal cardiac abnormalites,and is usually performed at 18-22 weeks gestation.when the risk of a fetal cardiac anomaly is particularly high, an earlier evaluation,at around 13-15 weeks, by either transabdominal or vaginal sonography, may be considered, as many caardiac anomalies are already demonstrable at this stage.this early examination should, however, be corroborated by a repeat evaluation around mid-gestation.

A complete fetal echocardiographic examination should incorporate the following Standard views:a demonstration of the visceral and cardiac situs,a four chamber view,ventriculoarterial connections, and course of the great arteries.Real-time examination of cardiac structures is enhanced by the use of color Doppler.

A baby's heart begins to develop at conception, but is completely formed by eight weeks into the pregnancy. Congenital heart defects happen during this crucial first eight weeks of the baby's development. Specific steps must take place in order for the heart to form correctly.

2. Indications for fetal echocardiography

2.1 Maternal indications fetal indications

- Family history of CHD
- Abnormal obstetrical ultrasound screen
- Metabolic disorders (eg,diabetes, PKU)
- Extracardiac abnormality
- Exposure to teratogens
- Chromosomal abnormality
- Exposure to prostaglandin synthetase inhibitors (eg,ibuprofen, salicylic acid, indomethacin)
- Arrhythmia
- Rubella infection
- Hydrops
- Autoimmune disease (eg,SLE, Sjogren's)
- Increased first trimester nuchal translucency
- Familial inherited disorders (Ellisvan Creveld, Marfan, Noonan's, etc)
- Multiple gestation and suspicion of twin-twin transfusion syndrome
- In vitro fertilization CHD, Congenital heart disease; PKU, phenyl ketonuria; SLE, sytemic lupus erythematosus.

While there are risk factors for congenital heart defects, over 90% of heart malformations have no known cause. For this reason researchers have classified most heart defects as multifactorial, meaning that there is no known explanation for the problem other than the possible interaction between hereditary and environmental factors. For this reason, many physicians have suggested examining all fetuses for heart defects, since most defects arise from pregnancies with no risk factors. The following lists factors associated with an increased risk for congenital heart defects. If any of these are present, the patient should be referred for Fetal Echocardiography at 18 to 24 weeks of gestation. In some cases the patient may desire first-trimester

- Fetal Echocardiography performed between 12 and 14 weeks of gestation.
- Maternal Drug Exposure and Diseases Women with seizure disorders taking anti-convulsants
- Women taking lithium for depression
- Women taking insulin for diabetes
- Women who have phenylketonuria

- Women exposed to Rubella
- Family History of Congenital Heart Disease
- Previous child with CHD, new risk is 1 in 20 to 1 in 100
- Previous two children with CHD, new risk is 1 in 10 to 1 in 20
- Mother has CHD, new risk is as high as 1 in 5 to 1 in 20
- Father has CHD, new risk 1 in 30
- Increased Maternal Risk for Down Syndrome and Other Chromosomal Defects
- Advanced maternal age (>35)
- Abnormal maternal serum screening increasing risk for Downy syndrome or Trisomy 18
- Chromosome abnormalities and CHD
- Down syndrome
- Trisomy 18 and Trisomy 13
- Turner's syndrome
- Cri du chat syndrome
- Wolf-Hirshhorn syndrome
- DiGeorge syndrome (deletion 22q11)
- Other Rare Genetic Diseases
- Marfan syndrome
- Smith-Lemli-Opitz syndrome
- Ellis-van Creveld
- Holt-Oram syndrome
- Noonan syndrome
- Mucopolysaccharidoses
- Goldenhar syndrome (hemifacial microsomia)
- William's syndrome
- VACTERL association (tracheal and esophageal malformations associated with vertebral, anorectal,
- cardiac, renal, radial, and limb abnormalities).
- Ultrasound -Identified Fetal Birth Defects of the Current Pregnancy

When a birth defect is detected during an ultrasound examination, there is a higher risk for an associated defect of the fetal heart. Therefore, a fetal echocardiogram should be performed.

2.2 Cardiovascular anatomy and fetal circulation

After birth the circulation is divided into two separate sides that are not connected. The left side of the heart consists of the pulmonary veins, left atrium, left ventricle, and aorta. The right side of the heart consists of the superior and inferior vena cava, the right atrium, the right ventricle, and the pulmonary artery. These two circulations are independent of each other and do not connect.

However, the fetal circulation is different. The right and left sides of the heart connect at the level of the foramen ovale and the ductus arteriosus. Because of these connections fetuses can develop serious heart defects and live while in the uterus, only to be severely compromised or die because of the circulatory changes that occur following birth. To understand the effect of certain types of heart defects it is therefore important to review fetal circulation.

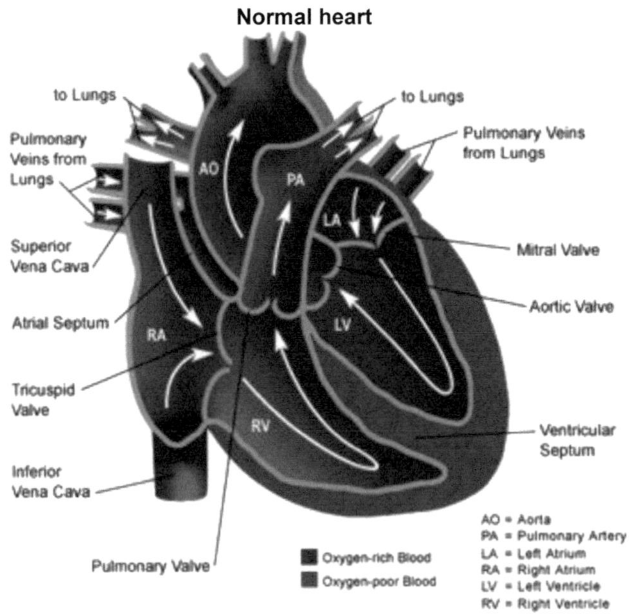

Fig. 1. Right Side of the Heart

1. Blood from the placenta returns to the fetus by the umbilical vein.The umbilical vein enters the fetal abdomen where blood continues through the intra-abdominal portion of this vessel.
2. Once inside the abdomen blood flows through the ductus venosus and is directed into the right atrial chamber. Because this blood has been enriched with oxygen and nutrients that it has picked up from the placenta, it is directed primarily through the foramen ovale into the left atrium. The foramen ovale is a small hole in the wall that separates the right and left atrial chambers. There is some mixing of blood within the right atrium.
3. The majority of blood enters the right atrium from the superior and inferior vena cava, as well as some blood from the ductus venosus (see above). The superior vena cava brings blood back from the head and upper extremities to the heart while blood from the inferior vena cava brings it back to the heart from the remainder of the body.
4. Blood is pumped from the right atrium into the right ventricle.
5. Blood from the right ventricle is pumped through the pulmonary valve into the main pulmonary artery. From here it is distributed to the lungs and to the ductus arteriosus.
6. The ductus arteriosus distributed blood to the entire body (excluding the head and upper extremities) as well as returns blood back to the placenta through the two umbilical arteries.

Left Side of the Heart

1. Blood from the placenta returns to the fetus by the umbilical vein. The umbilical vein enters the fetal abdomen where blood continues through the intra-abdominal portion of this vessel.
2. Once inside the abdomen blood flows through the ductus venosus and is directed into the right atrial chamber.Because this blood has been enriched with oxygen and nutrients that it has picked up from the placenta, it is directed through the foramen ovale into the left atrium.The foramen ovale is a small hole in the wall that separates the right and left atrial chambers
3. Once inside the left atrium the blood mixes with blood returning from the lungs and then enters the left ventricle.
4. Blood from the left ventricle is pumped into the aorta, which distributes blood to the brain and upper extremities.

Ultrasound examination of the fetal heart was first reported in the early 1980's when 2D technology allowed the examiner to identify the four-chambers of the fetal heart.Although the value of prenatal detection of heart defects was appreciated in a theoretical sense, it has only recently been realized as a benefit. The reason for this is that the ability to detect heart defects by the physician and/or sonographer has improved as the result of training and experience COLOR DOPPLER examination of the Heart Color Doppler ultrasound is a technique that enables the physician to identify the direction and speed of blood flow within a vessel or heart chamber. Color Doppler is not part of the Standard Examination of the heart, but is used by a specialist with special training in fetal echocardiography.

The use of color Doppler ultrasound for evaluation of the fetal heart and detection of birth defects was first reported by Dr. DeVore in 1987. Since this first publication over 200 articles have been published in the medical literature describing the use of this technology for evaluating the fetal heart. Color Doppler displays the flow of blood based upon its direction of flow; red-orange towards to top of the transducer, blue away from the transducer.

The transducer is always located at the top of the image. Therefore, when blood flow is towards the transducer it is depicted in red, and away from the transducer in blue. The different hues of red-orange and blue-green indicate the different velocities or speed that blood is flowing. For example, if the color Doppler display is yellow then it is flowing towards the transducer faster than if it is deep red.

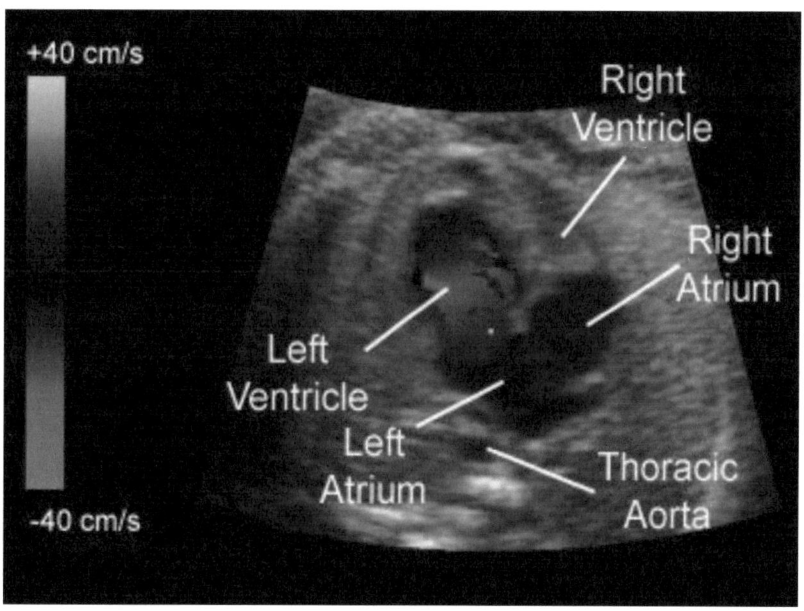

Fig. 2. This illustrates the use of color Doppler to identify the flow of blood into the ventricles.

3. Doppler waveforms analyzed

Measurement of the Doppler waveforms is compared to the age of the fetus. The following graphs illustrate the normal distribution of measurements for the waveforms recorded from the fetal heart.

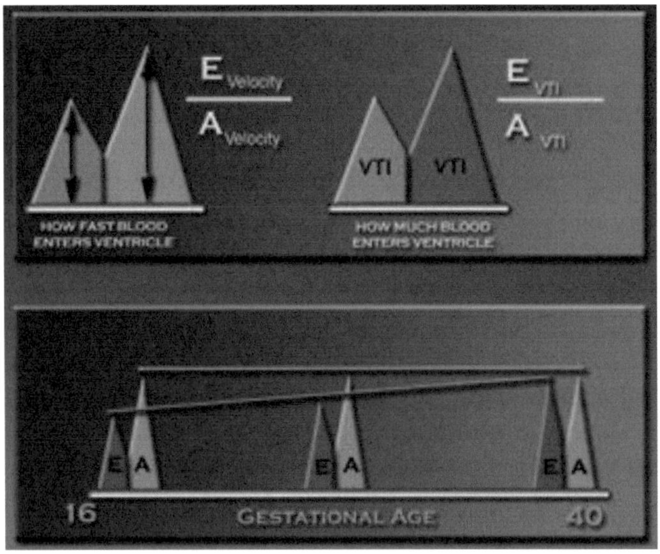

Fig. 3. This illustrates changes in the E and A waves as a function of the age of the fetus. As the fetus ages, the E wave form increases in height, representing an increase in speed as blood enters the ventricular chambers during the early filling phase of diastole. However, the A wave form does not increase in speed as the fetus ages. This suggests that the speed of blood resulting from atrial contraction remains unchanged, irrespective of the age of the fetus.

3.1 E/A ratio

This is a measurement of the compliance or stiffness of the ventricles as blood enters the chamber during diastole. In certain fetal conditions the measurement of this ratio may be altered.

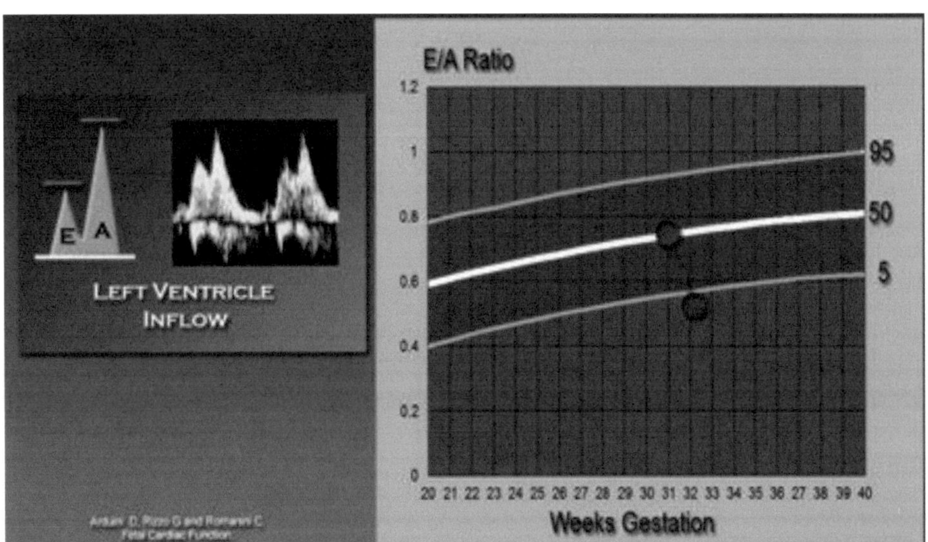

Fig. 4.

3.2 Peak velocity

This measures the speed at which blood is ejected from the ventricles. When the heart is not functioning properly,then the peak velocity may decrease.

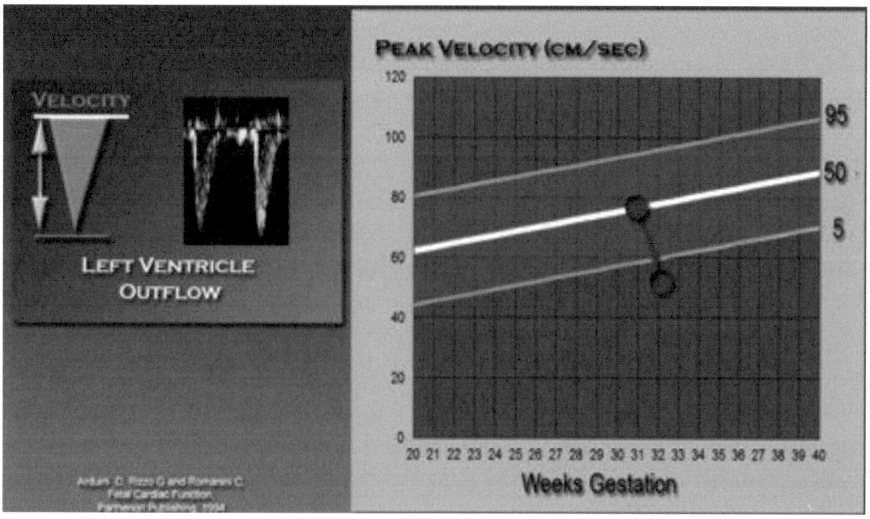

Fig. 5. This illustrates the normal range for the peak velocity of the aorta. If this decreases, this suggests cardiac dysfunction.

3.3 Time-to-peak velocity

This is a measure of how much resistance there is to blood as it is being pumped out of the ventricle. If the value increases, this means there is less resistance than normal. If it decreases, this means that there is more resistance to blood flow. This is often observed in fetuses with abnormal growth in which the fetus is smaller than normal.

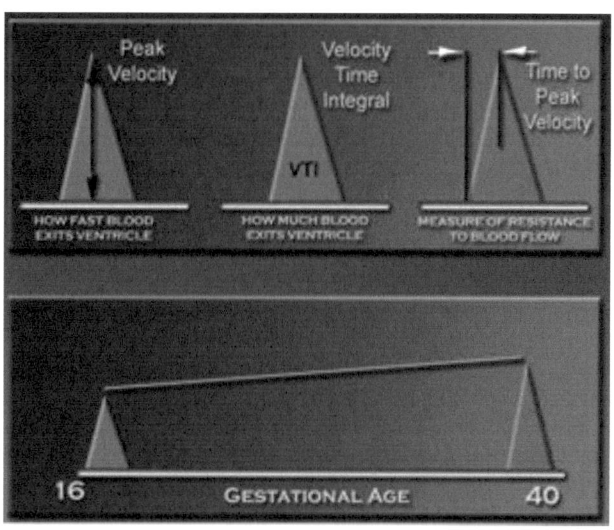

Fig. 6.

3.4 Pulsed doppler ultrasound examination of the heart

Pulsed Doppler ultrasound consists of displaying the blood flow patterns in a waveform. The pulsed Doppler enables the physician to record different flow patterns during the cardiac cycle from specific parts of the heart. From these waveforms measurements can be made to assist the physician in the interpretation of blood flow into and out of the heart.

3.4.1 Pulsed doppler relate to the electrocardiogram

The electrocardiogram, also known as an EKG, is a recording of the electrical activity of the heart during the cardiac cycle. To understand the pulsed Doppler waveform recorded from the heart researchers have compared it to the EKG.

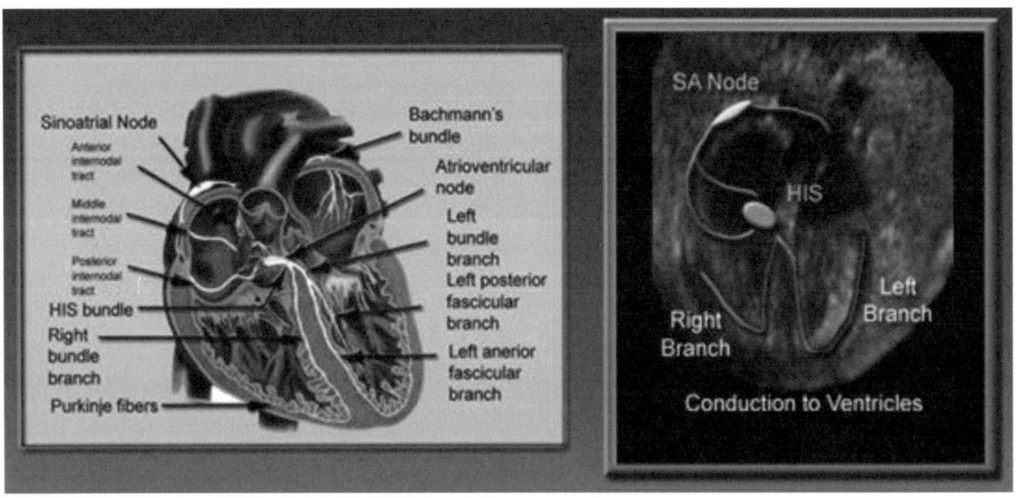

Fig. 7. This illustrates the electrical conduction of the heart.
The electrical signal originates in the SA Node located near the right atrium. It is first sent the atrial walls, resulting in contraction of the atrial chambers. The signal then is transmitted to the AV Node (green) to the ventricles. When this occurs the ventricles contract.

3.4.2 Doppler waveforms different when recorded from the right and left sides of the heart

Yes, the waveforms are different. For example, when the pulsed Doppler is recorded from the left ventricle the diastolic and systolic waveforms can be recorded at the same time. The reason for this is because the mitral and aortic valves are next to each other. However, these valves are not close together for the right ventricle and the waveforms must be recorded separately from different locations within the heart.

This compares the pulsed Doppler waveforms recorded from within the left and right ventricles (inflow) and the pulmonary and aortic outflow tracts (outflow). The waveforms from the inflow tracts are different because the left ventricle displays two waveforms. This is because the mitral and aortic valves are adjacent to each other, resulting in both waveforms being recorded simultaneously.

However, the aortic waveform within the left ventricle represents the flow exiting the left ventricle before it exits through the aortic valve.

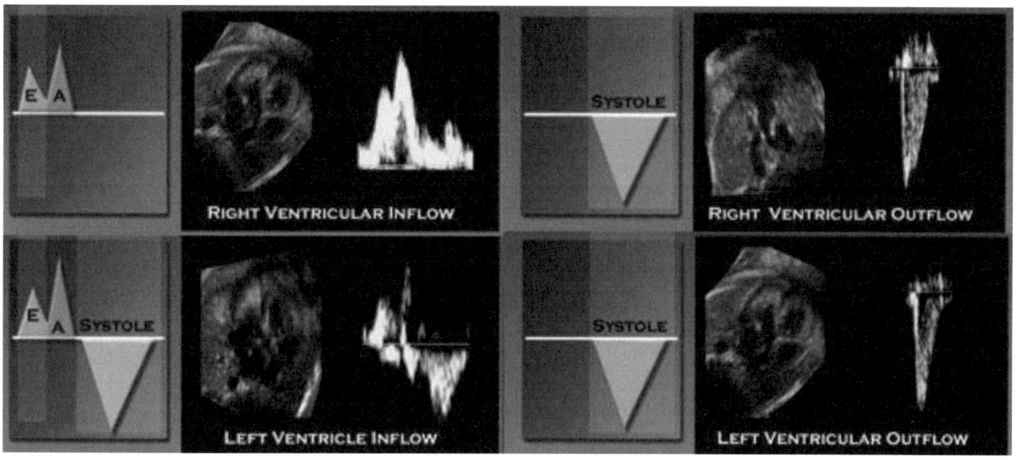

Fig. 8.

3.5 Equipment

Ultrasound systems used for fetal echocardiography should have capabilities for performing 2-dimensional,M-mode, and Doppler imaging.The requirements of fetal echocardiography are more stringent than for an infant or child with congenital or acquired heart disease .This is due to the increased demands for both spatial and temporal resolution.Anatomic surveys require axial resolution of 1mm or less and thiss is particularly important given the small size of critical fetal cardiac structures.Frames rates of 80to 100 Hz are frequentlyneeded to view important events occuring at heart rates in excess of 140 beats per minute.TO meet these requirements,imaging systems need to be optimally configured.In general,system settings are adjusted to minimize persistence and spatial averaging and to increase frame rate.All modalites of Doppler including color, pulse, high pulse repetition frequency, and continuous wave should be available.Tissue Doppler imaging has been recently applied in the assessment of fetal arrhythmania.Harmonic imaging is useful when acoustic penetration is diffucult such as in the presence of maternel obesty.Phased array transducers with fundamental frequencies between 4 and 12MHz are geberally used.Curvilinear ear probes may be helpful given the wider near-field of wiev.High frequency transducers with a narrower footprint commonly used in echocardiography of infants may also be helpful.

3.6 Examination technique

Although the goal is to achieve visualization of each of the essential components,not all will be visualized in every fetus at every examination.Fetal position in the uterus or increased activity may limit the ability to ontain visualization of each of the components.The number of vessels in the umblical cord is counted and Doppler sampling of the umblical artery and umblical vein is performed.After establishing the position of the fetus and the right/left and anterior/posterior orientation, and initial survey of the fetus is used to estimate the gestational age and to establish abdominal situs and cardiac position.The presence or absence of fluid in the pericardial,pleural, or peritoneal space should be noted.The position of the inferior vena cava and descending aorta at the level of of the diaphragm are established.Multiple scanning positions and sweeps are necessary to adequately image the fetal heart.Suggested views are described below with a brief explanation of how to achieve the view an the structures generally well seen.Reference sources are available, which illustrate these views in detail.The authors recognize that based on operator style, alternative or additional sweeps and views may be utilized to image the various structures of the fetal heart and still accomplish a comprehensive fetal echocardiogram.

3.7 Essential components of the fetal echocardiogram

3.7.1 Feature essential component

- Anatomic overview Fetal number and position in the uterus
- Establish stomach position and abdominal situs
- Establish cardiac position
- Biometric examination Cardiothoracic ratio
- Biparietal diameter
- Femur length
- Cardiac imaging views/sweeps Four-chamber view
- Four-chamber view angled towards great arteries ("Five-chamber" view)
- Long-axis view (left ventricular outflow)
- Long-axis view (right ventricular outflow)
- Short-axis sweep (cephalad angling includes "3 vessel"view
- Caval long-axis view
- Ductal arch view
- Aortic arch view
- Doppler examination Inferior and superior vena cava
- Pulmonary veins
- Hepatic veins
- Ductus venosus
- Foramen ovale
- Atrioventricular valves
- Semilunar valves
- Ductus arteriosus
- Transverse aortic arch
- Umbilical artery
- Umbilical vein
- Measurement data Atrioventricular valve diameter
- Semilunar valve diameter
- Main pulmonary artery
- Ascending aorta
- Branch pulmonary arteries
- Transverse aortic arch
- Ventricular length
- Ventricular short-axis dimensions
- Examination of rhythm and rate M-mode of atrial and ventricular wall motion
- Dopplerexamination of atrial and ventricular flow patterns

Structures viewed in the 4- and 5- chamber view

- Atrial and ventricular size
- Atrial and ventricular septae
- Atrioventricular size and function
- Coronary sinus
- Ventricular function in long axis
- Semilunar valve function (may not, however, be optimal to differentiate aorta from main pulmonary artery)
- Pulmonary veins

Structures viewed in the cardiac short-axis sweep

- Pulmonary venous return
- Inferior vena cava and hepatic veins
- Ventricular short-axis dimensions
- Ventricular-arterial relationship
- Right ventricular outflow tract
- Branch pulmonary arteries and origin
- Caval connections
- Innominate vein
- Ductus arteriosus
- Determination of arch sidedness and branching

Structures viewed in the cardiac long-axis sweep

- Superior and inferior vena cava
- Left ventricular outflow tract
- Ascending aorta
- Great vessel connection and size
- Ductus arteriosus and proximal ductal arch

Structures viewed in the caval long-axis view

- Superior vena cava
- Inferior vena cava and eustachian valve
- Patent foramen ovale
- Right pulmonary artery

Structures viewed in the ductal and aortic arch views

- Main pulmonary artery
- Branch pulmonary arteries
- Patent ductus arteriosus and direction of flow
- Aortic arch dimension (ascending, transverse, isthmus, and descending)
- Direction of flow in the aortic arch

Journal of the American Society of Echocardiography

808 Pediatric Council of the American Society of Echocardiography July 2004

4. Coarctation of aorta

The narrowed segment called coarctation can occur anywhere in the aorta, but is most likely to happen in the segment just after the aortic arch. This narrowing restricts the amount of oxygen-rich (red) blood that can travel to the lower part of the body. Varying degrees of narrowing can occur.

The more severe the narrowing, the more symptomatic a child will be, and the earlier the problem will be noticed. In some cases, coarctation is noted in infancy. In others, however, it may not be noted until school-age or adolescence. Seventy-five percent of children with coarctation of the aorta also have a bicuspid aortic valve - a valve that has two leaflets instead of the usual three. Coarctation of the aorta occurs in about 8 percent to 11 percent of all children with congenital heart disease. Boys have the defect twice as often as girls do.

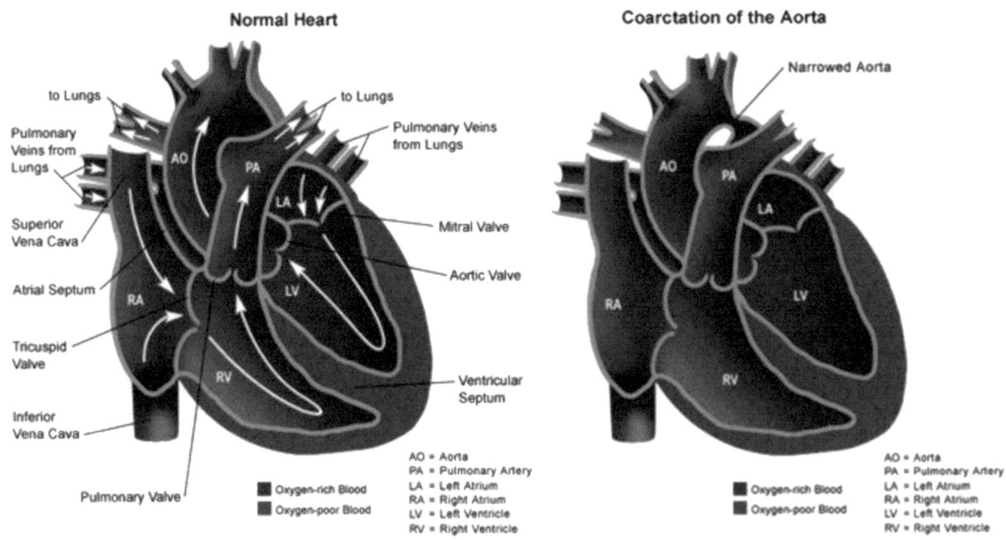

Fig. 9.

5. Hypoplastic left heart syndrome

Hypoplastic left heart syndrome (HLHS) is a combination of several abnormalities of the heart and great blood vessels. It is a congenital (present at birth) syndrome, meaning that the heart defects occur due to abnormal underdevelopment of sections of the fetal heart during the first 8 weeks of pregnancy. In the normal heart, oxygen-poor (blue) blood returns to the right atrium from the body, travels to the right ventricle, then is pumped through the pulmonary artery into the lungs where it receives oxygen. Oxygen-rich (red) blood returns to the left atrium from the lungs, passes into the left ventricle, and then is pumped out to the body through the aorta.

6. Transposition of the great arteries

In transposition of the great arteries, the aorta is connected to the right ventricle, and the pulmonary artery is connected to the left ventricle - the exact opposite of a normal heart's anatomy. Oxygen-poor (blue) blood returns to the right atrium from the body, passes through the right atrium and ventricle, then goes into the misconnected aorta back to the body. Oxygen-rich (red) blood returns to the left atrium from the lungs, passes through the left atrium and ventricle, then goes into the pulmonary artery and back to the lungs. Two separate circuits are formed - one that circulates oxygen-poor (blue) blood from the body back to the body, and another that recirculates oxygen-rich (red) blood from the lungs back to the lungs.

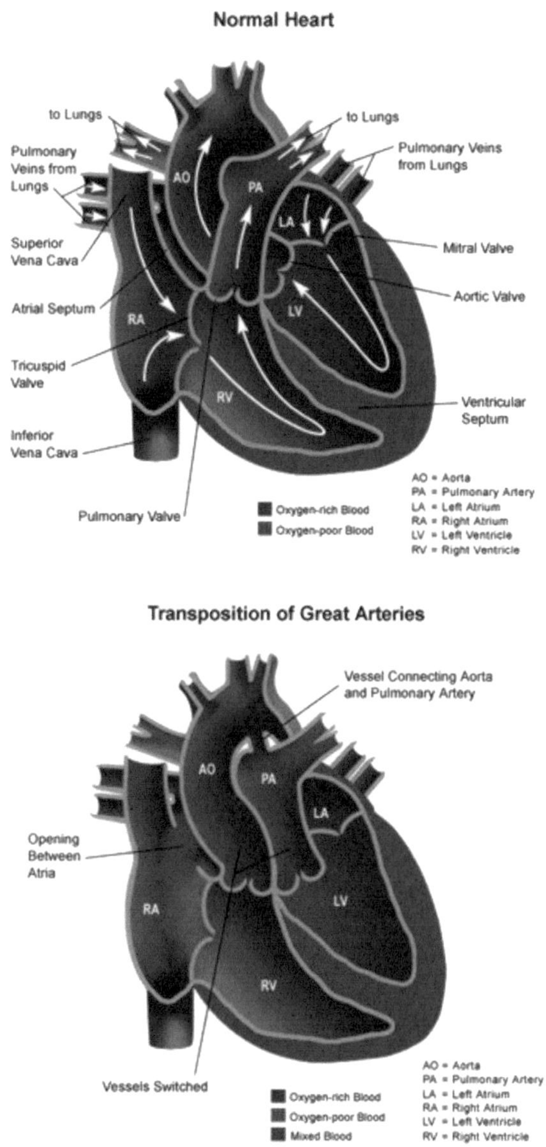

Fig. 10.

7. Pulmonary stenosis and atresia

Pulmonary stenosis and pulmonary atresia with intact ventriculer septum represent 9% and about %2 off all cardiac anomalies,respectively. The most common form of pulmonary stenosis is the valvar type,due to the fusion of the pulmonary leaflets.Hemodynamics are altered proportionally to the degree of the stenosis.The work of the right ventricle is increased,as well as the pressure,leading to hypertrophy of the ventriculer walls.

Pulmonary atresia with intact ventriculer septum in infants is usually associated with a hypoplastic righy ventricle.Prenatal diagnosis of pulmonary atresia with intact ventriculer septum relies on the demonstration off a small pulmonary artery with an atreticpulmonary valve.

8. Ebstein’s anomaly

The color Doppler defines the underlying pathology by demonstrating abnormal blood flow back into the right atrium from the right ventricle. The abnormal flow originates from a displaced tricuspid valve which is located lower in the ventricle than it should be. This is called Ebstein's malformation often seen in women who take anti-depressants such as Lithium.

9. Aortic stenosis

In general, the narrowing is found at the level of the aortic valve and a simple stenosis is rarely detected in the four-chamber view. However, a critical aortic stenosis is associated with a dilated and hypokinetic left ventricle with an echogenic endocardium, as a sign of endocardial fibroelastosis. Simple aortic stenosis can be detected only by using color Doppler. Antegrade turbulent flow (aliasing) is a characteristic finding in the five-chamber view. Pulsed Doppler analysis shows high velocities (more than 2 m/s) and a characteristic aliasing pattern. Continuous wave Doppler is therefore necessary to confirm the diagnosis. In critical aortic stenosis, there is antegrade turbulent flow across the aortic valve, but peak systolic velocities can vary from more than 2 m/s to values within the normal range, as an expression of left ventricular dysfunction. Due to the high pressure in the left ventricle, both a mitral regurgitation and a left to- right shunt at the level of the foramen ovale are found. In severe left ventricular dysfunction, a retrograde flow is seen within the aortic arch.

10. Hypoplastic right ventricle

In this condition, the aortic valve is generally atretic or severely stenotic and the left ventricle diminutive and non-contractile. The mitral valve is either atretic or stenotic. Color Doppler demonstrates reduced or absent diastolic filling of the left ventricle . In the four-chamber view, there is unilateral perfusion of the right ventricle. Often, there is mild tricuspid regurgitation. Careful examination of the intra-atrial communication shows an abnormal left-to-right shunt. In hypoplastic left heart syndrome, there is retrograde perfusion of the neck vessels and coronary arteries which can also be used for the differential diagnosis. Using color Doppler, it is then possible to confirm the diagnosis by demonstrating, in the three-vessel view, the retrograde perfusion in the hypoplastic aortic arch.

The color Doppler defines the underlying pathology by demonstrating the flow patterns within the heart.This is the labeled image of the pathology demonstrating several features. When the heart fills with blood (diastole) blood is observed filling only the left ventricle. When the heart begins to contract (systole) blood is observed going across the ventricular septal defect to fill the smaller right ventricle.

The arrows illustrate the ventricular septal defect (VSD). RA=right atrium, LA=left atrium, RV=right ventricle, LV=left ventricle.

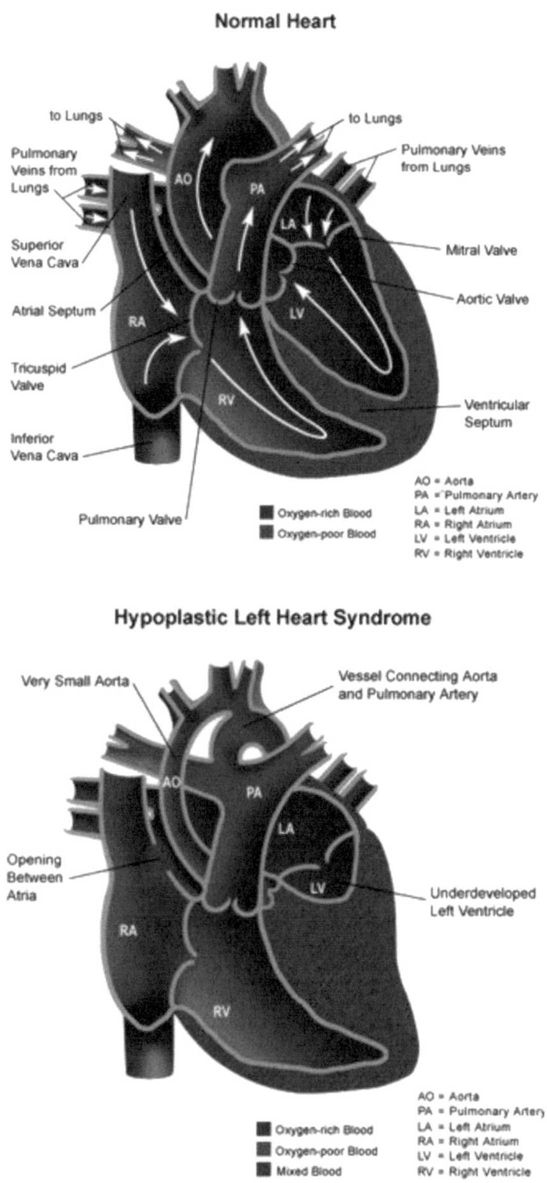

Fig. 11.

11. Tricuspid regurgitation

This image illustrates the four-chamber view using 2D ultrasound on the left and color Doppler on the right. Tricuspid regurgitation cannot be demonstrated using 2D ultrasound. This finding is important because tricuspid regurgitation is associated with an increased risk for Down syndrome when it is observed during the first or second trimeters of pregnancy.

RA=right atrium, LA=left atrium, RV=right ventricle, LV=left ventricle.

The right atrium is enlarged with what appears to be an abnormal triccolor Doppler on the right. Tricuspid regurgitation cannot be demonstrated using 2D ultrasound. This finding is important because tricuspid regurgitation is associated with an increased risk for Down syndrome when it is observed during the first or second trimeters of pregnancy.

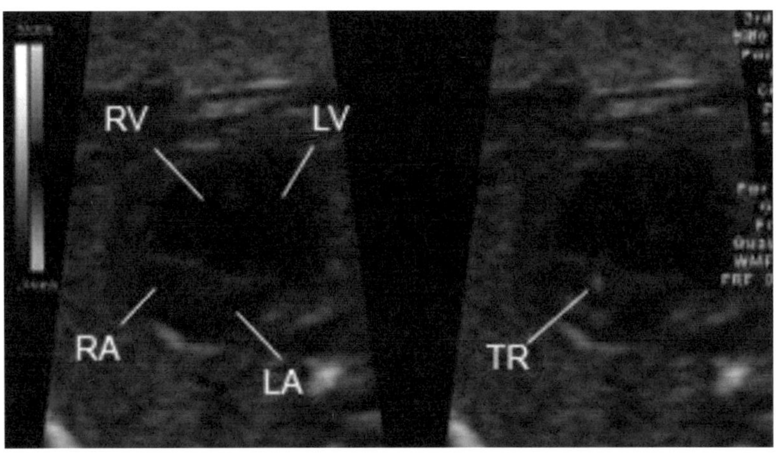

Fig. 12. RA=right atrium, LA=left atrium, RV=right ventricle, LV=left ventricle.

12. Ventricular septal defect

The defect can be either situated in the inlet, in the muscular part or, most commonly, in the perimembranous part of the ventricular septum. The defect can be suspected by two-dimensional ultrasound examination if it is larger than 3 mm. Color Doppler can help to identify small muscular septal defects. Although right and left ventricular pressures are quite equal prenatally, a bidirectional shunt across the defect is present. The best approach to examine a septal defect with color Doppler is the perpendicular insonation of the interventricular septum. In cases of an obstruction of an outflow tract, there is an unidirectional shunt to the contralateral side; in a ventricular septal defect with aortic stenosis, there is a left-to-right shunt.

This is the labeled image of the pathology demonstrating the shunting ventricular septal defect (VSD) easily identified with color Doppler ultrasound RA=right atrium, LA=left atrium, RV=right ventricle, LV=left ventricle.

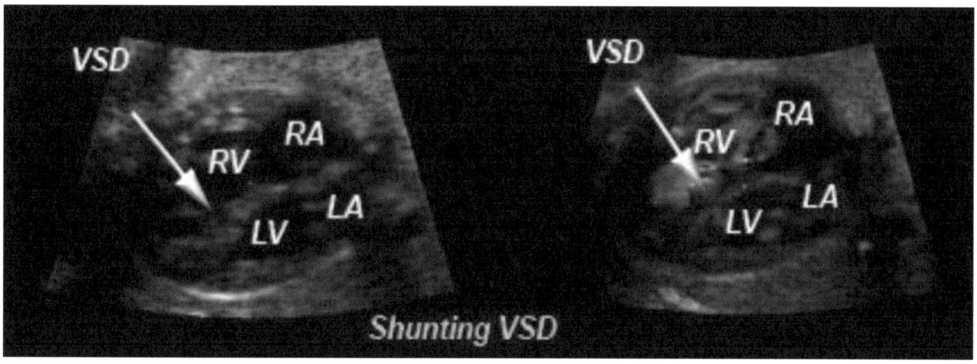

Fig. 13.

13. Other cardiac anomalies and arrhythmias

- Atrioventricular septal defects are a more relevant entity mostly because of the very frequent association with other anomalies such as trisomy 21;diagnosis of this defect is simpler although false-negatives may occur.
- Tricuspid dysplasia and Ebstein's malformation of the tricuspid valva may be complicated by severe tricuspid insufficiency ,cardiomegaly,and hydrops;such combination is most frequently lethal,with very few infants surviving.
- Irreguler paterns of fetal heart rhythms are frequent.short periods of tachycardia,braycardia,and ectopic beats as well are very commonly seen,and in the vast majority of cases have no clinical significanca.A sustained bradycardia of less than 100 bpm, a sustained tachycardia of more than 200 bpm and irregular beats occuring more than 1in 10 should be considered obnormal and require further investigation.The techniques of choice for the diagnosisof fetal dysrhythmias are M-mode and/or spectral Doppler ultrasound.
- premature atrial or ventriculer beats are by far the most frequentfetal arrhythmias.They are benign ,are not associated with an increased risk of cardiac malformations , and tend to disapper throughout gestation.Serial monitoring has been recommended because,thet sometimes can evolve toward fetal tachycardia.
- fetal tachycardias are potentially serious dysrhythmias that may cause fetal hydrops and perinatal death.
- congenital heart block may accur either as a consequence of a cardiac malformation or because of transplacental passage of maternal autoimmune antibodies.

14. Summary

The fetal echocardiogram is a unique ultrasound examination, which differs from the antenatal obstetrical ultrasound and from conventional echocardiogram in the infant,child,or adult.A unique ,high level set of skills and knowledge is required in order to perform this test.Diagnosis of cardiac defect is posibble ;however,a spesific examination is required (fetal echocardiogram)and this usually performed in pregnancies with an increased risk.The sensivity is in range of 80%..Most of the severe cardiac anomalies can be recognized by at least mid-gestation.While performing a standard sonogram from mid-gestation on,it is recommended to obtain a four-chamber view of the heart ;the sensitivity of this approach varies in different studies,but the general consensus is that is an acceptable approach.

15. References

Abramowicz JS, Kossoff G, Marsal K, Ter Haar G. Literature review by the ISUOG bioefects and safety committee. Ultrasound Obstet Gynecol 2002;19:318-9.

Allan L, Hornberger L, Sharland G, editors. Textbook of fetal cardiology. London: Greenwich Medical Media; 2000.

Berning RA, Silverman NH, Villegas M, Sahn DJ, Martin GR, Rice MJ. Reversed shunting across the ductus arteriosus or atrial septum in utero heralds severe congenital heart disease. J Am Coll Cardiol 1996;27:481-6.

Buskens E, Grobbee DE, Frohn-Mulder IME, Stewart PA, Juttmann RE, Wladimiroff JW, et al. Efficacy of routine fetal ultrasound screening for congenital heart disease in normal pregnancy. Circulation 1996;94:67-72.

Carvalho JS, Mavrides E, Shinebourne EA, Campbell S, Thilaganathan B. Improving the effectiveness of routine prenatal screening for major congenital heart defects. Heart 2002;88:387-91.

Deane C, Lees C. Doppler obstetric ultrasound: a graphical display of temporal changes in safety indices. Ultrasound Obstet Gynecol 2000;15:418-23.

Fouron JC, Zarelli M, Drblik SP, Lessard M. Normal flow velocity profile of the fetal aortic isthmus through normal gestation. Am J Cardiol 1994;74:483-6.

Ghi T, Huggon IC, Zosmer N, Nicolaides KH. Incidence of major structural cardiac defects associated with increased nuchal translucency but normal karyotype. Ultrasound Obstet Gynecol 2001;18:610-4.

Glickstein JS, Buyon J, Friedman D. Pulsed Doppler echocardiographic assessment of the fetal PR interval. Am J Cardiol 2000;86:236-9.

Hansen M, Kurinczuk JJ, Bower C, Webb S. The risk of major birth defects after intracytoplasmic sperm injection and in vitro fertilization. N Engl J Med 2002;346:725-30.

International Society of Ultrasound in Obstetrics and Gynecology (ISUOG). Safety statement, 2000. Ultrasound Obstet Gynecol 2000;16:594-6.

Journal of the American Society of Echocardiography Volume 17 Number 7 Pediatric Council of the American Society of Echocardiography.

Kleinman C, Donnerstein R, Jaffe C, DeVore G, Weinstein EM, Lynch DC, et al. Fetal echocardiography. A tool for evaluation of in utero cardiac arrhythmias and monitoring of in utero therapy. Am J Cardiol 1983;51:237-43.

Kurjak A. Are color and pulsed Doppler sonography safe in early pregnancy? J Perinat Med 1999;27:423-30.

Miller MW, Brayman AA, Abramowicz JA. Obstetric ultrasonography: a biophysical consideration of patient safety-the "rules" have changed. Am J Obstet Gynecol 1998;179:241-54. 1. Hoffman JI, Kaplan S. The incidence of congenital heart disease. J Am Coll Cardiol 2002;39:1890-900.

Nelson NL, Filly RA, Goldstein RB, Callen PW. The AIUM/ ACR antepartum obstetrical sonographic guidelines: expecta- Journal of the American Society of Echocardiography Volume 17 Number 7 Pediatric Council of the American Society of Echocardiography indications for detection of anomalies. J Ultrasound Med 1993;4:186-96.

Phillipos EZ, Robertson MA, Still KD. The echocardiographic assessment of the human foramen ovale. J Am Soc Echocardiogr 1994;7:257-63.

Quinones MA, Douglas PS, Foster E, Gorcsan J, Lewos JF, Pearlman AS, et al. ACC/AHA clinical competence statement on echocardiography: a report of the American College of Cardiology/American Heart Association/American College of Physicians-American Society of Internal Medicine task force on clinical competence (committee on echocardiography). J Am Coll Cardiol 2003;41:687-708.

Rein AJ, O'Donnell C, Geva T, Nir A, Perles Z, Hashimoto I, et al. Use of tissue velocity imaging in the diagnosis of fetal cardiac arrhythmias. Circulation 2002;106:1827-33.

Schmidt KG, Silverman NH, Van Hare GF, Hawkins JA, Cloez JL, Rudolph AM. Two-dimensional echocardiographic determination of ventricular volumes in the fetal heart. Circulation 1990;81:325-33.

Sharland GK, Allan LD. Normal fetal cardiac measurements derived by cross-sectional echocardiography. Ultrasound Obstet Gynecol 1992;2:175-81.

Sklansky M, Tang A, Levy D, Grossfeld P, Kashani I, Shaughnessy R, et al. Maternal psychological impact of fetal echocardiography. J Am Soc Echocardiogr 2002;15:159-66. American College of Radiology Standard for the Performance of Antepartum Obstetrical Ultrasound.

Standards for the Performance of the Antepartum Obstetrical Ultrasound Examination. Copyright 1994, by the American Institute of Ultrasound in Medicine.

Stumpflen I, Stumpflen A, Wimmer M, Bernaschek G. Effect of detailed fetal echocardiography as part of routine prenatal ultrasonographic screening on detection of congenital heart disease. Lancet 1996;348:854-7.

Tan J, Silverman NH, Hoffman JIE, Villegas M, Schmidt KG. Cardiac dimensions determined by cross-sectional echocardiography in the normal human fetus from 18 weeks to term. Am J Cardiol 1992;70:1459-67.

Tworetzky W, McElhinney DB, Reddy VM, Brook MM, Hanley FL, Silverman NH. Improved surgical outcome after fetal diagnosis of hypoplastic left heart syndrome. Circulation 2001;103:1269-73.

Verheijen PM, Lisowski LA, Stoutenbeek P, Hitchcock JF, Brenner JI, Cope JA, et al. Prenatal diagnosis of congenital heart disease affects preoperative acidosis in the newborn patient. J Thorac Cardiovasc Surg 2001;121:798.

Fetal Cardiac Magnetic Resonance (CMR)

Sahar N. Saleem
Radiology Department-Faculty of Medicine Kasr Al-Ainy-Cairo University
Egypt

1. Introduction

Congenital heart disease (CHD) is present in 0.8% of all live births and is therefore one of the most common congenital malformations (Fyler et al., 1980). The spectrum of congenital heart defects is significantly higher in fetuses than in live born infants because of their reduced viability (Tennstedt et al., 1999). The prognosis of congenital heart disease can be poor; almost one third to one half of congenital heart defects are severe and lethal unless an intervention is done early (Hoffman & Kaplan, 2002). Prenatal diagnosis of congenital heart disease results in referral of mothers with affe1cted fetuses to equipped centers where all facilities for neonatal cardiac care are available. The diagnosis of a congenital heart disease in a fetus should also prompt evaluation for genetic syndromes and associated non cardiac malformations (Cohen, 2001). Improvements in diagnosis and treatment have lead to more patients surviving to adulthood (Carvalho et al., 2002).

Echocardiography is the gold standard diagnostic imaging tool for prenatal detection of cardiac malformations (Kleinman et al., 1980). Fetal echocardiography combines the benefit of accurate assessment of cardiac anatomy and function probability (Carvalho et al., 2002). However, Ultrasonography (US) is occasionally limited by acoustic window, poor images of the distal vasculature, fetal position, maternal adipose tissue, abdominal wall scar form previous abdominal or pelvic surgery, and is user dependent (Forbus et al., 2004). As a consequence, there remains room for other modalities in studying the fetal cardiovascular system.

Cardiac Magnetic Resonance imaging (CMR) proved unequivocal advantages over other cardiac imaging modalities (Prakash et al., 2010). Technical advances during the last decade have brought CMR into the mainstream of noninvasive cardiac imaging. The clinical applications of CMR are well-established in pediatrics and adults patients. CMR is employed in clinical practice of congenital heart disease, cardiac masses, the pericardium, right ventricular dysplasia, and hibernating myocardium. Role of CMR includes anatomic and functional assessment of the cardiovascular system (Finn et al., 2006). Fetal MRI proved valuable in defining the details of fetal anatomy especially the central nervous system (Frates et al., 2004; Levine, 2006; Saleem et al., 2009) and potentially the heart (Gorincour et al., 2007; Saleem, 2008). However, CMR has not been thoroughly investigated in-utero.

2. Fetal Cardiac Magnetic Resonance (CMR)

The intent of this chapter is to serve as a primer for fetal Cardiac Magnetic Resonance (CMR) based on our clinical cases of normal and abnormal fetal hearts. The chapter will include discussion of fetal Magnetic Resonance Imaging (MRI); fetal CMR technical aspects; MRI anatomy of the fetal heart; in-utero diagnosis of CHD and associated fetal syndromes; and future of fetal CMR.

2.1 Fetal Magnetic Resonance Imaging (MRI)

2.1.1 Fetal MRI: Safety and ethics

Magnetic Resonance Imaging (MRI) is a non-invasive diagnostic examination that does not involve ionizing radiation with no known associated negative side effects or delayed sequels to date (Clements, 2000). However, because of the potential risk of MR imaging to the developing fetus it is always prudent to follow MR imaging ethics. The American College of Radiology (ACR) white paper on MR safety states that Fetal MR imaging is indicated if the risk-benefit ratio to the patient warrants that the study be performed (Kanal et al, 2002). According to The Safety Committee of the Society of MRI, fetal MRI is only indicated if other non-ionising diagnostic imaging methods are inadequate. It is also prudent to wait until after the first trimester before performing fetal MRI. (Glenn & Barkovich, 2006).

2.1.2 Fetal MRI: General indications

Fetal MRI is indicated to evaluate abnormalities and underlying etiologies that are not as readily depicted with Ultrasonography (US). In contradistinction to US, MRI visualization of the fetus is not significantly limited by maternal obesity, fetal position, or oligohydramnios and visualization of the brain is not restricted by the ossified skull (Levine, 2006). MRI provides superior soft tissue contrast resolution and the ability to distinguish individual structures such as brain, lung, liver, kidney, and bowel. MRI provides multiplanar imaging as well as a large field of view, facilitating examination of fetuses with large or complex anomalies, and visualization of the lesion within the context of the entire body of the fetus (Frates et al, 2004).

2.1.3 Fetal MRI: Technical aspects

MRI is performed on 1.5 T superconducting magnet and a phased-array surface coil. The mother lies supine during the examination. If the mother does not tolerate the supine position, MRI should be performed in the left lateral decubitus. No special preparations, fasting, or sedation are required (Levine, 2006).

Initial attempts at MRI of the fetus were challenging because of fetal motion and altered fetal position which produced significant imaging artefacts. Development of fast MRI sequences significantly decreased motion artifacts and eliminated the need for fetal sedation (Levine, 2006).

A variety of fast MRI sequences are currently available including single-shot fast spin echo (SSFSE) or half Fourier acquired single shot turbo spin echo (HASTE) to obtain T2-weighted images, fast gradient echo sequences with low flip angle shot (FLASH) to obtain T1-weighted images, and steady state free precession sequence (balanced fast field echo b-FFE) to obtain a balanced image (Brugger et al, 20006; Chung et al, 2000).

In young fetuses (less than 16 weeks' gestation) fetal movements will reduce the conspicuity of fetal anatomy. Small structures are especially difficult to identify early in gestation. With advancing gestation, the reduced fetal motion and the increased size of fetal structures will progressively enhance anatomical visualization (Frates et al, 2004). In addition, the general limitations of fetal MRI include the high costs, the limited availability, in addition to MRI-specific absolute contraindications like maternal pacemakers and ferromagnetic implants. Claustrophobia can be an additional issue, especially as pregnant women can have difficulties lying on their back, mainly in the third trimester (Saleem et al, 2009).

2.2 In-utero MR imaging of the fetal heart

2.2.1 Feasibility and patients' selection

MRI of the fetal heart is feasible (Saleem, 2008); however, it has not been thoroughly investigated with only few reports in literature most of them in the form of case reports or preliminary experiences (Gorincour et al, 2007; Kivelitz et al, 2004; Manganaro et al, 2008). We will depend in discussion of MRI of fetal heart in this chapter on findings from our study of 298 pregnancies at high risk for CHD that were enrolled sequentially from September 2003 to August 2010 in our institutional review board-approved study. The mean gestational age was 24 weeks with a range of 16-36 weeks.

Patients were eligible for enrolment if they were at possible risk for CHD or for an abnormality detected in fetal echocardiography. Risk factors for CHD were combination of history of previous pregnancies with CHD, a parent with CHD, maternal Rubella infection, maternal collagen disease, maternal Diabetes Mellitus, maternal exposure to a possible teratogen (Phenytoin medication), or abnormal findings in prenatal echocardiography. Written informed consent was obtained from all of the expectant mothers before MRI.

2.2.2 Technique

MRI was performed with a 1.5-T superconducting magnet (Gyroscan Intera, Philips Healthcare) and a phased-array surface coil. No maternal sedation, fetal sedation or paralysis, fetal cardiac gating, or controlled maternal breathing was used. The imaging time for the examination ranged between 15-45 minutes (20 minutes in average).

MR sequences include (Fig. 1):

a. **Bright blood sequences** using balanced steady-state-free-precession sequences (balanced-SSFP). Balanced SSFP sequences (Repetition time TR/Echo time TE, 3.5–4/1.7–2; flip angle FA, 60–90°; slice thickness, 3–5 mm; gap, 1 mm to section overlap of –3 mm) were performed for all patients. The thin overcontiguous sections are used for evaluation of small fetuses. The field of view FOV (205–350 mm2) is adjusted to increase or decrease in the fetal or maternal dimensions or when aliasing artifact is a problem. The matrix size is 183 x 256 or 256 x 256 according to the selected FOV; reduction of FOV compelled reduction of matrix size in some cases. One to three signals are averaged. The imaging time for each sequence depends on the number of slices and number of signals averaged.

b. **Dark blood sequences** using T2-weighted single-shot fast spin echo sequences (TR/TE 1000/151, Matrix 256 × 134, slice thickness 3 mm, FOV (205–350 mm2).
c. **Additional T1** Fast gradient echo sequence with low Flip angle shot was: TR/TE of 100-140/4.2 ms, 70-90° FA, 256x160-256 matrix, one signal acquired, slice thickness 4-6 mm with an inter-slice gap of 0.2-0.4 mm.

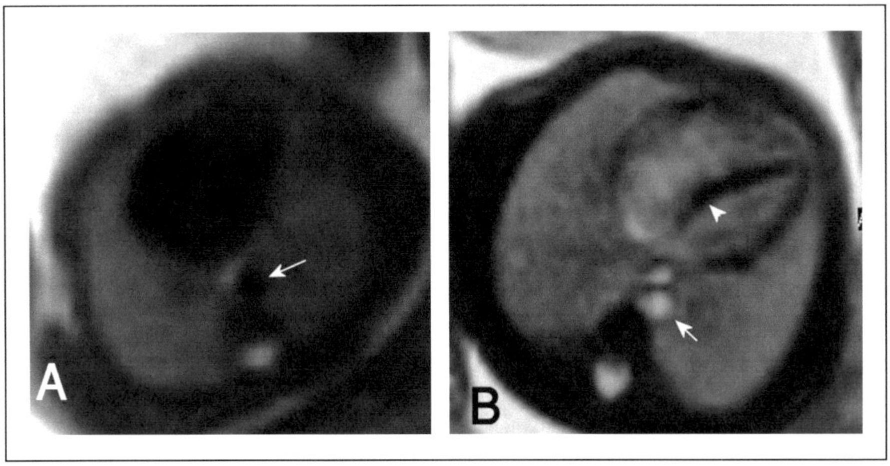

Fig. 1. Axial MR images of fetal thorax at 24 weeks' gestation using dark blood sequence single shot fast spin echo (SSFSE) (A) and bright blood sequence steady state free precession (SSFP) (B). SSFP is superior in visualizing cardiac morphology, interventricular septum (arrowhead) and thoracic aorta (arrows).

Planes:

A scout acquisition is performed (single shot fast spin echo: TR/TE 10000/100 msec, 4 mm slice thickness, matrix 196x256x256) is taken on maternal coronal or axial planes to determine fetal position for situs assessment. Series of images are then taken along the three fetal body planes and cardiac planes using mainly balanced SSFP (Fig. 2).

a. **Fetal body planes:** A series of images are taken along the three fetal body planes (axial, sagittal, and coronal). Each new acquisition is prescribed by use of images from the immediately previous acquisition to avoid misregistration caused by fetal movement. Additional images are obtained along the planes of the brain and any other suspected extra-cardiac region.
b. **Cardiac axes:** MR imaging are also attempted along cardiac axes. A representative image from each sequence is used as a scout to align the subsequent acquisition. From the coronal plane, the long-axis view is obtained along a line that extended from the cardiac apex to the middle of the left ventricle. A short-axis view perpendicular to the long axis also is obtained. In the short-axis view, the image in which the left ventricle is concentric and the right ventricle is crescent-shaped is chosen to align the plane for the four-chamber view. The plane for the four-chamber view extends along the center of the left ventricle and the farthest corner of the right ventricle. From the four-chamber image, the two-chamber view is obtained along the right and left sides of the heart (Saleem, 2008).

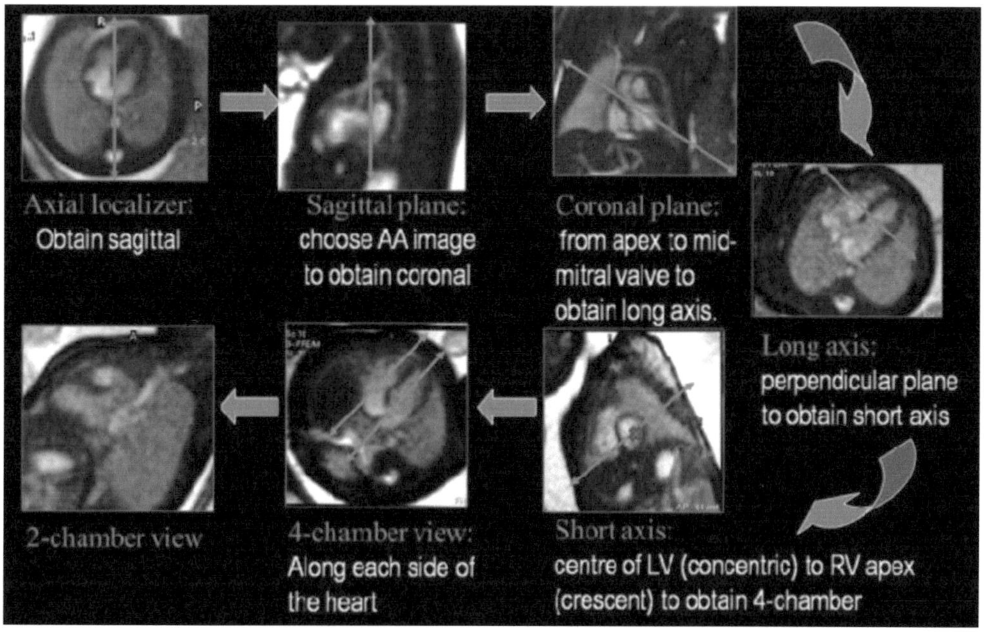

Fig. 2. MR imaging of fetal heart along three fetal body planes as well as cardiac axes.

2.2.3 MRI anatomy of the fetal heart

MRI anatomy of fetal heart in Axial plane: The figure (Fig.3) shows axial MR images (upper row) of a fetal heart in comparison to equivalent echocardiographic views (lower row) arranged from caudad to cephalad. At the level of the four cardiac chambers (Fig. 3A), the interventricular septum is central, cardiac axis is 45 degrees; both atria and both ventricles have comparable size. Atrio-ventricular and great arteries valves are occasionally seen. At a superior level (Fig. 3B), the left ventricular outflow tract (LVOT) can be seen. At the level of the right ventricular outflow tract (Fig. 3C), images show bifurcation of the main pulmonary artery to right and left pulmonary arteries. MR image can show the main bronchi in relation to the pulmonary artery branch which helps in assessment of the viscero-atrial situs; tracheobronchial tree cannot be seen on echocardiography. The three-vessel-view (Fig.3D) shows the aorta winds around the trachea as well as the left brachiocephalic vein which meets the right to form superior vena cava (SVC).

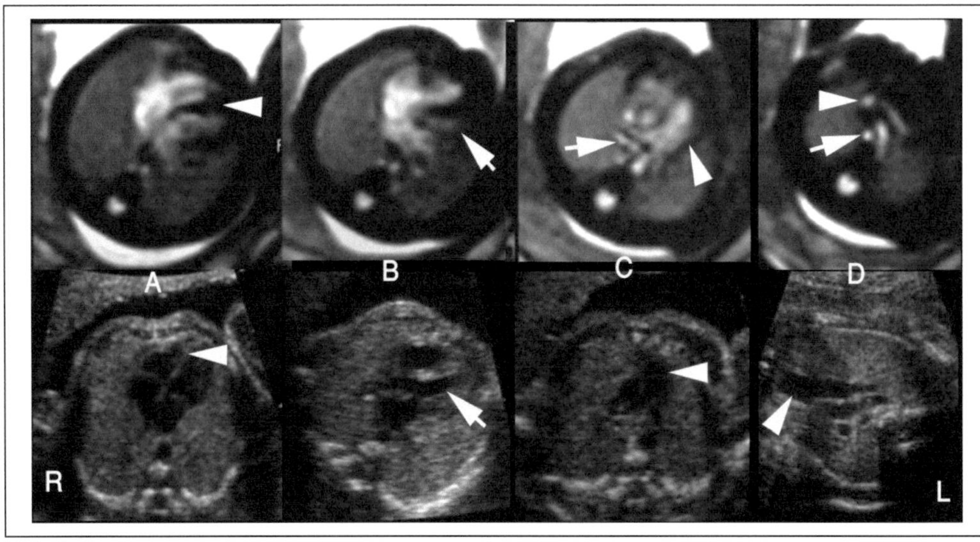

Fig. 3. Comparable axial anatomy of the fetal heart (at 26 weeks' gestation) in MRI (upper row) and echocardiography (lower row) from caudad to cephalad; R: right, L: left. (A) Four-cardiac-chamber view: arrowheads point to interventricular septum. (B) Left ventricular outflow tract (LVOT) view: arrows point to (LOVT). (C) Right ventricular outflow tract (RVOT) view: arrowheads point to the bifurcating main pulmonary artery; arrow in upper MR image points to the right main bronchus posterior to the right pulmonary artery. (D) Three-vessel-view: arrowheads point to the right brachiocephalic vein which meets its left counterpart to form superior vena cava (SVC). Aorta winds around the trachea (arrow in upper MR image points to fluid-filled trachea).

MRI anatomy of fetal heart in Coronal plane: In this plane, MRI shows cardiac apex, left ventricle, LVOT, inflow systemic veins and their tributaries drain to the right atrium, brachiocephalic veins join to form SVC, and hepatic veins drain to inferior vena cava (IVC) (Fig. 4).

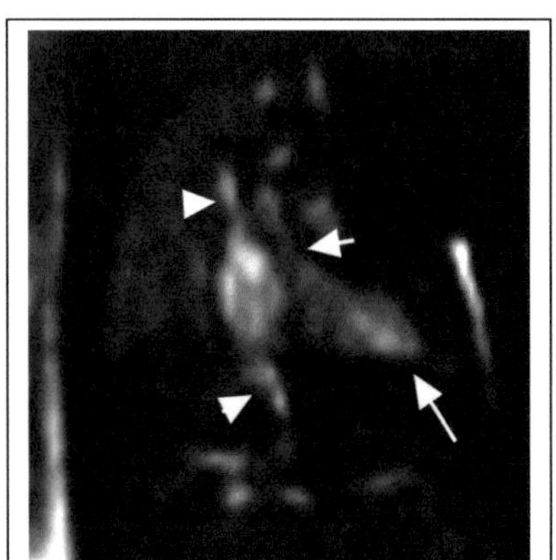

Fig. 4. Coronal MRI of normal fetal heart at 24 weeks' gestation shows SVC and IVC (arrowheads) draining into right atrium, cardiac apex (long arrow), and LVOT (short arrow)

MRI anatomy of fetal heart in sagittal plane: MRI shows in sagittal plane (Fig. 5) systemic inflow veins and connection between right ventricle and its outflow tract.

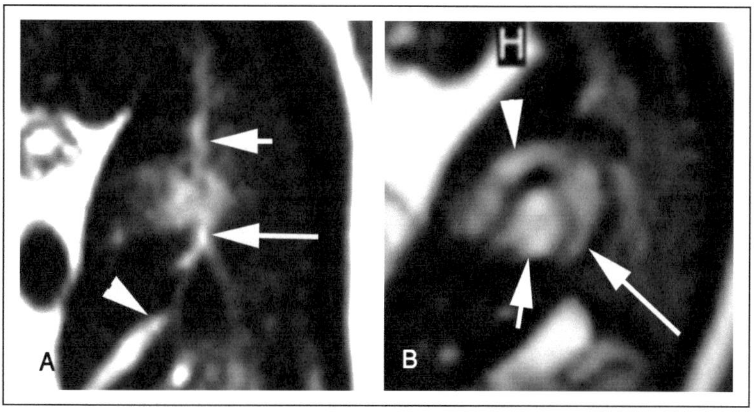

Fig. 5. Sagittal anatomy of normal fetal heart at 24 weeks' gestation obtained from right to left direction. (A) The image shows superior (short arrow) and inferior (long arrow) venae cave draining to right atrium. Umbilical vein (arrowhead) is also seen draining into IVC. (B) The image shows the pulmonary artery (arrowhead) originating from the right ventricle. Short arrow points to the left ventricle, and long arrow points to the left atrium.

MRI anatomy of fetal heart along cardiac axes (Fig.6 & Fig. 7). MR imaging along different cardiac axes reveals details of the fetal cardiac structures. Imaging along the long cardiac axis (Fig. 6A) and four cardiac chamber view (Fig. 6B) can show detailed morphologic features of the cardiac chambers namely the moderator band, atrial septal duct valve, foramen ovale, and pulmonary veins.

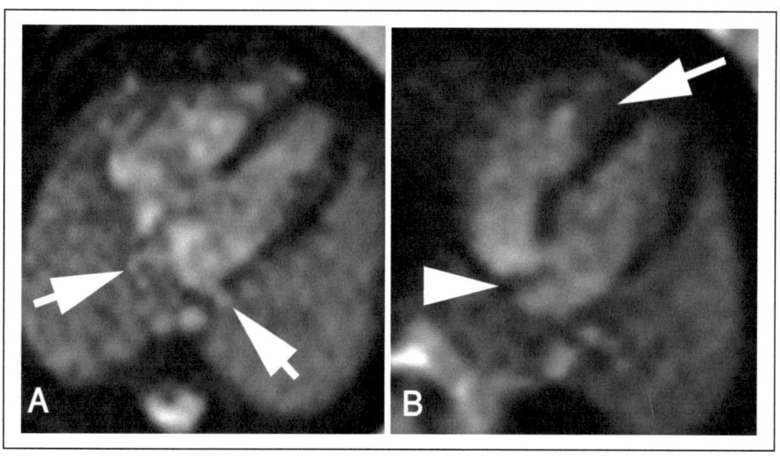

Fig. 6. MRI anatomy of fetal heart at 28 weeks' gestation along long cardiac axis (A) and 4-chamber view (B). In (A), arrows point to pulmonary veins. In (B), moderator band (arrow) appears as low signal intensity structure between the apical right ventricular septum and free right ventricular wall. Atrial septal duct valve (arrowhead) is directed to the left indicating the normal blood direction across the foramen ovale in fetal life from right to left

MR imaging along the short axis plane (Fig.7A) and two-cardiac-chamber view (Fig. 7B) of the fetal heart can show well the connection between the ventricles and great vessels.

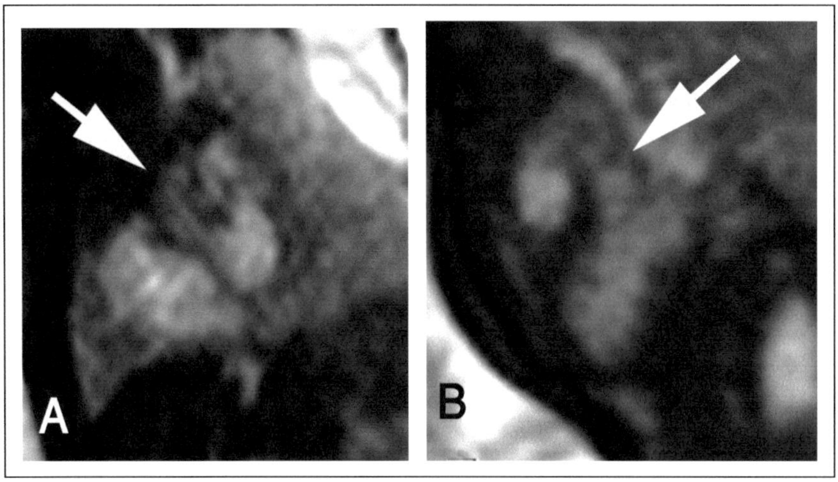

Fig. 7. MRI anatomy of fetal heart at 28 weeks' gestation displayed in short cardiac axis (A) and two-cardiac chamber view along the left heart (B) using b-SSFP sequence. Arrows in both views point to left ventricular outflow tract originating from the left ventricle

2.2.4 Image interpretation of fetal CMR

Prenatal echocardiographic images are analyzed with anatomic segmental approach to congenital heart disease (Carvalho et al, 2005). A modified segmental approach can be used to analyze MR images of the fetal heart (Saleem, 2008) that includes the following:

Visceroatrial situs: The stomach is normally on the left side, IVC on the right side, the embryologic left bronchus is long with no early division and runs under the left pulmonary artery, and the right bronchus is short and runs behind the right pulmonary artery.

Cardiac position: Most of the heart occupies normally the left side of the thorax with the cardiac apex to the left.

Cardiac size: The heart occupies normally one third of the thorax.

Cardiac axis: The cardiac axis is the angle between the true sagittal plane (between the spine and the anterior chest wall) and a plane along the interventricular septum.

Cardiac chambers: The cardiac chambers are evaluated for number (normally four), arrangement (left atrium normally is close to the fetal spine), relative size of both atria (normally equal in size), and relative size of both ventricles (normally equal in size). Moderator band identifies the morphological right ventricle. Foramen ovale and atrial septal duct valve location (presence in the left atrium indicates normal right-to-left blood flow). Intactness of interventricular septum and appearance of valves (atrioventricular and great arterial).

Ventricular looping: In a normal D-loop, the more anterior ventricle is the embryologic right one.

Inflow veins: Superior and inferior venae cavae normally connect to the right atrium. Two right and two left pulmonary veins normally join the left atrium; at least one pulmonary vein can be visualized in fetal CMR.

Outflow vessels: The left and right ventricular outflow tracts (aorta and pulmonary arteries) are evaluated for relative size (normally equal) and relative position in relation to each other (normally cross perpendicular in relation to their origin).

Ventriculoarterial concordance: Normally the aorta arises from the left ventricle. It can be traced in a regular arch that gives rise to three neck vessels. The pulmonary artery normally arises from a morphologic right ventricle and bifurcates at its distal end.

Side of the aortic arch: The side of the aortic arch is defined according to the main bronchus, above which it crossed the mediastinum posteriorly (Saleem, 2008).

2.3 Abnormal findings in fetal CMR

We include abnormal fetal cardiac findings detected upon using a modified segmental approach in analysis of CMR from our series of 298 pregnancies.

Viscero-atrial situs

MR imaging along maternal coronal or axial planes enables determination of fetal position for situs assessment. In situs inversus totalis, cardiac apex and stomach are detected on the right of the fetal body on coronal MR images (Fig. 8A). In heterotaxy, fetal CMR can detect a combination of cardiac, vascular and visceral abnormalities. In left atrial isomerism where left-sided organs are paired and right-sided structures may be absent, fetal MRI detected dextrocardia, central liver, polysplenia, and interrupted inferior vena cava with azygous continuation (double vessel sign) (Fig. 8B).

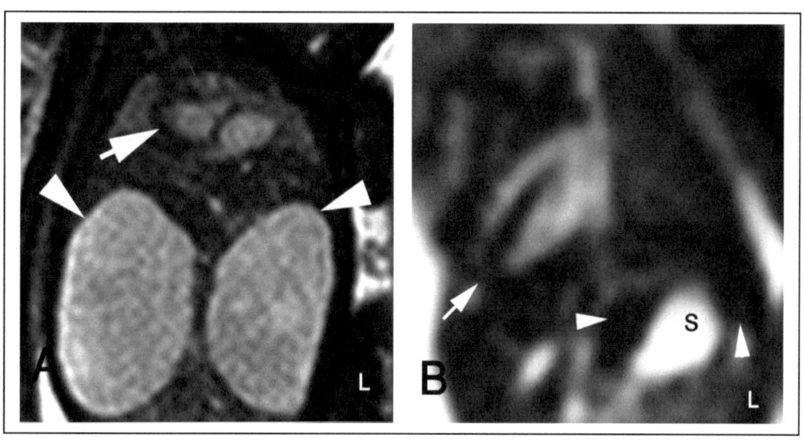

Fig. 8. Viscero-atrial situs abnormalities can be detected in fetal CMR in coronal (T2-SSFP) image. (A) In a 27 weeks' gestation fetus with situs inversus totalis, arrow points to right-sided cardiac apex and arrowheads point to associated hepatic cysts. (B) In a 20 weeks' gestation fetus with left atrial isomerism the cardiac apex points to the right (dextrocardia) (arrow). The fluid-filled stomach (s) occupies the left upper abdomen and is surrounded by multiple widely-spaced masses with low signal intensity characteristic for polysplenia

Cardiac Position and axis

In four-chamber transverse MRI view, most of the fetal heart normally occupies the left side of the thorax with the cardiac apex to the left. In a previous study of normal fetal hearts using MRI, the cardiac axis measurement (37.25° ± 7.15°) (Saleem, 2008) was in comparable with sonographic norms of (43° ± 2°) (Smith et al, 1995). When the axis of the heart is not within the normal range, the fetus is at increased risk of heart malformation or abnormal intrathoracic anatomy (Cohen, 2001). MRI axial four-chamber view depicts the fetal cardiac position and enables measurement of cardiac axis. Placement of the heart outside the chest (ectopia cordis) is a rare extreme cardiac position abnormality (Fig.9).

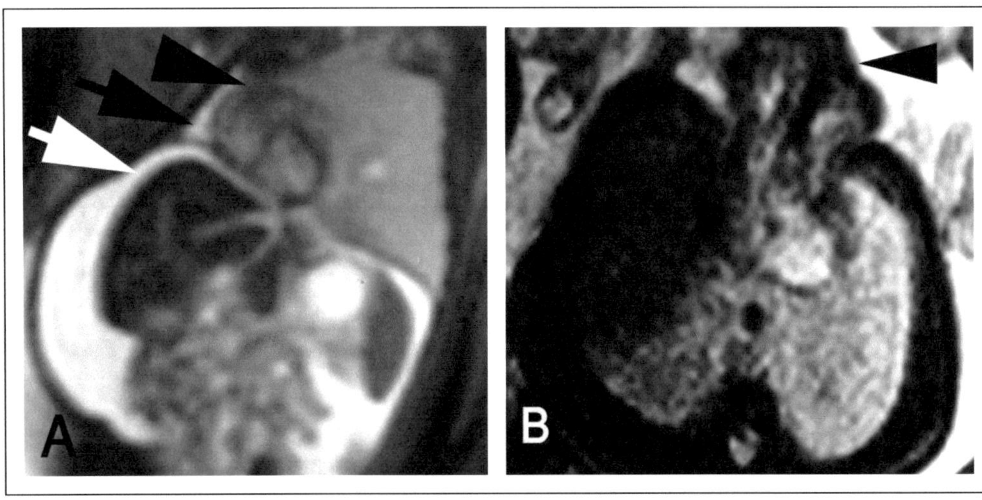

Fig. 9. Cardiac position abnormalities detected in fetal CMR. (A): Coronal T2-weighted SSFP image of a torso of 27 weeks' gestation fetus with cardiac position abnormality due to intrathoracic lesion. Arrowhead points to a deviated heart to the right hemithorax caused by intrathoracic abnormalities (hypoplastic right lung). Black arrow points to right pleural effusion and white arrow to associated ascites. (B): Axial T2-weighted SSFP of chest of 28 weeks' gestation fetus with ectopia cordis as part of Pentalogy of Cantrell. The axial image shows well the herniating heart (arrowhead) through the defective anterior chest wall

Balanced cardiac chambers

Four-cardiac-chamber and long-axis-cardiac MR views are valuable in assessing the number of chambers (normally four) of fetal heart as well as in comparing the sizes of both atria and both ventricles (normally have comparable sizes).

Detection of a balanced four-cardiac chamber view allows exclusion of odd number of chambers and unbalanced abnormalities of atrioventricular valves such as atresia (Saleem, 2008). In our experience, CMR allowed detection of imbalanced cardiac chambers in-utero (Fig.10). Abnormal decrease in size of cardiac chambers was detected by fetal CMR in cases such as hypoplastic left heart and hypoplastic right heart. In our series, fetal CMR also depicted abnormal increase in the size of individual fetal cardiac chamber such as dilatation of right atrium in Ebstein's anomaly and dilated right atrium in fetuses with partial anomalous pulmonary venous drainage.

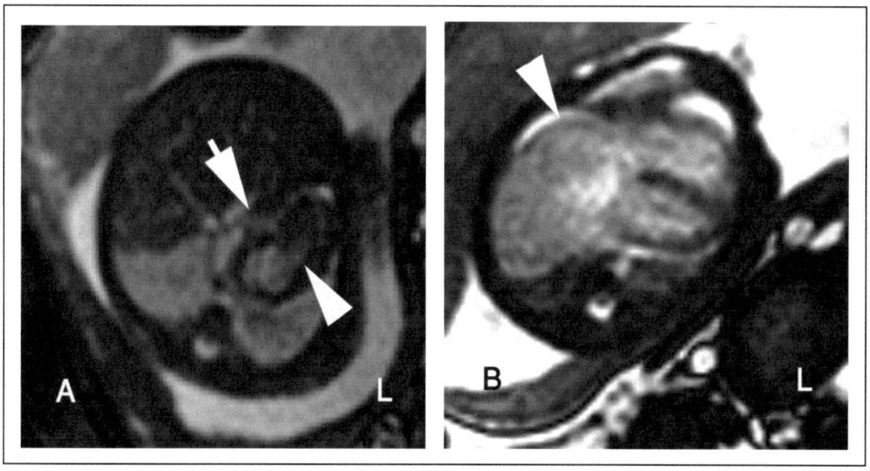

Fig. 10. Imbalanced fetal cardiac chambers detected four-chamber T2- SSFP CMR image. (A): A 24 weeks' gestation fetus with hypoplastic right heart (arrow) shows discrepancy in size with the normal left heart (arrowhead). (B) A 28 weeks' gestation fetus with Ebstein's anomaly shows aneurismal dilatation of the right atrium (arrowhead).

Intactness of interventricular septum: Interventricular septum appears in T2-SSFP fetal MR images as thin low signal intensity structure that separates the right and left ventricles (Fig.1B). Transverse four-chamber and long axis MR images are valuable in assessment of interventricular septum of fetal heart. Defects in the interventricular septum can be detected in fetal CMR as an isolated cardiac abnormality or part of a more complex heart anomaly (Fig.11).

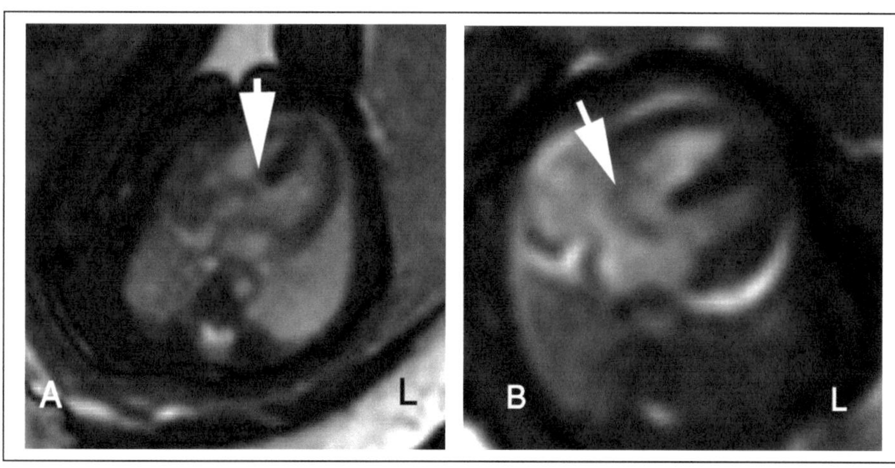

Fig. 11. Interventricular septal defects are detected in four-chamber T2-SSFP fetal CMR. (A) In a 25 weeks' gestation fetus with Trisomy 13, MR image shows a small high interventricular septal defect (VSD). (B). In a 30 weeks' gestation fetus, MR image shows a large atrioventricular septal defect (AV canal) (arrow) as part of a complex cardiac anomaly in association with transposition of great arteries (TGA) (not shown).

Inflow vessels: Superior and inferior venae cavae (SVC, IVC) can be detected draining to right atrium on coronal and sagittal fetal CMR. Normally, at least one pulmonary vein can be visualized in 4-chamber view draining to the left atrium (Saleem, 2008). Fetal CMR can diagnose inflow vessels abnormalities such as persistent left SVC (Fig.12) as well as anomalous pulmonary venous drainage.

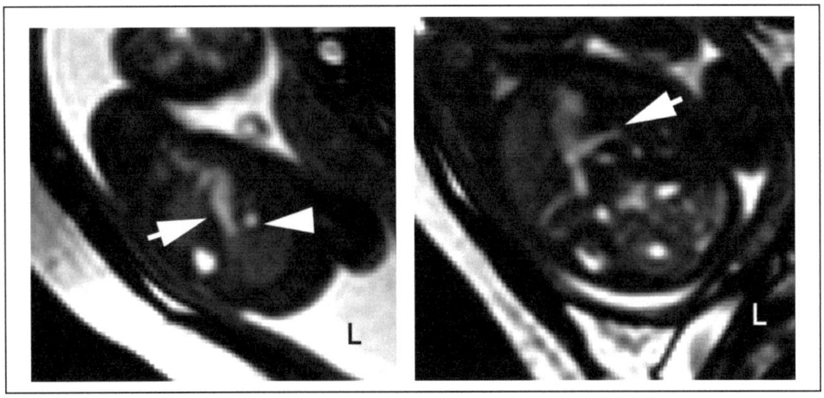

Fig. 12. Left superior vena cava (SVC) diagnosed by axial T2- SSFP MRI at 26 weeks' gestation. (A) Three-vessel axial image documents absent right and persistent left SVC (arrowhead) as well as right sided aortic arch (arrow). (B) Axial MR image caudad to (A) shows left SVC (arrow) draining into a dilated right coronary sinus.

Outflow vessels: In fetal CMR, left ventricular outflow tract (Aorta) can be detected on axial, coronal, and short axis views. Right ventricular outflow (pulmonary artery) tract can be identified on axial, sagittal and short axis views. Outflow vessels are normally equal in size and cross at their origin. Fetal CMR can detect conotruncal abnormalities (Fig. 13) such as transposition of great arteries (TGA), truncus arteriosus, Fallot's, and coarctation of aorta.

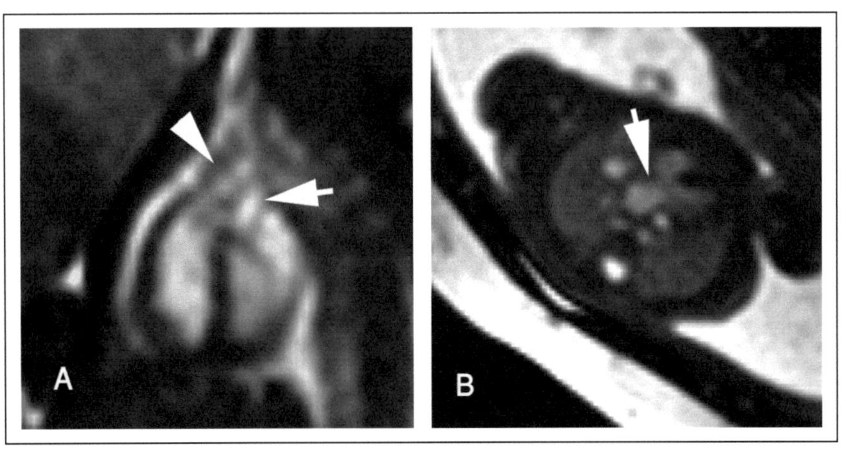

Fig. 13. T2-SSFP CMR diagnoses outflow vessels abnormalities in-utero. (A) Sagittal MRI of 30 weeks' gestation fetus with TGA shows parallel course of Pulmonary artery (arrowhead) and aorta (arrow) at their origin (Same fetus in Fig.11A). (B) Axial MRI of 26 weeks' gestation fetus shows a single outflow tract (truncus arteriosus) (arrow) over-rides VSD

Ventriculoarterial concordance: Fetal CMR using T2-SSFP can identify the morphological right ventricle through identification of the moderator band (Fig. 6B). The pulmonary artery normally arises from a morphologic right ventricle and bifurcates at its distal end. While the aorta arises from the left ventricle and can be traced in a regular arch that gives rise to three neck vessels.

Side of the aortic arch: The side of the aortic arch is defined according to the main bronchus, above which it crossed the mediastinum posteriorly (Saleem, 2008). The aortic arch is usually on the left. Right sided aortic arch can be detected on fetal CMR as an isolated finding or part of a complex cardiac malformation (Fig. 12A).

Cardiac masses and pericardial fluid: primary cardiac tumors are rarely diagnosed in utero and are usually seen on prenatal echocardiography. Few cases of cardiac rhabdomyomas have been reported in-utero by MRI (Kivelitz et al, 2004). On T2-SSFP sequence, fetal cardiac rhabdomyomas appear as low signal intensity masses in contrast with the high signal intracardiac blood. On T2-SSFSE, cardiac rhabdomyomas are less conspicuous as they appear of intermediate signal intensity against the low signal intensity intracardiac blood. Fetal CMR enabled precise detection of size and location of cardiac rhabdomyomas in multiple planes as early as 16 weeks' gestation (Fig. 14). Fetal CMR can identify well pericardial effusion as an isolated finding or in association with structural cardiac anomalies or hydropes fetalis (Fig. 14B).

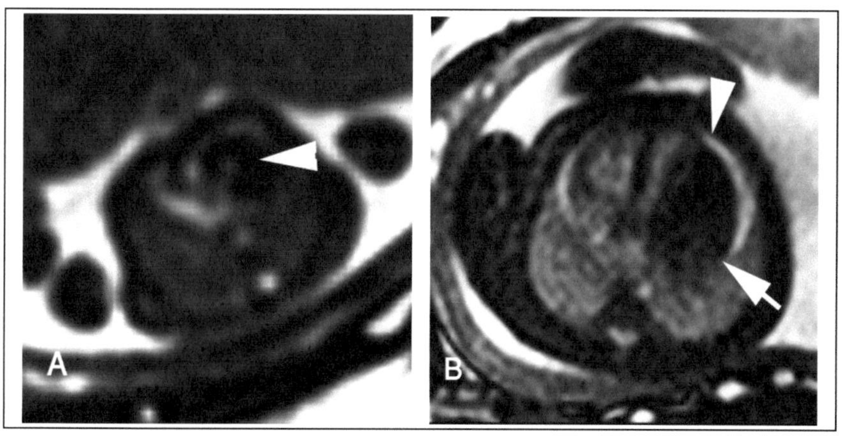

Fig. 14. In-utero MR imaging of cardiac rhabdomyomas. (A) Axial T2-SSFP four-chamber view of 16 weeks' gestation fetus show low signal intensity rhabdomyoma of the free left ventricular wall and interventricular septum (arrowhead). (B) Axial T2- SSFP four-chamber view of 26 weeks' gestation fetus shows a large intracardiac mass (rhabdomyoma) within the left ventricle (arrow). Note the associated high signal intensity rim of pericardial effusion (arrowhead).

2.4 Fetal CMR findings in complex congenital heart disease (CHD), CHD associated with extra-cardiac abnormalities and fetal syndromes

Multiple cardiac abnormalities can be concomitant in complex congenital heart diseases (Cohen et al, 2001). In our experience, in-utero MRI using SSFP sequence was useful in assessment of fetal heart anatomy and depiction of multiple cardiac structural abnormalities in complex congenital heart diseases in CHD. E.g., in Fallot's disease, fetal CMR identified septal defects (ventricular septal defect (VSD) in Fallot's tetralogy and atrioventricular (AV) canal in Fallot's pentalogy respectively) in association with overriding of aorta and stenotic pulmonary artery. CMR diagnosed a fetus with Transposition of great arteries (TGA) (Fig.13A) in concomitant with AV canal.

Complex congenital cardiac anomalies can be seen in the rare conjoined heart twins. Conjoined twins result from a separation defect in the embryonic plaque between the 13th and 17th days of gestation. Cardiac fusion is a very rare malformation that can be seen in twins conjoined at the level of the chest (Thoracopagus). Detailed evaluation of the degree of union and number of shared organs is required to predict the viability and prognosis of fetuses (O'Neill et al, 1988). In our series, fetal CMR helped in conjunction with ultrasonography in prenatal assessment of a thoracopagus conjoined twins with a shared eight-chamber heart and in a dicephalic twin with a shared 4-chamber heart (Fig. 15).

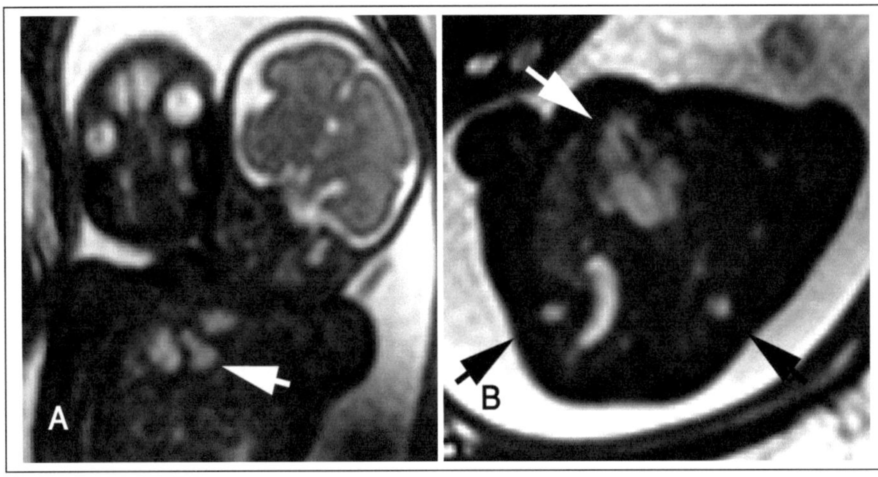

Fig. 15. In-utero CMR of dicephalic twin with a shared 4-chamber heart (A) Coronal T2-SSFP identifies dicephalic tripus dibrachius twin with single heart (arrow). (B). Axial T2-SSFP shows double spine (black arrows) and a single four chamber heart (white arrow).

Complex cardiac anomalies are frequently associated with extra-cardiac malformations (Prakash et al, 2010). The diagnosis of a congenital heart disease in a fetus should include prompt evaluation for associated non cardiac malformations and diagnosis of genetic syndromes (Carvalho et al, 2002). In-utero MRI can depict extracardiac anatomy and abnormalities of fetal brain, spine, lungs, liver, spleen, kidneys, and gastro-intestinal tract (Frates et al, 2004; Levine, 2006, Saleem et al, 2009). In our series, fetal MRI detected extracardiac abnormalities in association with cardiac structural abnormalities that helped in prenatal diagnosis of fetal syndromes. Extracardiac abnormalities associated with CHD include central nervous system, cranio-facial, urinary tract, lungs, gastrointestinal tract, liver, spleen, skeletal system, and miscellaneous abnormalities such as nuchal thickening and ascites. Examples from our cohort included: presence of cerebral subependymal tubers and giant cell astrocytoma in association with cardiac rhabdomyomas in fetuses with tuberous sclerosis (Fig.16). Prenatal detection of a tumor in the region of foramen of Monro should raise the suspicion of congenital subependymal giant cell astrocytoma associated with tuberous sclerosis (Mirkin et al, 1999).

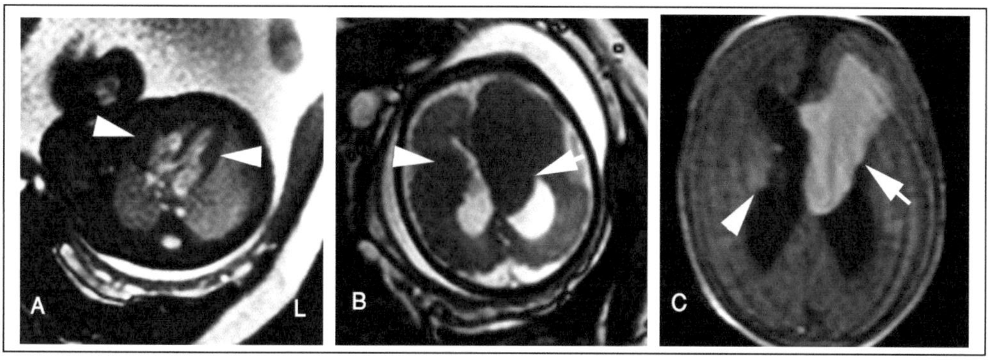

Fig. 16. Subependymal lesions in association with cardiac masses suggest the prenatal diagnosis of tuberous sclerosis. In-utero MRI using T2-SSFP at 29 weeks' gestation, of the chest (A) revealed multiple cardiac rhabdomyomas (arrowheads) associated with multiple cerebral subependymal masses (B) along the right lateral ventricle (arrowhead) as well as a large giant-cell astroytoma of the left foramen of Monro (arrow). Postnatal axial post-contrast MRI of the brain of the same case at the age of 7 days (C) documents enhancing congenital subependymal astrocytoma of foramen of Monro (arrow) as well as the non-enhancing subependymal tubers at the right lateral ventricle (arrowhead).

In our series, MRI documented the association of urinary tract dilatation with hypoplastic right heart in a fetus. These findings suggested the prenatal diagnosis of Kashani syndrome (Kashani et al, 1984). Identification of microcephaly, sacral agenesis in addition to Fallot's tetralogy, right sided aortic arch and aberrant left subclavian artery in another fetus suggested the prenatal diagnosis of cerebro-arthrodigital syndrome (Spranger et al, 1980) (Fig. 17).

In chromosomal abnormalities, fetal MRI identified Dandy Walker malformation in association with AV canal in a fetus with Trisomy 21 and holoprosencephaly in association with VSD (Fig.11A) in a fetus with trisomy 13.

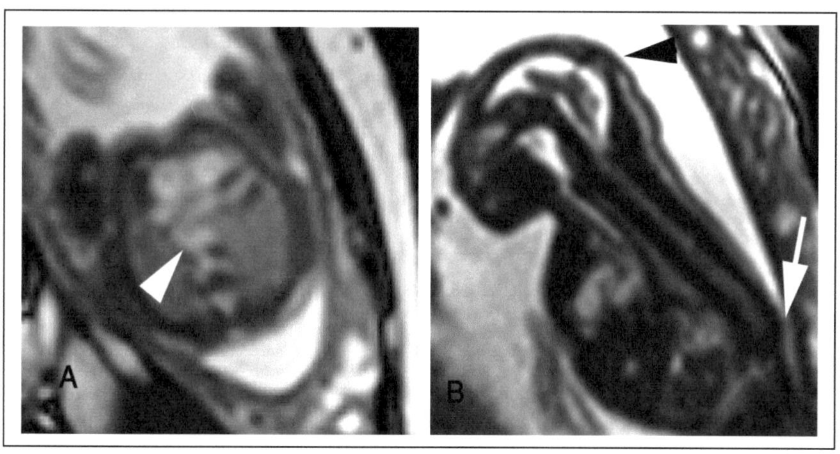

Fig. 17. Fetal MRI of a cerebro-arthrodigital syndrome at 20 weeks' gestation. (A) Axial T2-SSFP of heart shows right sided aortic arch with aberrant left subclavian artery (arrowhead) in association with Fallot's tetralogy. Sagittal MRI of the fetal body of the same fetus shows associated microcephaly (arrowhead) and sacral agenesis (arrow).

Fetal MRI documented prenatal ultrasonographic findings of AV canal defect, cerebral ventriculomegaly, and micromelia in a fetus with Fryns and Moerman syndrome (Fryns & Moerman, 1993). According to a report of 32 fetuses assessed for congenital heart disease, fetal MRI permitted identification of extracardiac anomalies associated with cardiac abnormalities. The authors document that MRI detected adjunctive fetal anomalies (particularly in CNS and neck) that US did not depict (Manganaro et al, 2008).

2.5 Fetal CMR limitations and future

Quantitative analysis of CMR was feasible in two fetuses with cardiac malformations by Fogel and colleagues. They found that measurements of ventricular volume could be obtained with MRI but not with fetal echocardiography. Both fetuses, however, were at advanced ages of gestation (34.5 and 36 weeks), and fetal sedation was necessary in one case. (Fogel et al, 2005).

Although cine MRI with the SSFP sequence is an established method of evaluation of cardiac function, imaging of a beating heart in a moving fetus is more complicated. The normal fetal heart rate of 120–160 beats per minute and unpredictable fetal body motion impair image quality owing to motion artifacts during MRI acquisition in utero (Guo et al, 2006). However, with the advent of parallel MRI technique, acquisition time is markedly reduced, yet image quality meets clinical requirements. Studies have shown that cine MRI in utero with steady-state acquisition and parallel imaging may be useful in the assessment of fetal body and cardiac movements. (Guo et al, 2006).Cine MR sequences for the evaluation of the contractile function of the fetal heart was attempted recently in fetuses with congenital heart diseases, yet it did not provide real-time images due to the high fetal heart rate and lack of fetal cardiac triggering (Manganaro et al, 2008).

Future fetal MRI sequences can take advantage of the improvement in radiofrequency and computing technology to decrease acquisition time and increase signal-to-noise ratio and image resolution. Fetal cardiac gating was attempted in sheep (Yamamura et al, 2010). As MRI technology advances, images of the heart are expected to be much clearer and to be acquired in a shorter time, allowing dramatic improvement in anatomic and functional MRI of the fetal heart. Reliable cardiac imaging in utero may have implications in the management of congenital heart disease, opening the possibility of fetal surgery (Saleem, 2008).

3. Conclusion

Fetal CMR facilitates visualization of the cardiac structures in multiple fetal body planes as well as cardiac axes. Fetal MR image analysis is possible using the anatomic segmental approach to congenital heart diseases. These features are potentially helpful for further characterization of cardiovascular abnormalities in utero. This chapter discusses the potentials of CMR in demonstrating normal and abnormal fetal heart rather than comparing it to echocardiography. Further studies are needed to evaluate the diagnostic utility and accuracy of in utero MRI of normal and abnormal hearts in correlation with the reference standard technique, fetal echocardiography. Further work is needed to advance MR imaging of the fetal heart through improvement of the available MRI sequences as well as introduction of functional MRI sequences and fetal cardiac gating.

4. Acknowledgment

I acknowledge Miss Amal Mahmoud, MRI operator at Cairo University, Egypt.

5. References

Brugger, PC.; Stuhr, F.; Linder, C.; Prayer, D. (2006). Methods of fetal MR: beyond T2-weighted imaging. *Eur J Radiol* Vol.57, pp. 172-181, 0720-048X

Carvalho, JS.; Mavrides, E; Shinebourne, EA; Campbell, S; Thilaganathan, B. (2002). Improving the effectiveness of routine prenatal screening for major congenital heart defects. *Heart* Vol.88, pp. 387-391, 1355-6037

Carvalho, JS.; Ho, SY.; Shinebourne, EA. (2005). Sequential segmental analysis in complex fetal cardiac abnormalities: a logical approach to diagnosis. *Ultrasound Obstet Gynecol* Vol.26 pp. 105–111, 0960-7692

Chung, HW.; Chen, CY.; Zimmerman, RA.; Lee, KW.; Lee, CC.; Chin, SC. (2000). T2-weighted Fast MR imaging with true FISP versus HASTE comparative efficacy in the evaluation of normal fetal brain maturation. Am J Roentgenol Vol.275, pp. 1375-1480, 0361-803X

Clements, H.; Duncan, KR.; Fielding K.; Gowland, PA.; Johnson, IR.; Baker, PB. (2000). Infants exposed to MRI in utero have a normal paediatric assessment at 9 months of age. *Br J Radiol* Vol.73, pp. 190-194, 0007-1285

Cohen, MS. (2001). Fetal diagnosis and management of congenital heart disease. *Clin Perinatol* Vol.28, pp. 11-29, 0095-5108

Finn, JP.; Nael, K.; Deshpande, V.; Ratib, O.; Laub, G. (2006). Cardiac MR imaging: state of the technology. *Radiology* Vol.241, No.2, pp. 338 - 354, 0033-8419

Fogel, MA.; Wilson, RD.; Flake, A.; Johnson, M.; Cohen, D.; McNeal, G.; Tian, ZY.; Rychik, J. (2005). Preliminary investigations into a new method of functional assessment of the fetal heart using a novel application of"real-time"cardiac magnetic resonance imaging. *Fetal Diagn Ther* Vol.20, pp. 475–480, 1015-3837

Forbus, GA.; Atz, AM.; Shirali, GS. (2004).Implications and limitations of an abnormal fetal echocardiogram. Am J Cardiol Vol.94, pp. 688-689, 0002-9149

Frates, M.; Kumar, A.; Benson, C.; Ward, V.; Tempany, C. (2004). Fetal anomalies: comparison of MR imaging and US for diagnosis. *Radiology* 2004; Vol.232, pp. 398-404, 0033-8419

Fryns, JP.; Moerman P. (1993). Short limbed dwarfism, genital hypoplasia, sparse hair, and vertebral anomalies: a variant of Ellis-van Creveld syndrome?. *J Med Genet* Vol.30, pp.322-324, 0022-2593

Fyler, DC.; Buckley, LP.; Hellenbrand, WE.; Cohn, HE. (1980). Report of the New England Regional Infant Care Program. *Pediatrics* Vol.65, Suppl. 375-461, 0031-4005

Glenn, OA.; Barkovich, AJ. (2006). Magnetic Resonance Imaging of the fetal brain and spine: an increasingly important tool in prenatal diagnosis, Part 1. *Am J Neuroradiol* Vol.27, pp. 1604-161, 0195-6108

Gorincour, G.; Bourliere-Najean, B.; BONELLO, b.; Philip, N.; Potier, A.; Kreitann, B.; Petit, P. (2007). Feasibility of fetal cardiac magnetic resonance imaging: preliminary experience. *Ultrasound Obstet Gynecol* Vol.29, pp. 105-108, 0960-7692

Guo, WY.; Ono, S.; Oi, S.; Shen, SH.; Wong, T.; Chung, HW.; Hung, JY. (2006). Dynamic motion analysis of fetuses with central nervous system disorders by cine magnetic resonance imaging using fast imaging employing steady state acquisition and parallel imaging. *J Neurosurg* Vol. 105, pp. 94 -100, 0022-3085

Hoffman, JI; Kaplan, S. (2002). The incidence of congenital heart disease. *J Am Coll Cardiol* Vol.39, pp. 1890-1900, 0735-1097

Kanal, E.; Borgstede, JP.; Barkovich, AJ.; Bell, C.; Bradley, WG.; Etheridge, S.; Felmlee, JP.; Froelich, JW.; Hayden, J.; Kaminski, EM.; Lester, JW Jr.; Scoumis, EA.; Zaremba

LA.; Zinniger, MD.; American College of Radiology. (2002). American College of Radiology white paper on MR safety. *Am J Roentgenol* Vol.178, pp. 1335-1347, 0361-803X

Kashani, IA.; Strom, CM.; Utley, JE.; Marin-Garcia, J.; Higgins, CB. (1984). Hypoplastic pulmonary arteries and aorta with obstructive uropathy in 2 siblings. Angiology Vol.35, No.4, pp. 252-256, 0003-3197

Kivelitz, DE.; Muhler, M.; Rake, A.; Scheer, I.; Chaoui, R. (2004). MRI of cardiac rhabdomyoma in the fetus. *Eur Radiol* Vol.14, No. 8, pp. 1513-1516, 0938-7994

Kleinman, CS.; Hobbin, JC.; Jaffe, CC.; Lynch, DC.; Tlaner, NS. (1980). Echocardiographic studies of the human fetus: prenatal diagnosis of congenital heart disease and cardiac dysrrhythmias. *Pediatrics* Vol.65, pp. 1059-1067, 0031-4005

Levine, D. (2006). Obstetric MRI. *Top Magn Reson Imaging* Vol.24, No.1, pp. 1-15, 0899-3459

Manganaro, L.; Savelli s.; Di Maurizio, M.; Perrone, A.; Tesei, J.; Francioso, A.; Angeletti, A.; Coratella, F.; Irimia, D.; Fierro, F.; Vnetriglia, F.; Ballesio, L. (2008). Potential role of fetal cardiac evaluation with magnetic resoance imaging: preliminary experience. *Prenat Diagn* Vol.28, pp. 148-156, 0197-3851

Manganaro, L.; Savelli s.; Di Maurizio, M.; et al. (2009). Assessment of congenital heart disease (CHD): Is there a role for fetal magnetic resonance imaging (MRI)?*European Journal of Radiology Vol.*72, pp. 172-180, 0720-048X

Mirkin, LD.; Ey, EH.; Chaparro, M. (1999). Congenital subependymal giant-cell astrocytoma: case report with prental ultrasonogram. *Pediatr Radiol* Vol. 29, No. 10, pp. 776-780, 0301-0449

O'Neill, JA.; Holcomb, GWIII.; Schnauffer, L.; Templeton, JM Jr.; Bishop, HC.; Ross, AJ III.; Duckett, JW.; Norwood, WI.; Ziegler, MM.; Koop, CE. (1988). Surgical experience with thirteen conjoined twins. *Ann Surg* Vol. 208, pp. 299-312, 0003-4932

Prakash, A.; Powell, A J.; Geva, T. (2010). Multimodality Noninvasive Imaging for Assessment of Congenital Heart Disease. *Circ Cardiovasc Imaging* Vol.3, No.1, pp. 112–125, 1941-9651

Saleem, SN. (2008). Feasibility of Magnetic resonance imaging (MRI) of the fetal heart using balanced Steady-State-Free-Precession (SSFP) sequence along fetal body and cardiac planes. *AJR* Vol. 191, pp. 1208-1215, 0361-803X

Saleem, SN.; Said, A-H.; Abdel-Raouf, M.; El-Kattan, EA.; Zaki, MS.; Madkour, N.; Mostafa, S. (2009). Fetal MRI in the evaluation of fetuses referred for sonographically suspected neural tube defects (NTDs): impact on diagnosis and management decision. *Neuroradiology* 2009 Vol.51, No.11, pp. 761-772, 0028-3940

Smith, RS.; Comstock, CH.; Kirk, JS.; Lee, W. (1995). Ultrasonographic left axis deviation: a marker for fetal anomalies. *Obstet Gynecol* Vol. 85, pp. 187-191, 0029-7844

Spranger, JW.; Schinzel, A.; Myers, T.; Ryan, J.; Giedion , A.; Opitz, JM. (1980). Cerebroarthrodigital syndrome: a newly recognized formal genesis syndrome in three patients with apparent arthromyodysplasia and sacral agenesis, brain malformation and digital hypoplasia. *Am J Med Genet* Vol.5, No. 2, pp. 13-24, 1552-4825

Tennstedt, C.; Chaoui, R.; Korner, H.; Dietel, M. (1999). Spectrum of congenital heart defects and extracardiac malformations associated with chromosomal abnormalities: results of a seven year necropsy study. *Heart* Vol.82, pp. 34-39, 1355-6037

Yamamura, J.; Frisch, M.; Ecker, H.; Graessner, J.; Hecher, K.; Adam, G.; Wedegärtner, U. (2010). Self-gating MR imaging of the fetal heart: comparison with real cardiac triggering. *European Radiology* Vol.21, No.1, pp., 142-149, 0938-7994

11

Models of Perspective on Various Kinds of Complex Congenital Heart Defects

Huai-Min Chen
Department Cardiovascular Surgery,
Kaohsiung Medical University Hospital, Kaohsiung,
Assistant Professor of Surgery, School of Medicine,
Kaohsiung Medical University, Kaohsiung
Taiwan

1. Introduction

Understanding normal and abnormal cardiac structures is best achieved through pathological specimens. Some cardiologists or cardiac surgeons are fortunate enough to work at centers where hearts from autopsies are preserved and catalogued for teaching purposes, but most practitioners still need to form a mental picture of the cardiac pathology and morphology. Actually, specific anatomic and diagnostic issues often remain in question after cautious preoperative and serial studies, and some physicians frequently fail to perform this mental exercise consistently. If we have a model which presents the cardiac anatomy and segmental relationship in a perspective view with a simple hand-drawn three-dimensional model to improve the understanding of the complex heart, it will be accessible to inexperienced staff and medical students and also to patients' families, and it will also save the considerable cost of image reconstruction. Some cardiac defects such as ASD, VSD, PDA, or TAPVR are easily visualized after echocardiographic examinations, but others remain challenges, especially hearts with misaligned cardiac segments and hearts with a double outlet right ventricle. In order to classify and clearly understand the variants of congenital cardiac defects, Dr. Van Praagh introduced three cardiac segments to establish a cardiac set. He used the coding system of the atrium, ventricle and great vessel to describe the hemodynamics and relationships of cardiac anatomy. The first code represents the atrium status including situs solitus or inversus. The second code represents the ventricular status including ventricular D-loop and L-loop. The third code represents the relationships of the great arteries including the aorta located anteriorly to the pulmonary trunk (D-malposition or L-malposition), and the aorta located posteriorly to the pulmonary trunk (solitus or inversus position). The system clearly categorizes complex cardiac defects, but different cardiac anomalies can be present under the same coding conditions and the hemodynamics of the codes and the connections between ventricular-arterial segments are still not easily understood by inexperienced personnel because the system lacks stereotactic structures. This is why we wished to develop a simple three-dimensional model to depict complex hearts. Before creating the models of variant congenital cardiac defects, we needed to determine the stereography of anomaly heart. We found the transverse cross-section of heart at the atrio-ventricular junction offers the best reconstructive level for stereo-images because of its coverage of most cardiac structures and defects. From the picture, we can clearly visualize the heart with its specific relationships at the atrio-ventricular and ventricular-arterial segments. For the atrium, we used a broad-base triangular appendage to indicate the morphological right atrium; a finger and tube-like structure indicates the morphological left atrium. For the atrio-ventricular valves, we used the oval annulus with tri-leaflets, which indicates the atrio-ventricular valve of the morphological right ventricle; the bean-like structure with bi-leaflets indicates the atrio-ventricular valve of the morphological left ventricle; the aorta is indicated by the two coronary ostia. The tricuspid valves and pulmonary valves are separated by the ventricular infundibular fold (VIF) and infundibulum septum (crista supraventricularis).

2. The differentiation of great artery and aortic arch

The embryonic courses of the cardiovascular system from the beginning of the cardiac tube to differentiation into the atriums, the ventricles, and the great arteries, and the setup of the complete circulation are very complicated and delicate. We will discuss mainly the changes among the ventricles and the great arteries including the migration, septation and absorption of the truncus; the following development of aorta and pulmonary artery; and finally, the possible variants of connection between ventricle and corresponding great artery. Understanding such embryonic defects and anomalies are very helpful to interpret the hemodynamic and treatment of complex congenital cardiac defects, especially in the part of mal-connections of cardiac segments.

3. The setup of circulation

The initial circulation system is achieved by the almost simultaneous formation of the heart and three networks: intraembryonic, vitelline, and umbilico-allantoic. From the third week to the beginning of the second month of embryonic age, the embryo lives on its small reserves of yolk sac (the vitelline circulation); the primitive intraembryonic circulation and allantoic circulation are forming. At the end of the second month, the vitelline circulation disappears and the allantoic circulation becomes the placenta stage by connecting the umbilical vessels and placenta.

4. The transformation of aorta

The primitive arterial system undergoes numerous modifications in its development, which are quite complex in the anterior region where aortic arches are formed. The ventral arteries, the first aortic arches, and the dorsal aortas are continuous. In each branchial arch, 5 pairs of aortic arches are formed successively and join the ventral to the dorsal aortas. The dorsal aortas extend from the cranial region to the caudal region and develop paired segmental arteries to the somites. The left and right primitive ventral aortas and aortic arches arise from the dilated terminal region of truncus, known as aortic sac, and terminate in the primitive dorsal aorta of the corresponding side. The two dorsal aortas approach each other and fuse at about week 4 to form the adult descending aorta. During weeks 6 to 8, the primitive aortic arch pattern is transformed into the basic adult arterial arrangement. The details of differentiations of five paired arches are discussed as below:

5. Regression of aortic arch

In Fig.1 we demonstrate the regression of aortic arch. Six pairs of aortic arches in pharyngeal arches are theoretically formed; however, the fifth pair is essentially only a temporary doubling of the fourth pair, and the aortic arches are never all present at the same time. When the third and fourth arches appear, the first and second arches have disappeared (before 31 days of embryo age).

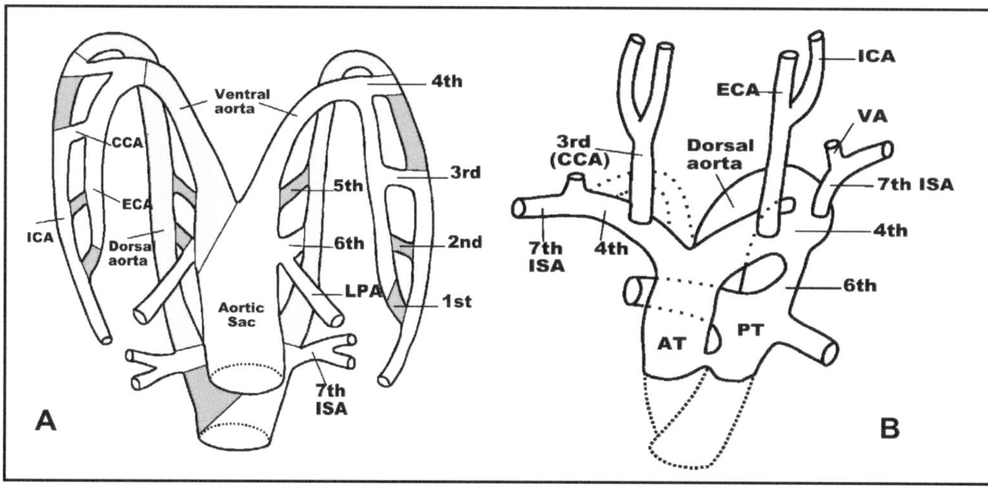

Fig. 1. The developments and regression of aortic arches from embryonic pharyngeal arches to adult aorta. Fig.1.A presents the primitive aorta in embryo stage, and the gray-colored area marks the regions will undergo regression and absorption. Fig.1-B presents the basic adult aorta. AT: aortic trunk; CCA: common carotid artery; ECA: external carotid artery; ICA: internal carotid artery; ISA: intersegmental artery; LPA: left pulmonary artery; PT:pulmonary trunk; VA: vertebral artery.

The first and second paired aortic arches are nearly complete regressed in the main except for the small part that develops into capillary structures of the maxillary artery; the dorsal aorta between the third and fourth paired aortic arches will be totally absorbed, making the bilateral third aortic arches form common carotid arteries and proximal part of internal carotid arteries (ICAs) on both sides, and its distal part of the primitive ventral aorta will form the external carotid artery (ECA) as well as the distal part of the primitive dorsal aortic forms the internal carotid artery (ICA); the fourth arch on the left forms the aortic arch which is located between the left common carotid artery (LCCA) and the left subclavian artery (LSCA), and the right one forms the right innominate artery and the proximal part of the right subclavian artery (RSCA); the fifth arch almost completely regresses before developing; the sixth arch appears during the middle period of the 5th week of embryo, the bilateral proximal parts (close to aortic sac) will form the left pulmonary artery (LPA) and the right pulmonary artery (RPA), but the distal part of the left side will form the ductal arteriosus, and the distal part of the right one will completely regress. The distal part of the pulmonary artery is derived by buds of the sixth arch and develops into the pulmonary system. Once the partitioning of the truncus finishes, the pulmonary arteries will arise from the pulmonary trunk. After the pulmonary vascularization completes, the primitive right dorsal aorta will totally and completely regress from the site of bifurcation.

Concerning the seventh intersegmental artery (ISA), its left part forms the LSCA, and the right part forms the distal RSCA, so the primitive dorsal aorta between the 4th arch and 7th ISA will totally disappear. The left dorsal aorta goes on remodeling by a wide margin making the left 7th ISA, while the ductus arteriosus and the left fourth arch link together in a very short distance.

6. Developments of Cono-Truncus-Aortic sac (aortic-pulmonary septum)

The vascular developments and changes we will state as follows:

From ventricular outflow tract to aortic sac, the truncus can be divided into three regions by the level. The proximal part of the conus is linked with the ventricle, followed successively by the truncus, and the distal part of the aortic sac. Finally the truncus will differentiate into the aorta and pulmonary artery by complex procedures. Firstly, the conus will undergo three stages of development including septation, migration and absorption. During conus septation, the conus will present 2 masses: Dextro-Dorsal Conal Crest (DDCC) and Sinistra-Ventral Conal Crest (SVCC). The DDCC extends to ventricular outflow tract and fuses with the Superior Endocardial Cushion (SEC)) and the Right Lateral Endocardial Cushion (RLEC) to form crista supraventricularis which will be a septum among the Tricuspid valve and pulmonary valve; SVCC extends to ventricular outflow tract and forms the left part of the outlet septum (conal septum) with some SEC, which becomes a part of the primitive interventricular septum (Fig.2).

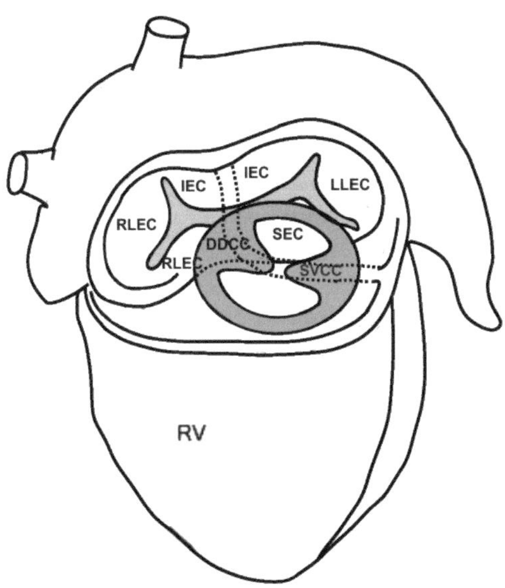

Fig. 2. The anatomic and structural relationships of endocardial cushion and conus-truncus at the level of atrio-ventricular and ventricular-arterial junctions. DDCC: dextro-dorsal conal crest; IEC: inferior endocardial cushion;; LLEC: lateral endocardial cushion ; RLEC: right lateral endocardial cushion ; SEC: superior endocardial cushion; SVCC: sinistra-ventral conal crest.

Two masses will present in truncal level, too. It is Dextro-Superior Truncal Swelling (DSTS) and Sinistra-Inferior Truncal Swelling (SITS) respectively. The DDCC will extend superiorly and fuse with the DSTS, and the SVCC also extends superiorly and fuses with SITS (Fig.3.1). During the fusion processes procession, two masses of right intercalated truncal swelling (RITS) and left intercalated truncal swelling (LITS) in the pulmonary conus and aortic conus will present between the conal and truncal levels, which will fuse with DSTS and SITS and form the future semilunar valves of the great arteries. From the above-mentioned discussion, we can observe the vascularities which form the pulmonary system are developed from the sixth paired arches and their buds. The arches are closed to the aortic sac and extended from ventral aorta to dorsal aorta, so the posterior cavity of the aortic sac will differentiate into the pulmonary trunk and fuse with the primitive pulmonary artery to become the pulmonary system (Fig.1). So after septation of the truncus, the pulmonary trunk, no matter whether right-sided or left-sided, will be at the rear of the aortic trunk at the level of terminal aortic sac (aortic-pulmonary septum). This concept is very important for us to realize the various types of ventricular-artery mal-connection and to judge the possible truncal positions.

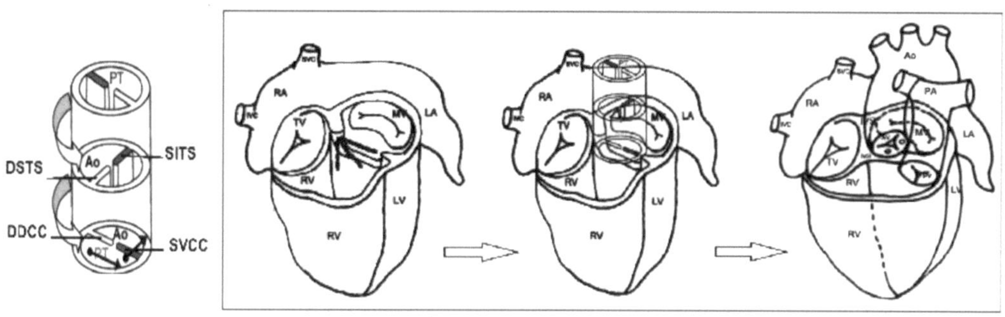

Fig. 3.1. The creation of cardiac perspective model step by step with the combination of truncus and heart with atrio-ventricular structures. There are three possibilities in direction of conal septum above the primitive interventricular septum. The conal septum is parallel to the IVS in this figure. The extension and spiral rotation of conal septum (DDCC-SVCC) to truncal septum (DSTS-SITS) and more extension to aorto-pulmonary septum result in the pulmonary artery rotates from right to left and from anterior to posterior. DDCC: dextro-dorsal conal crest ; DSTS: Dextro-Superior Truncal Swelling ; SITS: Sinistra-Inferior Truncal Swelling ; SVCC: Sinistra-Ventral Conal Crest.

7. Development of endocardial cushion

Before we study the field of ventricular-arterial connection and the atrioventricular septal defect (endocardial cushion defect), we should know the development and composites of the endocardial cushion (Fig.2). The endocardial cushion is fused by the inferior endocardial cushion (IEC), superior endocardial cushion (SEC), right lateral endocardial cushion (RLEC), left lateral endocardial cushion (LLEC), interatrial septum (IAS), primitive interventricular septum (IVS), dextrodorsal conal crest (DDCC), and sinistroventrol conal crest (SVCC). The DDCC and SVCC in Conal trunk (cavity) will fuse with the primitive interventricular septum and form the conal septum. The DDCC will extend to SEC and RLEC, which changes to the cristal supraventricularis. The cristal supraventricularis can be separated into the septal portion and parietal portion (ventricular infundibular fold, i.e., free wall between inferior vena cava and RV). The ventricular infundibular fold (VIF) is the main part to separate the tricuspid valve and the pulmonary valve. The SEC will develop into the free portion of anterior mitral leaflet, the left surface portion of the infundibular septum, the external wall of the left ventricular outlet tract (LVOT), and the left side surface of the outlet septum.

The IEC will develop into the septal portion of the anterior mitral leaflet, the septal leaflet of the tricuspid valve, and the inlet septum of the IVS. The IEC will fuse with the septum primum and close the foramen primum. The LLEC develops into the posterior mitral leaflet, and the RLEC develops into the posterior leaflet and the lateral portion of the anterior-lateral leaflet of the tricuspid valve. The DDCC differentiates into the median portion of anterior leaflet of the tricuspid valve, the right side surface of cristal supraventricularis and outlet septum. The secondary inter-ventricular foramen is closed by the fusion of the IEC, primitive IVS, DDCC, and SVCC (Fig.2). The fusion of DDCC and SVCC will become the conal septum, i.e. the parietal band of septal marginal trabecularis (SMT). It can extend anteriorly to form the anterior limb of SMT, and extend posteriorly to form the posterior limb of SMT. The portion above the two limbs is the septal portion of crista supraventricularis which is formed by the regression of DDCC and SEC, it also can be called as infundibular septum or outlet septum. The other part is the parietal portion of crista supraventricularis which is formed by the regression of DDCC and RLEC; it is located between the posterior limb of SMT, primitive IVS, and the free wall of right ventricle. It is also called as the ventricular infundibular fold (VIF). The parietal band (anterior limb and posterior limb) and the septal band of right ventricle we can group as the septal marginal trabecularis (Fig.3.2). That is to say, the conal crest of DDCC and SVCC inserts itself from the posterior limb of septal marginal trabecularis (SMT) to the anterior limb of SMT, and the conal septum is formed. The conal septum and the crista supraventricularis will separate the right and left ventricle. But before the conal septum does not completely fuse, the ventricle and truncus still link through the primitive interventricular foramen, so the free border of the primitive IVS and the endocardial cushion will be the margins of the primitive interventricular foramen. After the fusion processes of DDCC and SVCC are completed in upward and downward directions, the primitive interventricular foramen is then closed. The ventricle will link with its own trunk at this moment, and only the secondary interventricular foramen is left to communicate between two ventricles (Fig.6). If the secondary interventricular foramen is still open after birth, then it would be the so-called ventricular septal defect (VSD). Finally, the membrane septum will close the secondary interventricular foramen and the primitive IVS, and the course of ventricular septation is completed. The margins of the secondary interventricular foramen are as below: the posterior inferior margin is made up by the free border of IEC; the anterior margin is made up by the free border of primitive IVS; and the floor is supported by the conal septum.

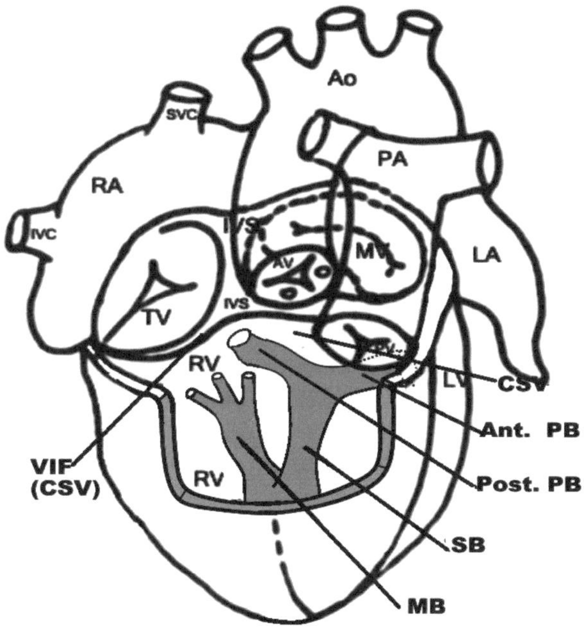

Fig. 3.2. The longitudinal cross-section of right ventricle to demonstrate the anatomies of right surface of inter-ventricular septum. CSV: cristal supraventricularis; MB: moderate band; PB: parietal band; SB: septal band; VIF: ventricular infundibular fold.

8. The spiral rotation of truncus and arrangement of great arteries

Most of the developmental defects of ventricular outflow tract are related with cardiac neural crest. During the course of embryonic development, neural crest provides the cells to differentiate into a septum to separate the aortic trunk and pulmonary trunk. In animal models, we can find the outflow tract defects in neural crest-resected embryos. These anomalies involve aorta, pulmonary artery, and mal-alignment or mal-connection of ventricles. From the outflow tract to the terminal of cardiac tube (Aortic sac) during the time of normal development, its endocardiac jelly inside will form a pair of cushions arranged in opposite directions, and these cushions will be twined spirally together in the course of extending, and run through the whole tract. The cells come from neural crest infiltration and migration to outflow tract and distal endocardial cushion at the same time, and the next is the integration of endocardial cushion. This course will begin from the distal part of truncus; the terminal outflow tract will be divided into aortic trunk and pulmonary trunk, and merge with meschymal cells of the posterior wall of aortic sac. The aortic trunk connects with the left 4th paired arch, and pulmonary truck connects with the left 6th paired arch.

From these models, we observe the septum will extend from ventricular outflow tract to conal and truncal septum, if posterior aspect of conal cavity can extend to anterior aspect of truncal cavity after spiral rotation, it will present a relative longer outflow tract. That is to say, there will be fibrous discontinuity (muscle band) between ventricle and great artery. But if it is anterior aspect of conal cavity extending to be the posterior aspect of truncal cavity during the septal rotation (such as the pulmonary artery in {S.L.D}-IAI), then it will have relatively short outflow tract, and may present fibrous continuity in ventricular-arterial connection. On the contrary, if it is the posterior aspect of conal cavity rotating to posterior aspect of truncal cavity, it will be the same situation with a relatively short outflow tract and fibrous continuity in ventricular-arterial connection (the aorta in {S.D.S}-normal heart). In the vertical conal septum, the direction of interventricular septum (ventricular looping status) and spiral rotation of truncal septum will be the key points, but the median cavity is the usual one with the fibrous continuity. The left one in D-looping status and the right one in L-looping status stands for the median conus respectively.

9. Built-up the perspective model

In Fig.3.1, we have reconstructed the perspective model with the combination of heart with atrio-ventricular structures and truncus step by step to exhibit the A-V and V-A relationships. Really, any model can be built by such a method. The first step is to define the ventricular looping status and the direction of IVS, which is right-posterior to left-anterior in D-looping ventricle and left-posterior to right-anterior in L-looping ventricle. The conal septum may be parallel to the IVS or not depending on the conal position and direction. There are three even four (horizontal) possibilities of different conal directions that could be considered. The second step is to determine the position and rotation of truncal cavity in individual great artery. Such a rotation can be counterclockwise or clockwise in direction or even with no rotation. I believe the counterclockwise rotation of the conal-truncal septum more easily happens in D-looping heart and the clockwise rotation of the conal-truncal septum more easily happens in L-looping heart. The final step is to put the pulmonary trunk in posterior position with the decision of aorta in rightward or leftward, and the descending aorta is located on the same side with the main pulmonary artery. In this figure we use the {S.D.S}-normal heart to demonstrate the procedures of how to build the perspective cardiac models.

10. Hypothesis of cardiac segmental connections

The heart is differentiated from a cardial tube into two atriums, two ventricles, and two trunks; how to guarantee its connection's exactness is very important for the survival of the organism after birth. How to keep its correct relationship after serial migration, septation, spiral rotation and absorption between the distinct ventricle and related trunk is the field that we still fail to understand in depth. Actually, among them, every step finishes under rigorous genetic regulation and control. Even so, the principle of hydromechanics must be followed in blood flow. So we put forward the following assumptions to explain the possible developments and variations from ventricle to conus, conus to truncus and to the aorto-pulmonary septum:

1. Just as in the previous discussion, the pulmonary trunk which arises from aortic sac, no matter whether left-sided or right-sided, will be in the posterior aspect.
2. From conal septum to truncal septum and truncal septum to aorto-pulmonary septum, the angle of spiral rotation between them should not be too wide.
3. From conal septum to truncal septum, and truncal septum to aorto-pulmonary septum, its direction of extension (i.e. spiral rotation) will be identical, and the pulmonary trunk after complete septation will be the location in posterior aspect.

4. The rotational direction of truncal septum will change the blood flow from ventricular outflow tract (ventricle-conus) and result in different hemodynamics (such as {S.D.L} which can be the anatomically corrected malposition (ACM), and can be the complete TGA (cTGA), which is decided by the rotational direction of truncal septum).
5. The conal septum and truncal septum are similar to water diversion boards which drain the blood flow from ventricle to its own circulation.

11. Variants of the septation and spiral rotation of Cono-Truncal septum

In Figs. 4.1 ~ 4.3, we have listed the different possible abnormalities of the truncus regarding the septal septation and spiral rotation. Discussed in aortic sac level as above, only the two kinds of right-posterior pulmonary trunk and left-posterior pulmonary trunk are possible; the DSTS and SITS also determine the truncal septum in the direction of left-posterior to right-anterior in truncal level, but sometimes may present Dextro-Inferior Truncal Swelling (DITS) and Sinistra-Superior Truncal Swelling (SSTS), then the truncal septum will be turned into right-posterior to left-anterior oblique direction.

So we can sort the relationships of the two great arteries as four groups by the position of aortic trunk in the truncal level according to the classification and coding system of Dr. Van Praagh, they are {--.--.S} (Ao is right posterior to PA),{--.--.I} (Ao is left posterior to PA), {--.--.D }(Ao is right anterior to PA), and {--.--.L}(Ao is left anterior to PA).

As for the direction of conal septum which is decided by DDCC and SVCC, the direction of conal septum is right-posterior to left anterior oblique direction and is identical to the interventricular septum in the normal D-looping ventricle. But this may present the abnormal conal septums with Dextro-Ventro Conal Crest (DVCC) and Sinistra-Dorsal Conal Crest (SDCC) and cause the direction of conal septum to become left-posterior to right-anterior oblique direction (alike as the direction of interventricular septum in L-looping ventricle). In addition, we also discuss the condition of side-by-side conal cavities, i.e. the situation of vertical conal septum.

The direction extended from conal septum to truncal septum may be a clockwise rotation, may be counterclockwise too, and may continue the same direction to extend to aorta-pulmonary septum. The course of such spiral rotation may stop, and cause conal septum, truncal septum or aorta-pulmonary septum to be all in the same direction (such as {S.D.D}-cTGA). But the location of the pulmonary trunk is posterior to the aortic trunk in the level of aortic sac, so aortic trunk and pulmonary trunk in conal level will be decided by the whirling direction of septums (conal and truncal septums), instead of deciding from its connected ventricle.

11.1 Direction of right-posterior to left-anterior conal septum

In Fig. 4.1 we list all possible relationships of two great arteries based on the direction of right-posterior to left-anterior conal septum. In accordance with the direction of truncal septum, we divide this group into three subgroups: no change in direction, counterclockwise rotation, and clockwise rotation in direction respectively. Each truncal subgroup can still be divided into two to three groups according to the direction of aorto-pulmonary septum: no change in direction, counterclockwise rotation, and clockwise rotation in direction, too.

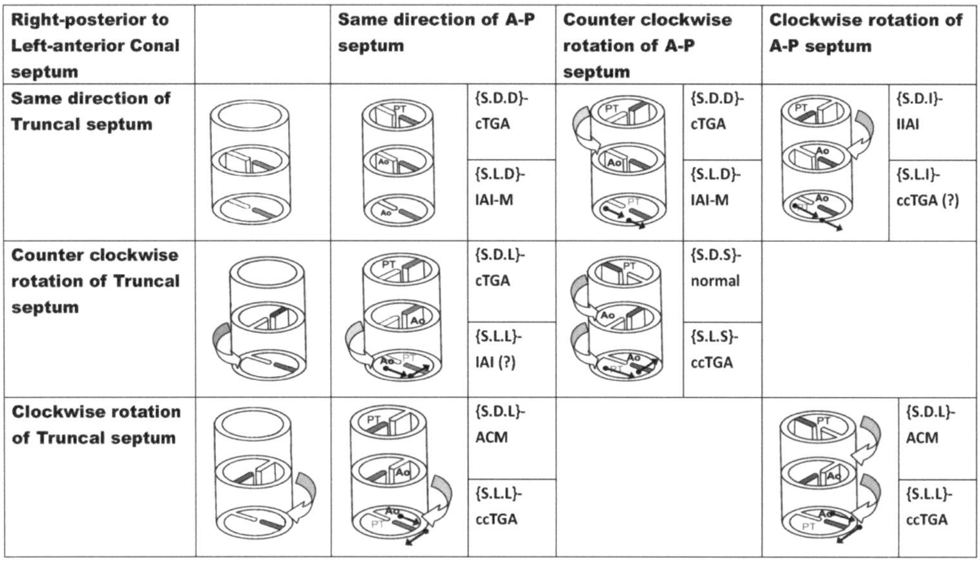

Fig. 4.1. All possibilities of different directions of conal -truncal – aortopulmonary Septum in the group of right-posterior to left-anterior conal septum. Three subgroups of same direction of truncal septum, counter clockwise rotation and clockwise rotation of truncal septums are listed. Two to three subtypes are included in each subgroup according to the direction of aortopulmonary septum. The anatomies and hemodynamic status are different between D-looping and L-looping ventricle in the same subtype. Arrow head presents the direction of spiral rotation from the lower truncus to the upper truncus. ACM: anatomically corrected malposition; cTGA: complete Transposition of Great Artery; ccTGA: congenital corrected TGA; IAI-M: isolated atrial inversion with malposition; IIAI: isolated infundibulo-arterial inversion.

Actually the hemodynamics are not really decided by the directions of the three septums, the atrio-visceral status and ventricular looping status play the most important parts. For example, if a heart possess the same direction of right-posterior to left-anterior in conal, truncal, and aorto-pulmonary septums, it can be the type of {S.D.D}-cTGA in D-looping status or the type of {S.L.D}-IAI-M (IAI with mal-position of great artery and we will discuss later) in L-looping status; but if we consider the more complex anomaly such as DORV, such a situation we have another section to discuss. This group can be classified into several subgroups such as {S.D.D}-cTGA, {S.D.I}-IIAI, {S.D.L}-cTGA, {S.D.S}-normal heart, and {S.D.L}-ACM in D-looping status; (S.L.D)-IAI-M, and {S.L.L}-ccTGA in L-looping status. Besides, there is the presence of two questionable arrangements as {S.L.I}-ccTGA, {S.L.L}-IAI, and we have marked them with question marks in Fig. 4.1. The hollow big arrow point means the direction of spiral rotation from lower (proximal) septum to upper (distal) septum, and the solid small arrow point means the direction of blood flow under the guide of conal septum and truncal septum. All types of perspective cardiac models we list in Figs .5.1~Fig.5.4, and the all cardiac models are discussed and set in situs solitus of atrial status ({S. --.--}).

11.2 Direction of left-posterior to right-anterior conal septum

Similarly we list all possibilities based on the direction of left-posterior to right-anterior conal septum in Fig. 4.2 and this group can be classified into several subgroups such as {S.D.L}-ACM, {S.D.S}-posterior TGA, {S.D.D}-cTGA, and {S.D.I}-posterior TGA in D-looping status; {S.L.L}-ccTGA, {S.L.S}-IVI, {S.L.D}-IAI-M, {S.L.D}-ccTGA, and {S.L.I}-IAI in L-looping status. There is a questionable arrangement in this group which is {S.D.D}-ACM.

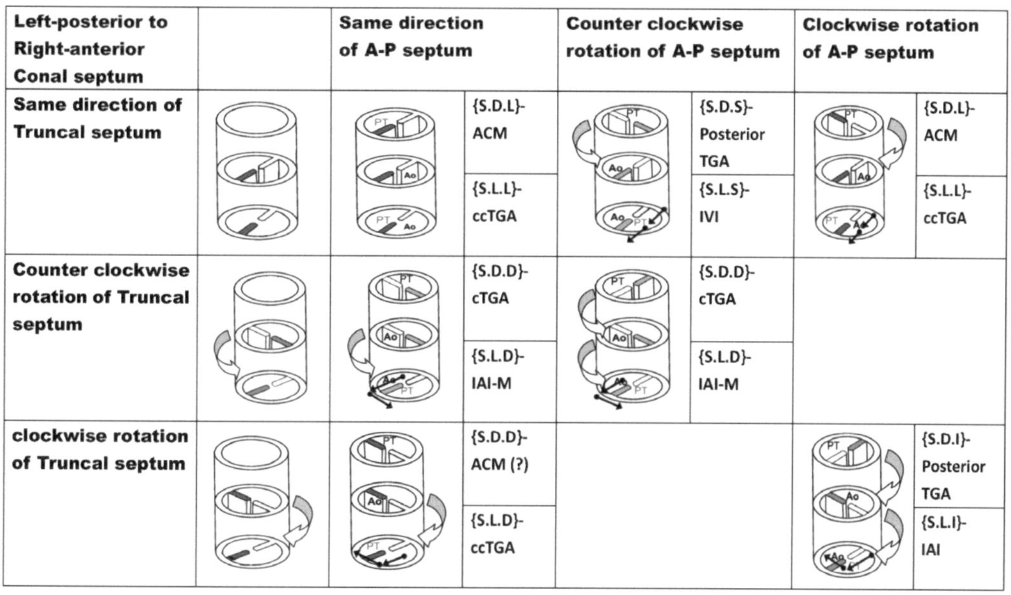

Fig. 4.2. Group of left-posterior to right-anterior conal septum. The detailed description is the same as in Fig. 4.1. ACM: anatomically corrected malposition; cTGA: complete transposition of great artery; ccTGA: congenital corrected TGA; IAI: isolated atrial inversion; IVI: isolated ventricular inversion.

11.3 Vertical truncal septum

In Fig. 4.3, we exclude the possibilities of vertical truncal septum because it is not addressed by Dr. Van Praagh. Two subgroups are listed with all types of {S.D.D}-cTGA and {S.D.L}-ACM in D-looping status; {S.L.D}-IAI-M and {S.L.L}-ccTGA in L-looping status. We also exclude the possibilities of horizontal conal septum because it more easily occurs in the conal truncal malformations such as DORV, so we discuss such condition in the section of DORV.

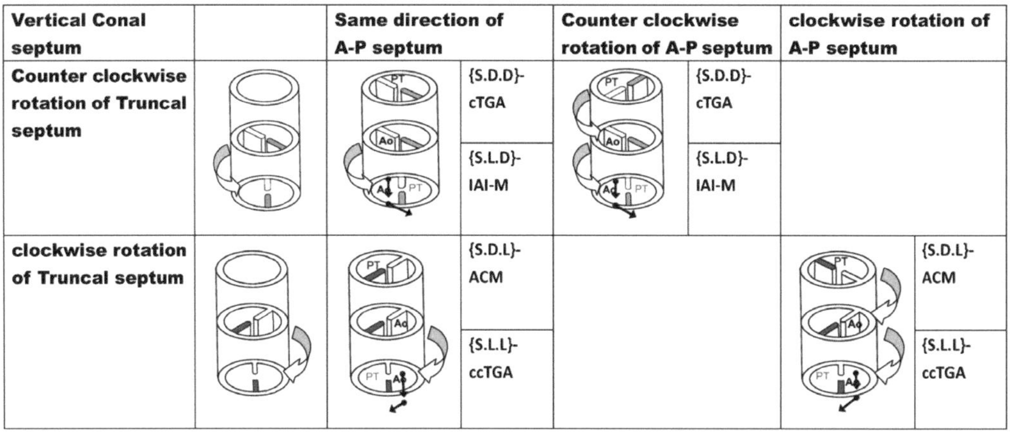

Fig. 4.3. Group of vertical conal septum. The detailed description is as in the Fig. 4.1. ACM: anatomically corrected malposition; cTGA: complete transposition of great artery; ccTGA: congenital corrected TGA; IAI-M: isolated atrial inversion with malposition.

12. Classification by ventricular looping

If we categorize the segmental mal-connections of the heart according to the ventricular looping status and the four relationships of truncal cavity, we can put several following groups in order.

In D-looping group there are the following possibilities:

1. [S.D.S]--- normal heart or posterior TGA
2. [S.D.L] --- cTGA or ACM (with six variants)
3. [S.D.D] --- cTGA (with six variants)
4. [S.D.I] --- Posterior TGA or IIAI

In L-looping group there also are the following possibilities:

1. [S.L.S] --- IVI
2. [S.L.I] --- IAI
3. [S.L.D] --- IAI-M (with six variants) or ccTGA
4. [S.L.L] --- ccTGA(with six variants)

The corresponding relationships of conal septum, truncal septum, and AP septum can refer to the Fig.4.1~Fig.4.3.

13. Atrio-Ventricular and Ventricular-Arterial relationship

According to the corresponding relations of their Atrial-Ventricular and Ventricular-Arterial connection again, we can divide segmental mal-connection of the heart into four groups as well. We also depict their unusual mechanisms and figure the perspective models in the following.

13.1 Atrio-Ventricular concordance with Ventricular-Arterial concordance

In the group of atrio-ventricular (A-V) concordance with ventricular-arterial (V-A) concordance (Fig.5.1), three subgroups of {S.D.S}-normal, {S.D.I}-IIAI, and {S.D.L}-ACM are included. In (S.D.S) the tricuspid valves and pulmonary valves are separated by the ventricular infundibular fold (VIF) and infundibulum septum (crista supraventricularis). The aorta is posterior and to the right of the main pulmonary artery at the level of the valves and it rotates 90 to 110 degrees in a counter clockwise direction which results in the aorta lying anteriorly to the pulmonary arteries at the level of the aorto-pulmonary trunk.

The {S.D.I} is characterized by the two great arteries normally related with inversion, with the result that there is no hemodynamic derangement in patients with IIAI. However, significant associated malformations often coexist including dextrocardia, criss-cross heart, large VSD, and conotruncal malformation of the inverted TOF. The aortic-mitral continuity excludes the other diagnostic possibility of an anatomically corrected malposition of the great arteries ({S.D.L}-ACM). ACM means that the great arteries are abnormally related to each other and to the ventricles, but they arise above anatomically corrected ventricles. The aorta arises anteriorly and to the left of the main pulmonary artery and the muscular subaortic conus separates the aortic and mitral valves, which may result in hypoplasia of the aorta. Both the aorta and subaortic conus are above the left ventricle. Twisting of the conus-truncus in one direction and of the ventricular loop in the opposite direction appears to be of central importance in the morphogenesis of ACM. The external morphology may be misdiagnosed as {S.L.L}-TGA, but from the epicardial course of coronary arteries and ventricular trabeculation, a differential diagnosis can be made between {S.L.L}-TGA and {S.D.L}-ACM. However, in a rare condition the {S.D.L}/{I.L.D} may present an anatomy other than ACM with the characteristics of TGA. That is to say, the {S.D.L}/{I.L.D} may have the anatomy of ACM or TGA. The conditions also happen in the type of {S.L.D} groups.

We will discuss why the two different hemodynamics can be present in {S.D.L} and {S.L.D}. In the six variants of {S.D.L}-ACM they can be divided into two groups based on the location of pulmonary trunk at the level of AP septum, one is right-posterior and the other is left-posterior respectively. Each group consists of three subtypes and they are different in the directions of conal septum which one is right-posterior to left-anterior conal septum, another is left-posterior to right-anterior conal septum, and the other is vertical conal septum. Although the conal septums are different in directions, the perspective cardiac models would be similar. In spite of the differences between their conal directions, they are consistent in the spiral rotation from conal septum to truncal septum and truncal septum to the AP septum (clockwise direction) respectively, and this is different from the {S.D.L}-cTGA which is in counterclockwise rotation from conal septum to truncal septum. Either left-posterior or right-posterior aspect of pulmonary trunk, the three subtypes of {S.D.L}-ACM we demonstrate with the similar cardiac model because we find the direction of truncal septum plays the role of guiding the blood flow by extension with the conal septum when the blood is pumped from ventricular outflow tract and conal cavity, and the site of conal cavity and the direction of conal septum will determine the constructions between the ventricle and the corresponding great artery such as mitral-aortic/ mitral-pulmonary/ tricuspid-aortic/ tricuspid-pulmonary fibrous continuity or discontinuity. The difference in the two subgroups of {S.D.L}-ACM is the further rotation between the truncal septum and the AP septum, and it leads the aortic conus and aortic trunk (level of AP septum) occupies on the opposite site which causes more degrees of spiral rotation on the external appearance of great arteries.

A-V concordance V-A concordance		Rt-posterior to Lt-anterior conus	Lt-posterior to Rt-anteror conus	Vertical conus
{S.D.S}-Normal	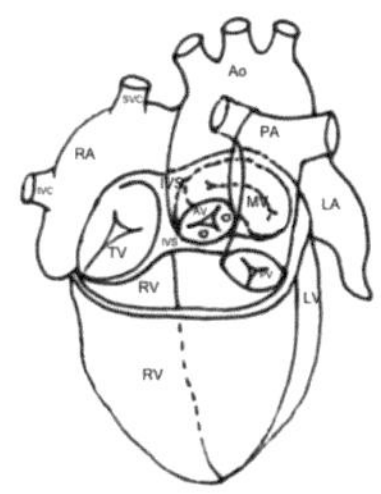	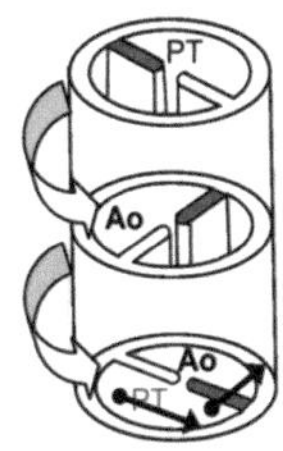		
{S.D.I}-IIAI	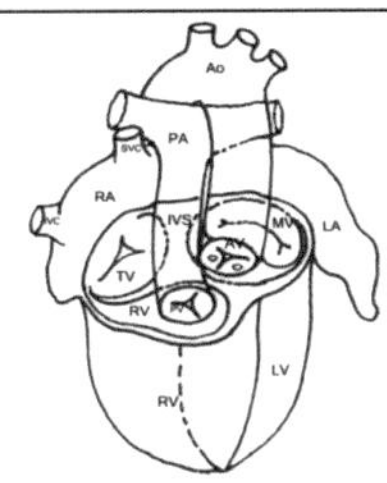	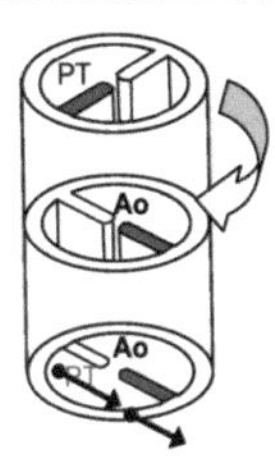		
{S.D.L}-ACM **Pulmonary trunk over right-posterior**	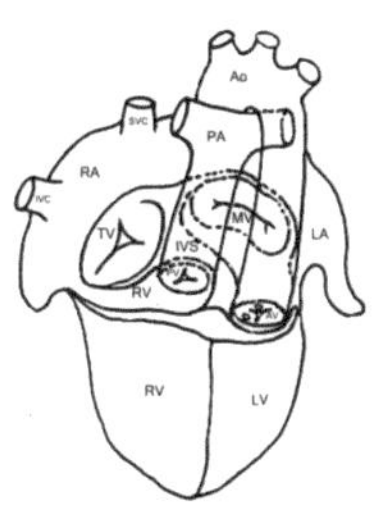	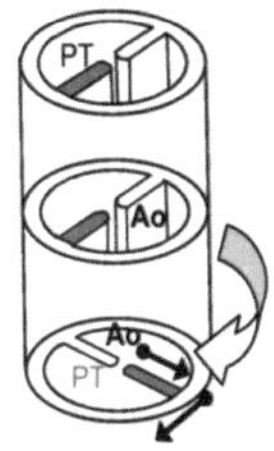	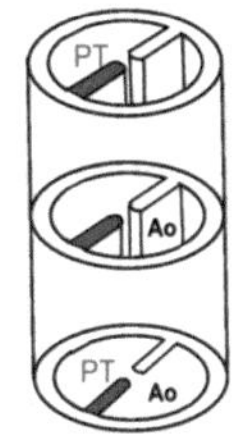	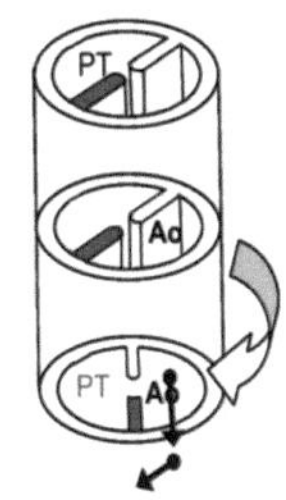
Pulmonary trunk over left-posterior	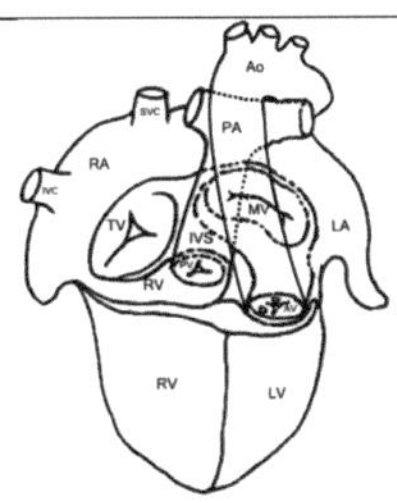	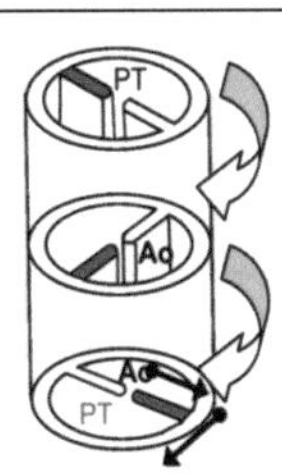	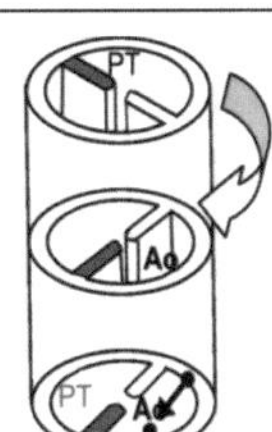	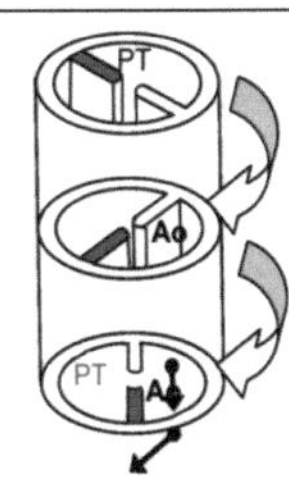

Fig. 5.1. The perspective cardiac models and corresponding truncus with the hemodynamic of atrio-ventricular concordance and ventricular-arterial concordance. Three subgroups, {S.D.S}-normal, {S.D.I}-IIAI, and {S.D.L}-ACM, are included. In the six variants of {S.D.L}-ACM they can be divided into two groups based on the location of pulmonary trunk at the level of AP septum. Each group consists of three subtypes and they are different in the directions of conal septum. Although the conal septums are different in directions, the perspective cardiac models would be similar. ACM: anatomically corrected malposition; IIAI: isolated infundibulo-arterial inversion.

13.2 A-V discordance with V-A concordance

In the group of A-V discordance with V-A concordance (Fig.5.2), three subgroups of {S.L.S}-IVI, {S.L.I}-IAI, and {S.L.D}-IAI-M are included. In {S.L.S}-IVI this rare cardiac malformation is characterized by atrio-ventricular discordance, ventricular-arterial concordance, and normally related great arteries in a spiral fashion, but the ventricles are inverted in relation to the normal heart. The conal crest develops abnormally with an abnormal direction of conal and inter-ventricular septum from right to left and anterior to posterior. The main pulmonary artery originates from the left-sided morphological right ventricle with a sub-pulmonary conus. The systemic venous return drains into a right-sided morphological left ventricle and also pumps the blood directly into the aorta in the same way as with {S.L.I}-IAI. The patient will suffer from cyanosis and could be treated with an atrial switch operation. The difference between {S.L.I}-IAI and {S.L.S}-IVI is the relationship of the great arteries and the orientation of the truncal septum (spiral rotation between conal-truncal level in {S.L.I}-IAI and the rotational direction between truncal -AP septum level).

The mirror image of {S.L.I} is {I.D.S} and it enables us to more clearly understand the hemodynamics of {S.L.I}/{I.D.S} present the characteristics of isolated atrial inversion. In this subgroup of {S.L.D} there also exist six variants with three of right-posterior aspect of pulmonary trunk and the other three of left-posterior aspect of pulmonary trunk. The hemodynamics in these six variants possess the same characteristics of systemic venous flow returns to right-sided left ventricle with pumping into aorta; the pulmonary venous flow returns to left-sided right ventricle with pumping into pulmonary artery. The aorta is located on right anterior to pulmonary artery which looks like anatomically corrected mal-position (ACM) or transposition of great artery (TGA) but is not, because their hemodynamics are not the ACM's A-V and V-A concordance nor the TGA's A-V concordance with V-A discordance, so they should be coded as the name of "isolated atrial concordance (IAC)" or the "IAI with mal-position of great artery (IAI-M)" instead of the ACM malformation. We favor the term of {S.L.D}/{I.D.L}-IAI-M. The differences between the {S.L.D}-ccTGA and {S.L.D}-IAI-M are the opposite spiral rotation of truncal septum (the direction of truncal extension), and the ventricle of subaortic conus connected (mitral-aortic discontinuity in {S.L.D}-IAI-M and tricuspid-aortic discontinuity in {S.L.D}-ccTGA). Without the intracardiac evaluation, the two external morphologies look alike especially the one of {S.L.D}-IAI-M with pulmonary trunk over left-posterior. Just the same as in {S.D.L}-ACM, the further rotation of truncal septum to AP septum cause the aortic conus and aortic trunk to be located on the opposite side. We also use the same perspective cardiac model to stand for each of the three variants in the two subgroups of {S.L.D}-IAI-M because they are just different in the directions of conal septum. Patients in this group will suffer from cyanosis due to the A-V discordance and V-A concordance, so the atrial switch operation is the option of treatment. Of course, the associated cardiac anomalies should be evaluated before intervention.

13.3 A-V concordance and V-A discordance

In the third group of A-V concordance and V-A discordance (Fig. 5.3), four subgroups of {S.D.S}-posterior TGA, {S.D.I}-posterior TGA, {S.D.L}-cTGA, and {S.D.D}-cTGA are included.

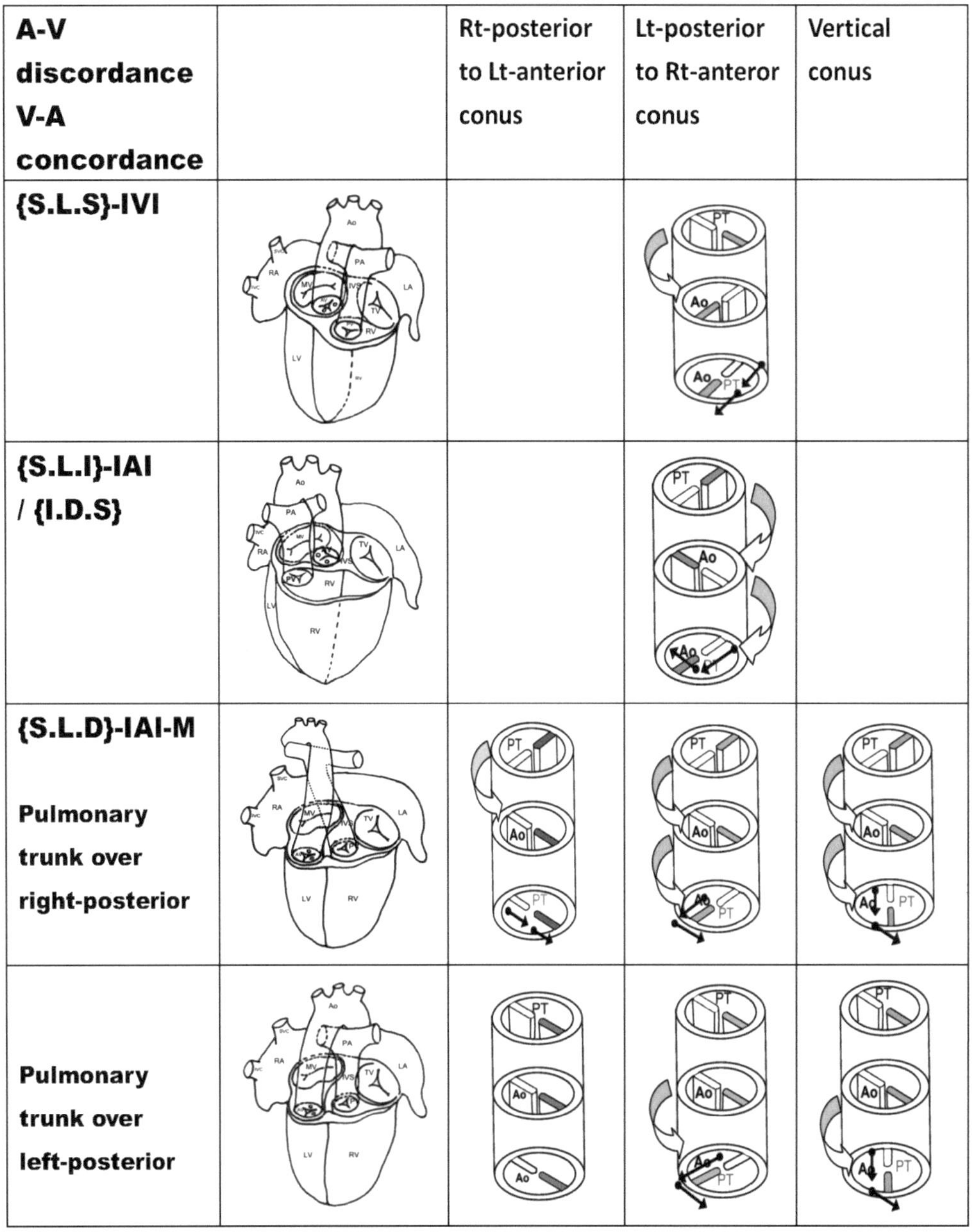

Fig. 5.2. The perspective cardiac models and corresponding truncus with the hemodynamic of atrio-ventricular discordance and ventricular-arterial concordance. Three subgroups, {S.L.S}-IVI, {S.L.I}-IAI, and {S.L.D}-IAI-M, are included. In the six variants of {S.L.D}-IAI-M they can be divided into two groups based on the location of pulmonary trunk at the level of AP septum. Each group consists of three subtypes and they are different in the directions of conal septum. Although the conal septums are different in directions, the perspective cardiac models would be similar. IAI-M: isolated atrial inversion with malposition. IVI: isolated ventricular inversion.

The patients will suffer from cyanosis but they should be treated with arterial switch operation. In {S.D.S}-posterior TGA the conal septum is reversed as compared with the {S.D.S}-normal heart and the other difference is the lack of the spiral rotation between the conal-truncal septum In {S.D.S}-posterior TGA. The external morphologies are similar regardless of atrial-ventricular appearance and the relationship between the great artery, nonetheless we can differentiate from the mitral-aortic fibrous continuity and tricuspid-pulmonary discontinuity in {S.D.S}-normal heart, but in {S.D.S}-posterior TGA the aortic valve is located right-posterior-inferior to the pulmonary valve and aortic-mitral fibrous continuity may persist through a high VSD or some present with aortic-tricuspid fibrous continuity because of the deficiency of the subaortic muscular conus. The greater part of the aortic orifice is above the right ventricle and the pulmonary artery arises to the left of the conal septum and is completely above the left ventricle. The two great vessels are in a spiral relationship rather than straight and parallel as in (S.D.D)-TGA or (S.L.L)-TGA. The flow of circulation is atrio-ventricular concordant and ventricular-arterial discordant in the same manner as in TGA. In {S.D.I}-posterior TGA, the aortic conus is located on the right-posterior aspect but the spiral rotation of the truncal septum results in the pulmonary trunk being more anterior and rightward, so the pulmonary valve is right-anterior to the aortic valve with the further extension of pulmonary trunk. The ventricular-arterial connections are mitral-pulmonary fibrous discontinuity and tricuspid-aortic fibrous continuity.

The type of {S.D.L}-cTGA possesses the same directions of truncal septum and AP septum and sometimes the conal septum as the type of {S.D.L}-ACM but the hemodynamic is really different just because the direction of spiral rotation is quite contrary. The two types are almost the same in the external morphology, besides, the subaortic conus is also present in the two types. So the major differences are the direction of the conal-truncal extension and the connections between ventricles and great arteries, which are the tricuspid-aortic discontinuity with subaortic conus in {S.D.L}-cTGA and mitral-aortic discontinuity with subaortic conus in {S.D.L}-ACM.

The fourth subgroup of {S.D.D}-cTGA can be classified into two groups by the location of pulmonary trunk as well. In each subgroup, the directions of conal septum in three variants may be different but the truncal septums have the same direction and the aortic trunk is right-anterior to the pulmonary trunk; the further rotation in level of truncal-AP septum makes the aorta rotate to the opposite side. The direction of the inter-ventricular septum is the same as that of the normal heart, running from right-posterior to left-anterior. Such a segmental arrangement causes the aorta to be located right-anteriorly (D-malposition) to the main pulmonary artery and to originate from the morphological right ventricle. Fibrous continuity exists between the mitral valve and the pulmonary valve, and the subaortic conus arises between the tricuspid and aortic valves.

In summary, besides the understanding of the hemodynamics traced by the models, the surgeons can delineate the course of the epicardial coronary arteries in spite of the possible variants of coronary anomalies and plan the surgery without difficulty, because patients in this group will suffer from cyanosis and the treatment is the arterial switch operation, of which the epicardial coronary arteries re-implantation is the most important and difficult procedure.

A-V concordance V-A discordance		Rt-posterior to Lt-anterior conus	Lt-posterior to Rt-anteror conus	Vertical conus
{S.D.S}-posterior TGA	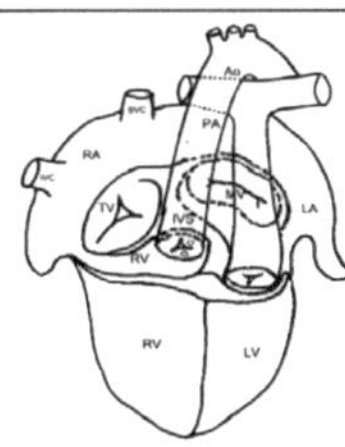		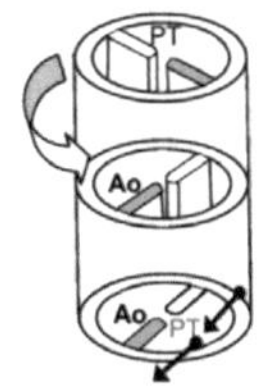	
{S.D.I}-posterior TGA	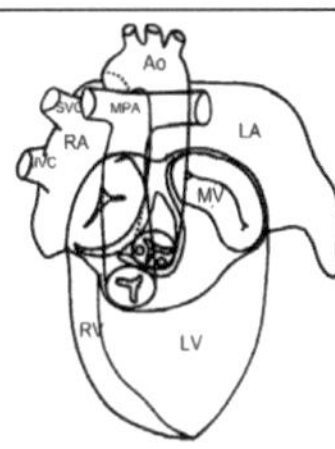		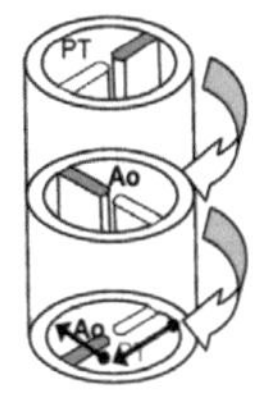	
{S.D.L}-cTGA	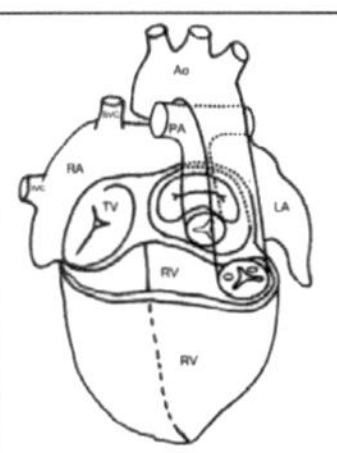	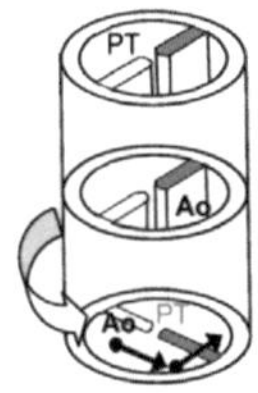		
{S.D.D}-cTGA **Pulmonary trunk over right-posterior**	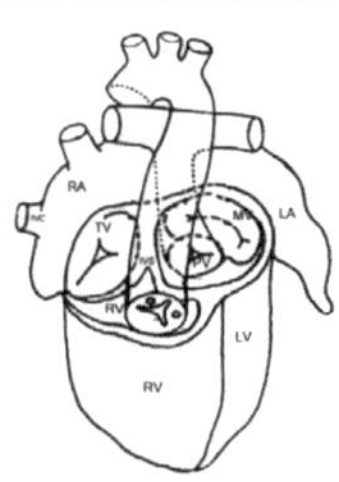	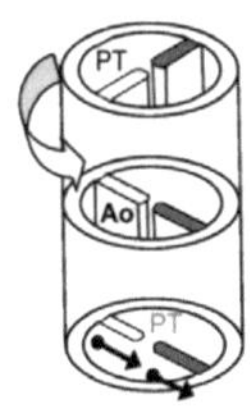	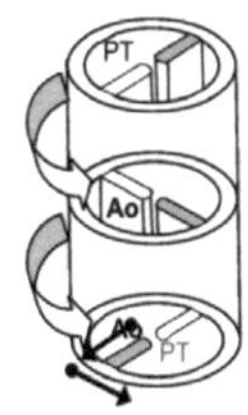	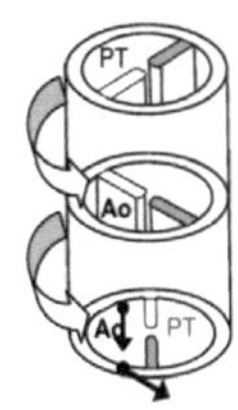
Pulmonary trunk over left-posterior	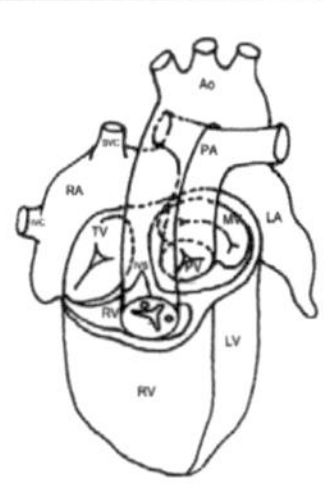	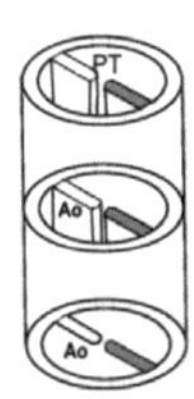	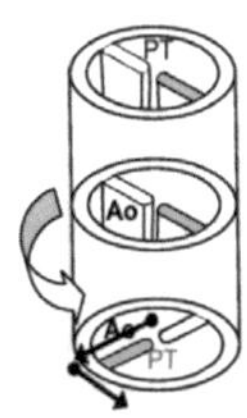	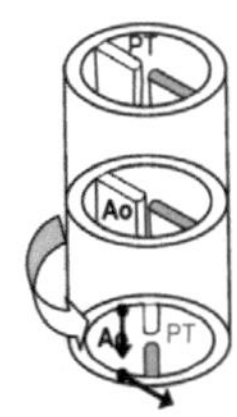

Fig. 5.3. The perspective cardiac models and corresponding truncus with the hemodynamic of atrio-ventricular concordance and ventricular-arterial discordance. Four subgroups, {S.D.S}-posterior TGA, {S.D.I}- posterior TGA, {S.D.L}-cTGA, and {S.D.D}-cTGA are

included. In the six variants of {S.D.D}-cTGA they can be divided into two groups based on the location of pulmonary trunk at the level of AP septum. Each group consists of three subtypes and they are different in the directions of conal septum. Although the conal septums are different in directions, the perspective cardiac models would be similar. cTGA: complete transposition of great artery.

13.4 A-V discordance and V-A discordance

Three subgroups are included in this category, one is {S.L.D}-ccTGA, another is {S.L.L}-ccTGA, and the other is {S.L.S}-ccTGA (Fig.5.4). In {S.L.D}-ccTGA the way of conal septum is the same as the inter-ventricular septum (L-looping). The truncal rotation is clockwise and makes the left-anterior aortic conus moving rightward and more anteriorly. The mitral valve is connected to the pulmonary valve with fibrous continuity and the aortic valve is disconnected from the tricuspid valve with the subaortic conus. If the spiral rotation extends to the level of AP septum, the type of {S.L.D}-ccTGA may shift to the {S.L.I}-IAI.

In (S.L.L)-ccTGA the inter-ventricular septum is directed from left-posterior to right-anterior as a mirror image of the normal heart. The main pulmonary artery is right-posterior to the aorta without a spiral relationship and it originates from right-sided morphological left ventricle with mitral-pulmonary fibrous continuity. Subaortic conus exists and causes discontinuity of the tricuspid-aortic valves. Some patients may have mal-alignment of the conal septum toward the right-sided left ventricle and this may cause subpulmonary stenosis which causes the effect of physiological pulmonary artery banding, so we can explain why some patients of (S.L.L)-ccTGA can tolerate such a cardiac anomaly over the longer term.

According to the location of pulmonary trunk, two subgroups are divided and three variants are included in each subgroup, and we still use the same perspective cardiac model to present the three variants. The trunk septums in the six variants are the same in the direction of left-posterior to right-anterior. The spiral rotation also proceeds in common with the clockwise direction but the further extension of rotation at the level of truncal-AP septum makes the left-lower aortic conus extending to right-upper aorta and the external relationship of great arteries shifts from the parallel shape to the crossing form. In {S.L.S}-ccTGA the truncal septum extends more left and anteriorly, which causes the left ventricle connects with the pulmonary artery with the conus formation and right ventricle connects with aorta in tricuspid-aortic fibrous continuity. The aorta locates posteriorly to the pulmonary artery, which is the same as posterior TGA but the hemodynamic is as congenitally corrected TGA, so we list the {S.L.S} in this group. The hemodynamic in this group is double discordance, so the picture of cyanosis is not the main symptom unless another cardiac anomaly exists such as pulmonary stenosis or TAPVR, unfortunately, cardiac anomalies usually occur. The patients require receiving operative correction because future miseries of right ventricular failure and pulmonary hypertension will happen. The definitive operation for the type of A-V discordance and V-A discordance is double switch operation (atrial switch and arterial switch), and any single switch procedure will make the patient more worse in cyanosis.

The Congenital Heart Surgery Nomenclature and Database Project published in the Annals of Thoracic Surgery in April 2000 classified six main anatomic types of TGA including

{S.D.D/A/L}, {S.L.L/D}, {I.L.L/D}, {I.D.D}, {A.D.D}, and {A.L.L}. Actually the {S.D.D} and {I.L.L}, {S.D.L} and {I.L.D}, {S.L.L},and {I.D.D} could be considered as mirror images of each other.

A-V discordance V-A discordance		**Rt-posterior to Lt-anterior conus**	**Lt-posterior to Rt-anteror conus**	**Vertical conus**
{S.L.D}-ccTGA	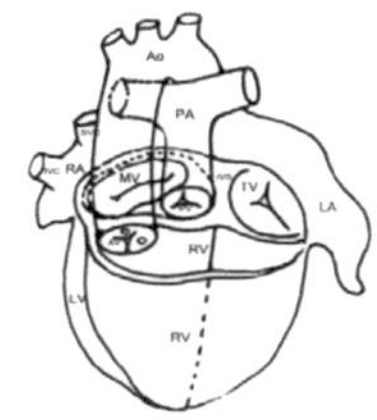		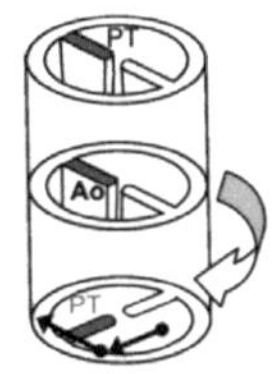	
{S.L.S}-ccTGA	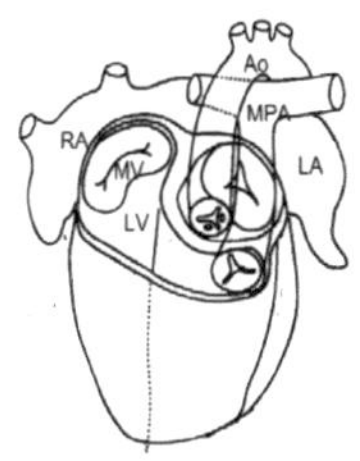	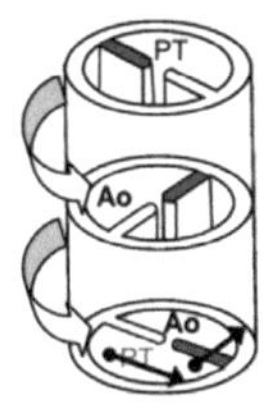		
{S.L.L}-ccTGA **Pulmonary trunk over right-posterior**	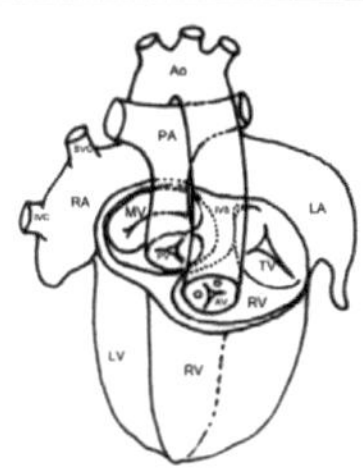	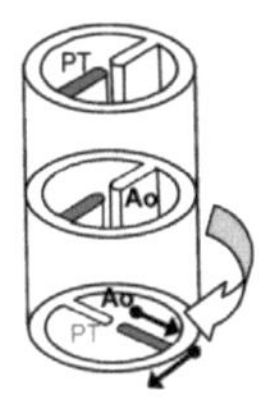	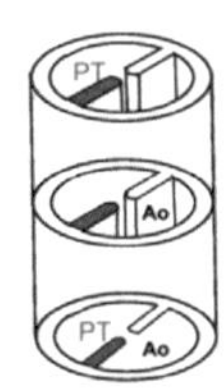	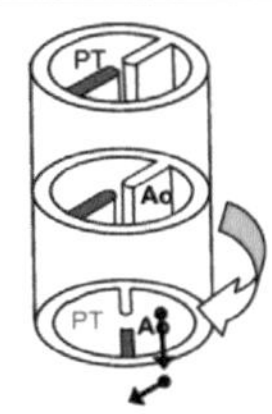
Pulmonary trunk over left-posterior	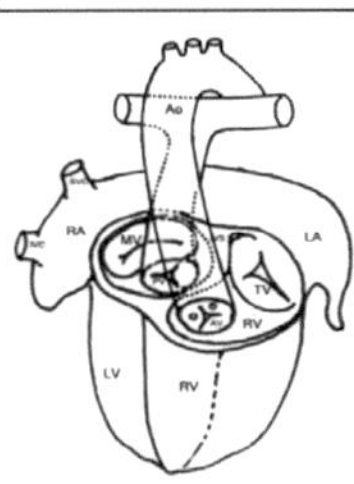	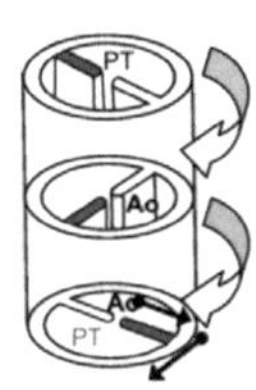	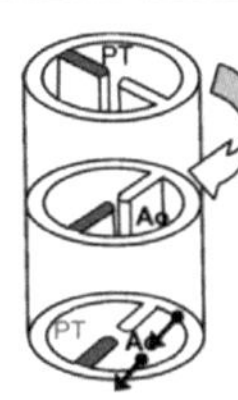	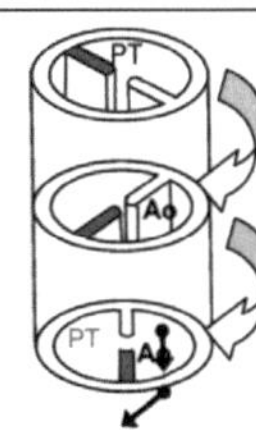

Fig. 5.4. The perspective cardiac models and corresponding truncus with the hemodynamic of atrio-ventricular discordance and ventricular-arterial discordance. Three subgroups, {S.L.D}-ccTGA, {S.L.S}- ccTGA, and {S.L.L}-ccTGA, are included. In the six variants of {S.L.L}-ccTGA they can be divided into two groups based on the location of pulmonary trunk at the level of AP septum. Each group consists of three subtypes and they are different in the directions of conal septum. Although the conal septums are different in directions, the perspective cardiac models would be similar. ccTGA: congenital corrected TGA.

All the types we discuss above are restricted to the atrial-visceral status in the situs solitus (morphologic right atrium, i.e. systemic venous atrium locates on the right-handed side; morphologic left atrium is on the left-handed side), the situs inversus can be considered as the mirror image of the corresponding type such as the {S.D.D} and {I.L.L} are mirror images, etc. According to the principles of such model, three kinds of situations would have conflicts with existing concepts, so we are not sure the three questionable types exist or not. One is {S.L.I} with right-posterior to left-anterior direction of conal and truncal septums and clockwise rotation of AP septum which is coded as ccTGA (Fig.4.1), another is {S.L.L} with right-posterior to left-anterior direction of conal septum and counter clockwise rotation of truncal septum with the same direction of AP septum which is coded as IAI-M (Fig.4.1), and the other is {S.D.D} with left-posterior to right-anterior conal septum and clockwise rotation of truncal septum with the same direction of AP septum which is coded as {S.D.D}-ACM (Fig.4.2). Further study is necessary to confirm the three models and their hemodynamic status.

14. Double outlet right ventricle

The meaning of DORV is the two great arteries completely or almost completely originating from the right ventricle, actually an infundibular malformation. During the development of embryo in DORV, its infundibular septum (outlet septum) was not going to participate in the formation of outlet portion of IVS, with instead positioning on morphologic RV and forming this anomaly. DORV includes a spectrum of cono-truncal malformation, may present from Tetralogy of Fallot to TGA, but there are still many assumptions that are proposed in the embryo evolution also. The assumptions include these below:

1. Failure of conal insertion.
2. Failure of absorption of bulbo-ventricular flange (BVF) or VIF.
3. Failure of absorption of posterior conus.
4. Mal-alignment between the conal septum and interventricular septum.
5. Failure of incorporation of anterior conus.
6. Anomalous development of conal-truncal and aorta-pulmonary septum.

But still no theory can explain all abnormal possibilities completely. Because of the variety of the complexities and associated anomalies, each case should also focus on the spatial relationship of great artery, inter-infundibular relationship, the location of VSD, and the stenosis of outflow tract; others such as visceral-atrial status, ventricular looping status, the cono-truncal relationship and the septation of aorta-pulmonary septum, etc. should be evaluated carefully. Fortunately, most DORV is situs solitus in visceral-atrial status, and atrial-ventricular concordance with D-looping ventricle ({S.D.X}) or atrial-ventricular discordance with L-looping ventricle ({S.L.X}), so the degrees of difficulties are decreased while we make diagnoses.

the development of IVS is incomplete, which causes the non-differentiation of membranous, inlet and trabecular portions, thus the infundibular septum (outlet septum) will separate the two ventricular outflow tracts. We use the hypothesis of Dr. Lilliam Valdes-Cruz to explain the mechanisms of DORV.

14.1 Classification of DORV

In Fig.6 we demonstrate the normal cardiac development in the level of atrio-ventricular-arterial junction (i.e. endocardial cushion). In Fig.6.A, we can notice the truncus migrates from right to left, and the DDCC and SVCC present in the conal cavity, which divides the conus into two coni, one antero-lateral and one postero-medial. Eventually the postero-medial conus will incorporate into the left ventricle and become the left ventricular outflow tract (LVOT). Before incorporation, the medial conus communicates with the left ventricle via the primitive interventricular foramen (blank asterisk). The DDCC and SVCC merge gradually with each other to be the conal septum, which moves leftward and downward close to the primitive IVS due to the absorption of the mid-portion of bulboventricular flange (BVF). This draws the aorta over the primitive left ventricle and finally completely locates above the left ventricle and becomes the aorta. In an approximately 32-day-old embryo, the bulboventricular flange (bulboventricular fold synonymous of cono-ventricular flange or bulbo-atrio-ventricular ledge) moves toward the superior endocardial cushion. Near the end of the fifth week, the posterior extremity of the flange terminates almost midway along the base of the superior endocardial cushion and is much less prominent than before (Fig.6.B,C). Finally the flange between the medial conus and the atrioventricular valve will disappear and result in the mitral-aortic fibrous continuity. Some authors consider that the persistence of BVF with the failure incorporation of medial conus into left ventricle are the mechanisms of DORV, and the good development of bulboventricular flange may be due to ineffective conal absorption.

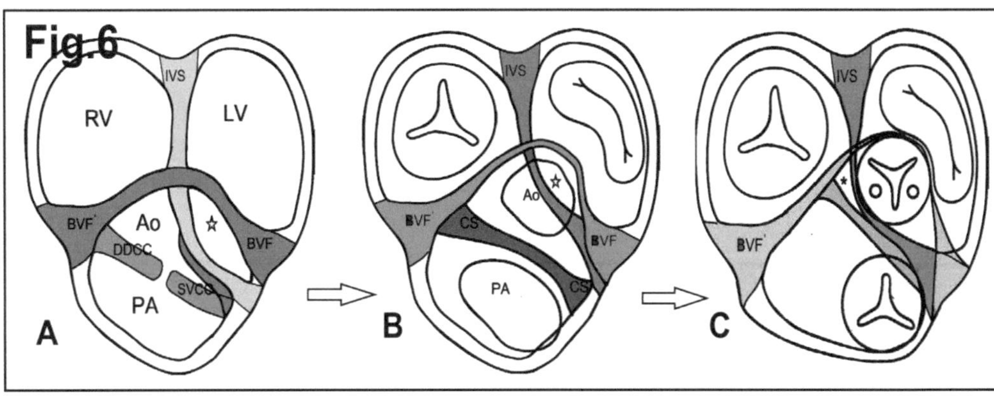

Fig. 6. Processes of Migration, septation, and absorption in atrio-ventricle-arterial junction. The conus cavity is divided into two coni by DDCC and SVCC, and the truncus and ventricles are separated by BVF in the level of endocardial cushion. Conal septum moves leftward and downward to close to the primitive IVS due to absorption of the mid-portion of BVF. This draws the aorta over the primitive left ventricle and finally completely locates above the left ventricle and becomes the aorta. BVF: bulboventricular flange; CS: conal septum; DDCC: dextro-dorsal conal crest; SVCC: sinistra-ventral conal crest. The blank asterisk indicates the primitive interventricular foramen, and the black one indicates the secondary interventricular foramen (VSD).

14.2 Modes of variant DORV

Based on this model, we can determine the spatial relationships of infundibular cavities (the conal cavities) according to the insertion and direction of its outlet septum:

1. Outlet septum insertion to anterior limb of SMT.
2. Insertion to the fusion point of posterior limb of SMT with VIF.
3. Insertion at region between posterior and anterior limbs of SMT.
4. Insertion to VIF itself.

And the relationship of its infundibular cavity, because of the difference of its septal direction, there are the following aspects:

1. Right-posterior to left-anterior outlet septum (antero-lateral with postero-medial infundibulum).
2. Horizontal outlet septum (strict anterior and posterior infundibulum).
3. Left-posterior to right-anterior outlet septum (antero-medial with postero-lateral infundibulum).
4. Vertical outlet septum (side-by-side relationship).

In each relationship of infundibulum, there are several variants could be listed. The two main subgroups are classified by the directions of truncal septum: one is right-posterior to left-anterior truncal septum and the other is left-posterior to right-anterior truncal septum as per the previous classification. There can be two different directions (clockwise and counterclockwise) of spiral rotation in the truncal septum and in the AP septum, so many variants can be found, and we list all in Fig. 7. In accordance with the insertion of outlet septum, we classify the anomalies of DORV into four groups as in the previous description.

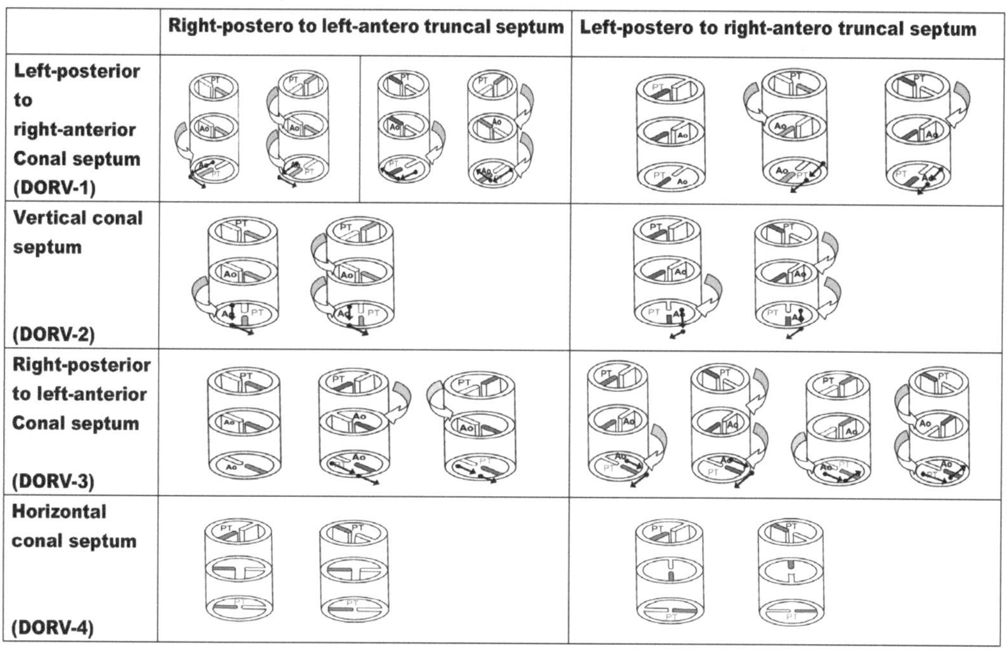

Fig. 7. All possibilities of arrangements of conal-truncal-AP septums in double outlet right ventricle. Four groups are categorized by different directions of conal septums. DORV-1: left-posterior to right-anterior conal septum; DORV-2: vertical conal septum; DORV-3: right-posterior to left-anterior conal septum; DORV-4: horizontal conal septum. Two subgroups are divided by the direction of truncal septum which are right-posterior to left-anterior truncal septum and left-posterior to right-anterior truncal septum.

14.2.1 Outlet septum insertion to anterior limb of SMT

The first one is outlet septum insertion to anterior limb of SMT (Fig.8.1). The direction of conal septum will greatly determine the degrees of outflow tract stenosis such as the conal septum extending from left-posterior to right-anterior would cause the compromise of lateral conal cavity and a larger connection between VSD and the medial conal cavity; but if the conal septum is in the direction of right-posterior to left-anterior, the compromised one would be the posteromedial conus. Although the direction of conal septum is important, the key points of hemodynamic decision are the size and the location of VSD (primitive interventricular foramen) and the VSD-related conal cavity. If the VSD is larger enough or is closer to the orifice of outflow tract, the corresponding great artery would develop more normally; if the VSD related artery is pulmonary artery rather than the aorta, the degrees of cyanosis and the operative procedures would be more complicated. In this group the VSD-related great artery is the one which locates on the posteromedial conal cavity. Three subgroups are divided by the conal direction, and several variants are included in each group which are DORV-3, DORV-4, and DORV-1 individually. The subgroups of DORV-1, 2, 3, and 4 are listed in Fig. 7.

Generally speaking, if the VSD appears as a muscular defect, we can think this is a DORV with noncommitted VSD; if the infundibular septum is hypoplastic or absent, we can think it is like a DORV with doubly committed VSD. Besides, the other associated anomalies, the size of VSD, and the degrees of ventricular hypoplasia are all required to be known before surgical intervention, not only because the decision of the two ventricular or single ventricular repairs is very important for the surgical outcomes, but because accurate decisions are dependent on detailed structural evaluation. Indeed, most of the DORV are repaired as single ventricle because of valvular dysfunction, ventricular hypoplasia, and great artery anomalies. Furthermore, the type of horizontal conal septum is included in DORV compares with the CHD of non-DORV with lack of the horizontal one.

14.2.2 Insertion to the fusion point of posterior limb of SMT

The second group (Fig. 8.2) is the type of conal septal insertion to the posterior limb of SMT. Three subgroups, the left-posterior to right-anterior direction of conal septum, the vertical conal septum, and the right-posterior to left-anterior conal septum, are included. The corresponding subgroups with variants of different truncal and AP septum are DORV-1, DORV-2, and DORV-3 respectively. In this group, the VSD-related great artery is the medial conal cavity, and the direction of conal septum can influence the stenotic degree of outflow tract. In the left-posterior to right-anterior direction and the vertical direction of conal septum, the lateral conal cavity will be compromised by the conal septum; on the contrary, the right-posterior to left-anterior conal direction will compromise the medial conal cavity. Actually the development and hypoplasia of great arteries are not entirely decided by the conal septum, the size and location of VSD, the degrees of valvular dysfunction, and the balance between two ventricles, etc. - all are decisive factors.

14.2.3 Insertion at region between posterior and anterior limbs of SMT

The third group (Fig. 8.3) has the type of conal septum insertion in the SMT (between SMT). Three subgroups can be noticed based on the direction of conal septum, too. One is right-posterior to left-anterior conal direction and its possible Truncal-AP septum variants are listed in DORV-3; another one is horizontal conal septum with the possible variants listed in DORV-4; and the other is left-posterior to right-anterior conal septum with the possible variants in DORV-1. The VSD may be more remote in this type because of the space occupied by the conal septum resulting in the non-committed type VSD, but if there is absence or hypoplasia of the conal septum, the VSD may present as the doubly committed type. In the first one, the postero-medial conus may be more restricted, but in the third one, the antero-lateral conus is more restricted.

14.2.4 Insertion to VIF itself

The fourth group (Fig. 8.4) is the type of conal septum insertion to VIF itself; there are three subgroups based on the direction of conal septum, too. First one is left-posterior to right-anterior conal direction and its possible Truncal-AP septum variants are listed in DORV-1; the second one is vertical conal septum with the possible variants listed in DORV-2; and the third one is right-posterior to left-anterior conal septum with the possible variants in DORV-3. The VSD related great artery is the one which locates on the medial conal cavity, and the restricted one is the lateral conal cavity.

No matter what the type is, the clinical importance of DORV is determined on the size and location of VSD, the position of VSD-related great artery, the balance between ventricles, the competence of valves, and other associated anomalies, etc..

In the clinical aspects, the most possibly confused cardiac anomalies with DORV are the Fallot type DORV, TOF, and TGA ({S.D.D}). They may look alike in external appearance but the internal structures possess some differences. Before talking about the Fallot type DORV, we need to know the basic concept of TOF:

15. Tetralogy of Fallot and related topics

According to Dr. Van Praagh's theory, the Tetralogy of Fallot results from a mal-development of the subpulmonary conus whereby the aortic valve comes to lie more anteriorly, superiorly and leftwards relative to the pulmonary valve than is normal. That is to say, the conal septum is shifted more anteriorly, superiorly and leftwards, causing right ventricular outflow tract (RVOT) obstruction, hypoplasia of the pulmonary artery and right ventricular hypertrophy. It is difficult to depict the anterior, superior, and leftward deviation of the conus without a three-dimensional representation. Using this figure, drawn in perspective, we can understand the impact of conus deviation on the development of the pulmonary artery and right ventricle, and see why an anterior malalignment of the VSD will cause RVOT obstruction, pulmonary hypoplasia and how the posterior malalignment of VSD will cause left ventricular outflow tract obstruction and hypoplasia of the left cardiac structures. With this depiction, the condition of TOF and the surgical methods can also be clearly represented to patients' families. In TOF, the aorta is located more anteriorly in position because of hypoplasia of pulmonary artery and anterior overriding of aorta (Fig.9.A). Such an appearance also can be seen in the type of {S.D.D}-TGA with pulmonary stenosis (Fig.9.B) or in the type of {S.D.D}-DORV with subpulmonary VSD (Fig.9.C).

	Conal septum insertion to anterior limb	
Right-posterior to Left-anterior Conal septum	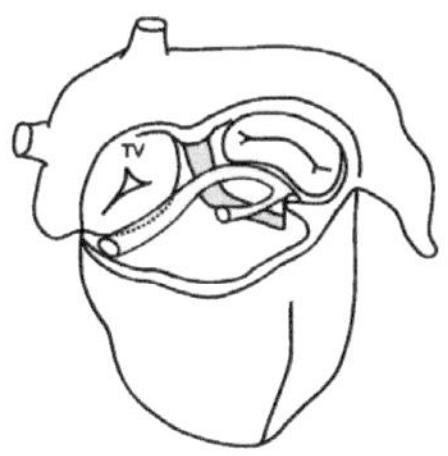	Variant types of Right-posterior to Left-anterior oblique direction of conal septum (Fig.7-DORV-3)
Horizontal conal septum	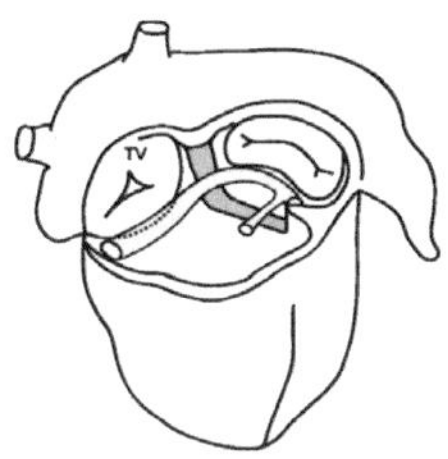	Variant types of horizontal conal septum (Fig.7-DORV-4)
Left-posterior to Right-anterior Conal septum	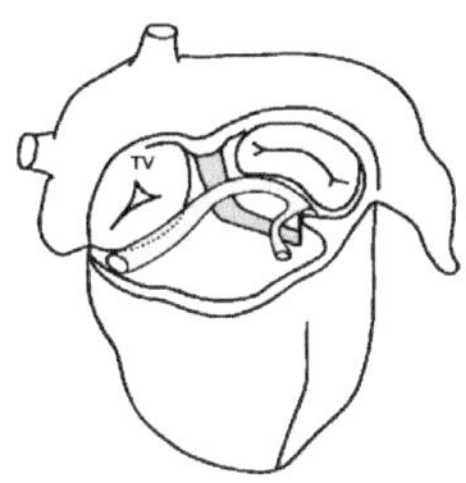	Variant types of Left-posterior to Right-anterior oblique direction of conal septum (Fig.7-DORV-1)
Model: **VSD is related with posteromedian conal cavity**	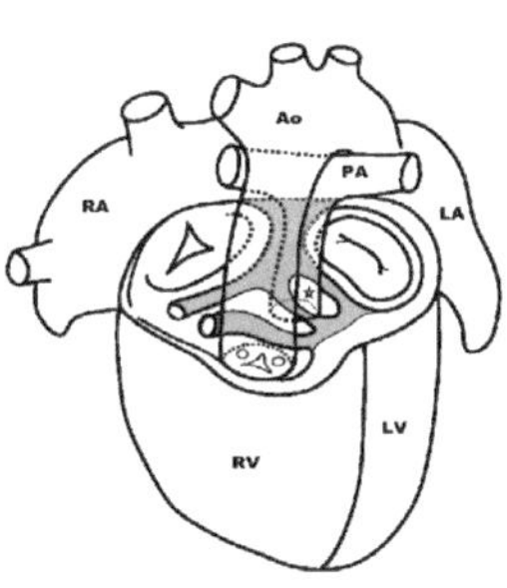 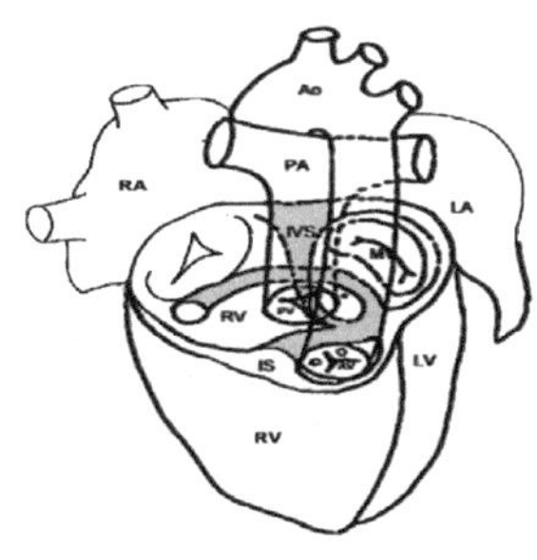	

Fig. 8.1. The group of DORV with conal septum inserts to anterior limb of SMT. Three subgroups are listed including the right-posterior to left-anterior conal septum, horizontal conal septum, and left-posterior to right-anterior conal septum. The corresponding variants of arrangements of conal-truncal-AP septum are Fig.7-DORV-3, Fig.7-DORV-4, and Fig.7-DORV-1 respectively. In the group the VSD is related with posteromedian conal cavity, such as {S.D.D}-DORV is a type of subpulmonary VSD.

	Conal septum insertion to posterior limb	
Left-posterior to Right-anterior Conal septum	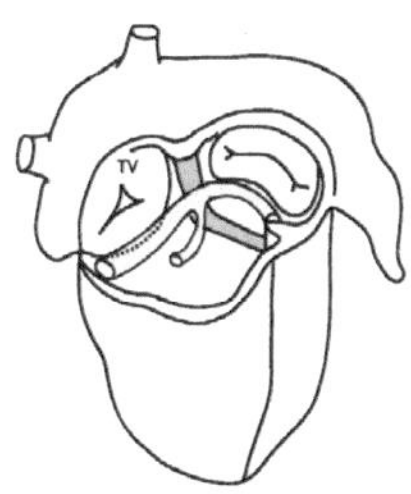	Variant types of Left-posterior to Right-anterior oblique direction of conal septum (Fig.7-DORV-1)
Vertical direction Conal septum	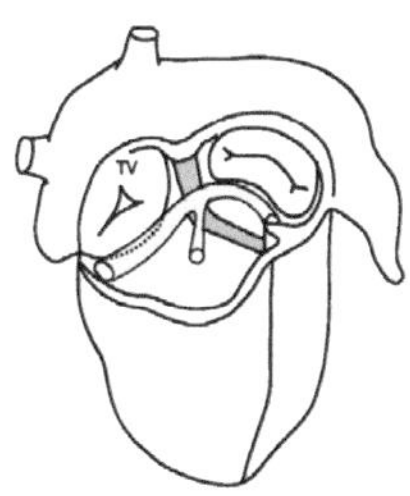	Variant types of vertical direction of conal septum (Fig.7-DORV-2)
Right-posterior to Left-anterior Conal septum	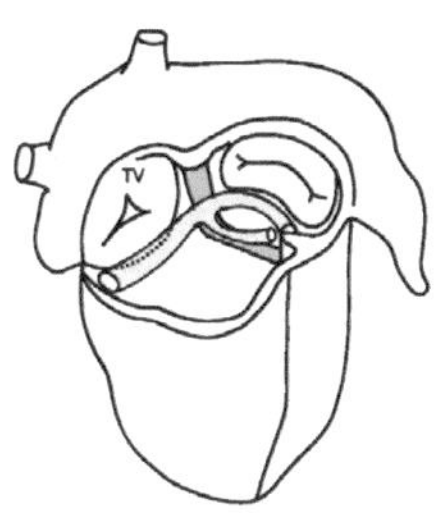	Variant types of Right-posterior to Left-anterior oblique direction of conal septum (Fig.7-DORV-3)
Models: **VSD is related with median conal cavity**	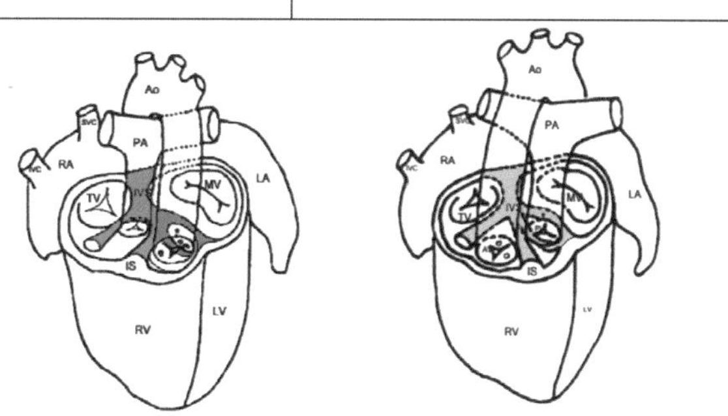	

Fig. 8.2. The group of DORV with conal septum inserts to posterior limb of SMT. Three subgroups are listed including the left-posterior to right-anterior conal septum, vertical conal septum, and right-posterior to left-anterior conal septum. The corresponding variants of arrangements of conal-truncal-AP septum are Fig.7-DORV-1, Fig.7-DORV-2, and Fig.7-DORV 3 respectively. In the group the VSD is related with median conal cavity, such as {S.D.D}-DORV is a type of subpulmonary VSD.

	Conal septum insertion between SMT	
Right-posterior to Left-anterior Conal septum	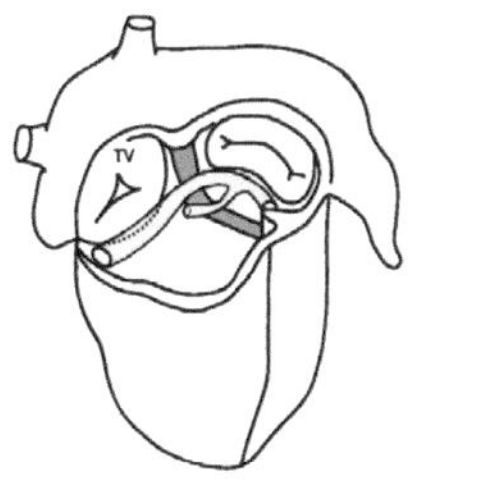	Variant types of Right-posterior to Left-anterior oblique direction of conal septum (Fig.7-DORV-3)
Horizontal conal septum	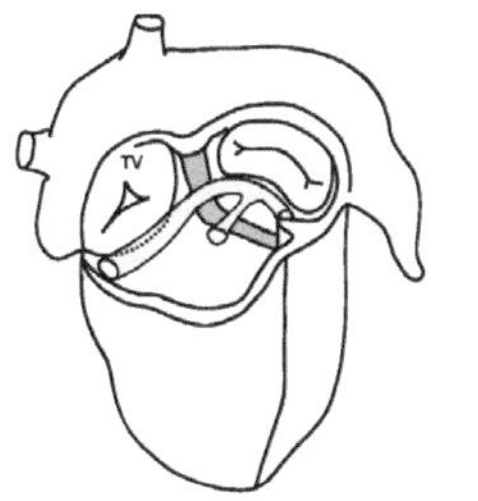	Variant types of horizontal conal septum (Fig.7-DORV-4)
Left-posterior to Right-anterior Conal septum	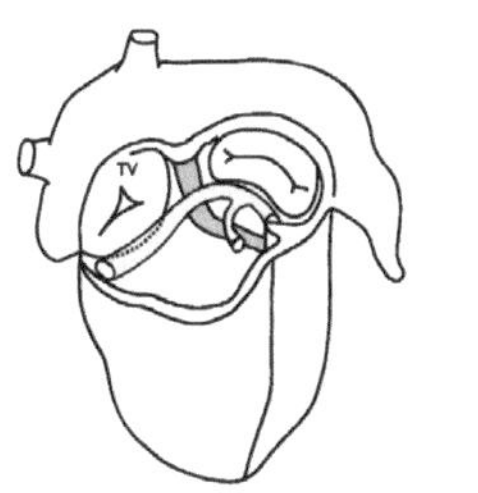	Variant types of Left-posterior to Right-anterior oblique direction of conal septum (Fig.7-DORV-1)
Model: Non-committed or Doubly committed VSD	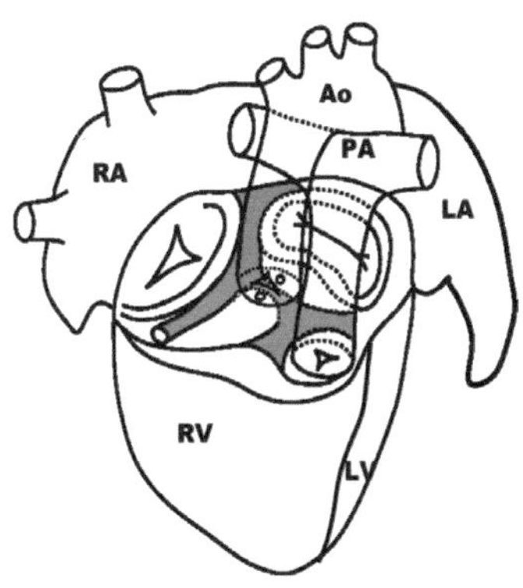	

Fig. 8.3. The group of DORV with conal septum inserts between SMT. Three subgroups are listed including the right-posterior to left-anterior conal septum, horizontal conal septum, and left-posterior to right-anterior conal septum. The corresponding variants of arrangements of conal-truncal-AP septum are Fig.7-DORV-3, Fig.7-DORV-4, and Fig.7-DORV-1 respectively. The VSD may be more remote in this type because of the space occupied by the conal septum and results in the non-committed type VSD, but if absence or hypoplasia of the conal septum, the VSD may present as the doubly committed type.

	Conal septum insertion to VIF itself	
Left-posterior to Right-anterior Conal septum	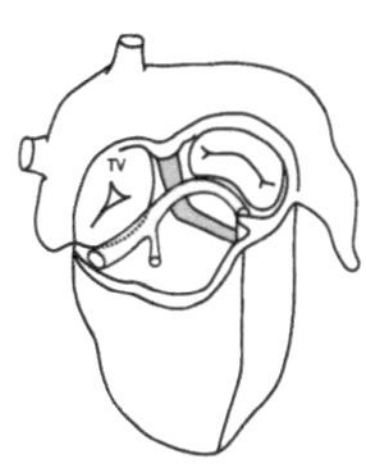	Variant types of Left-posterior To Right-anterior oblique direction of conal septum (Fig.7-DORV-1)
Vertical direction Conal septum	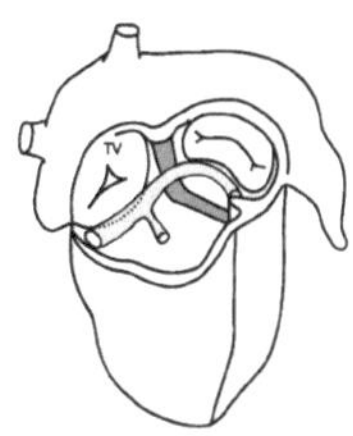	Variant types of vertical direction of conal septum (Fig.7-DORV-2)
Right-posterior to Left-anterior Conal septum	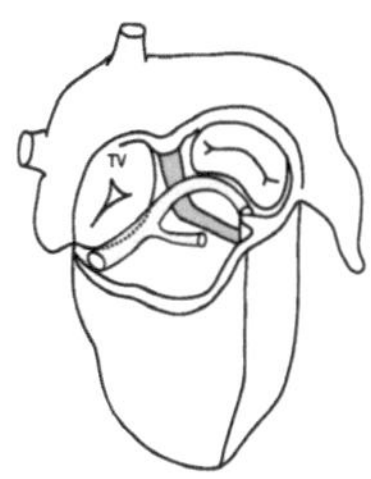	Variant types of Right-posterior To Left-anterior oblique direction of conal septum (Fig.7-DORV-3)
Models: **VSD is related with median conal cavity**	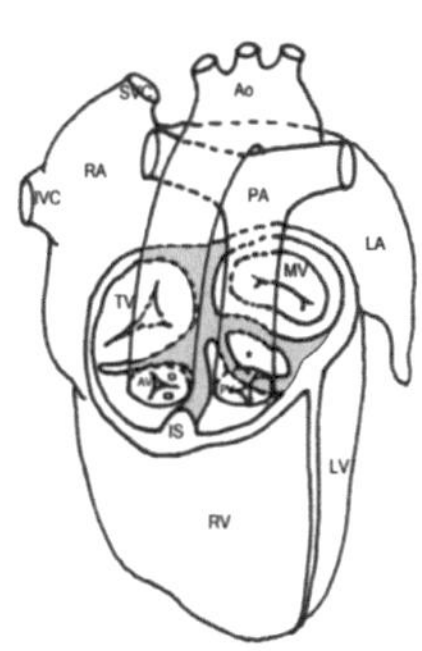 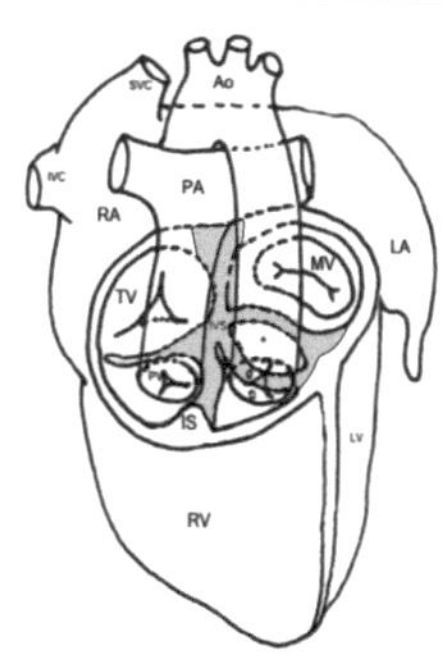	

Fig. 8.4. The group of DORV with conal septum inserts to VIF itself. Three subgroups are listed including the leftt-posterior to right-anterior conal septum, vertical conal septum, and right-posterior to left-anterior conal septum. The corresponding variants of arrangements of conal-truncal-AP septum are Fig.7-DORV-1, Fig.7-DORV-2, and Fig.7-DORV-3, respectively. The VSD is related with median conal cavity,too.

15.1 Fallot type v.s. TGA type DORV

Because external appearances cannot offer us a definitive diagnosis, echocardiographic evaluations become the gold standard of diagnosis. Establishing difference between the TOF and DORV has been disputed for a long time. The general concept is the 50 % rule of the aortic overriding over right ventricle in spite of the mitral-aortic continuity or discontinuity, that is to say the subaortic conus is not essential for the diagnosis of DORV. It means in TOF that the aorta overrides less than 50% above right ventricle, and in DORV the aorta overrides more than 50% above right ventricle. The Fallot type DORV (Fig. 9.D) means the two great arteries both originate from right ventricle with an anterior-positioned and hypoplastic pulmonary artery, and the TGA type DORV means the two great arteries both originate from right ventricle, too, but with an posterior-positioned pulmonary artery with a subpulmonary VSD ({S.D.D}-DORV).

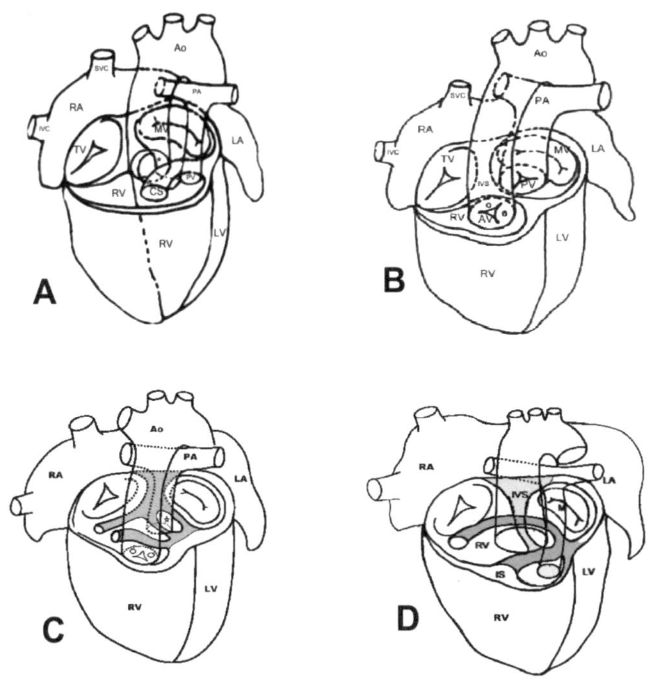

Fig. 9. Collections of DORV variants including the Fallot type DORV (Fig.9.D), the TGA type DORV (Fig.9.C) and the distinct similar models, TOF (Fig.9.A) and {S.D.D}-TGA (Fig.9.B).

15.2 TOF with AVSD

In the Finally, we wish to discuss the issue of TOF with AVSD because this type of CHD is more complicated and is poorly understood in morphology and surgical anatomy. In Fig. 10, we draw the pictures of preoperative (Fig. 10-A), postoperative (Fig. 10-B) models, and the bizarre patch we surgeons use to repair the VSD and to reroute the overriding aorta into left ventricle. The patch looks like a teardrop with a semicircle in one part and a tapering oval in another part. In the past, we didn't have the perspective model of AVSD with TOF, and this really was a concern for a long time as to understand why the patch would be such a shape.

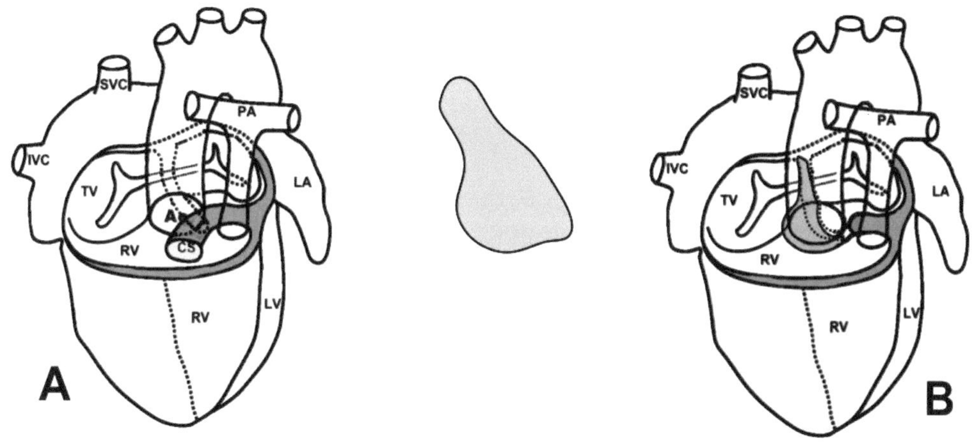

Fig. 10. Fallot type AVSD is delineated by the cardiac model to demonstrate how to repair the VSD and reroute the overriding aorta into left ventricle with the bizarre patch. The narrow part of patch is to repair the VSD and the wider part is for the subaortic rerouting. The patch repair follows conal septal resection. CS: conal septum.

16. Revised and summary of A-V & V-A segmental connections

The table has been modified in comparing with the one on earlier paper. We recode the type of {S.L.D}-ACM as {S.L.D}-IAI-M, we also add extra two types of {S.D.S}-posterior TGA and {S.D.I}-posterior TGA in the group of Atrio-Ventricular concordance with Ventricular-Arterial discordance, and {S.L.S}-ccTGA in the group of Atrio-Ventricular discordance with Ventricular-Arterial discordance.

	Ventricular-Arterial Concordance	Ventricular-Arterial Discordance
Atrio-Ventricular Concordance	{S.D.S} / {I.L.I} {S.D.L}-ACM / {I.L.D} {S.D.I}-IIAI / {I.L.S}	{S.D.D}-cTGA/{I.L.L} {S.D.L}-cTGA/{I.L.D} {S.D.S}-posterior TGA {S.D.I}-posterior TGA
Atrio-Ventricular Discordance	{S.L.S}-IVI / *{I.D.I}* {S.L.I}-IAI / {I.D.S} {S.L.D}-IAI-M/ {I.D.L}	{S.L.L}-ccTGA/{I.D.D} {S.L.D}-ccTGA/{I.D.L} {S.L.S}-ccTGA

Table 1. The summary of atrio-ventricular concordance/discordance and ventricular-arterial concordance/discordance. The table has been modified in comparing with the one published on earlier paper. ACM: anatomically corrected malposition; cTGA: complete transposition of great artery; ccTGA: congenital corrected TGA; IAI: isolated atrial inversion; IAI-M: isolated atrial inversion with arterial malposition; IVI: isolated ventricular inversion.

17. References

Anderson RH, Wilkinson JL, Arnold R, Becker AE. Morphogenesis of bulboventricular malformations II. Observations on malformed hearts. Brit Heart J 1974; 36: 948–970.

Anderson RH, Becker AE, Van Mierop LHS. What should we call the Crista? Br Heart J 1977; 39:856-859.

Anderson RH, Becker AE, Wilcox BR, Macartney FJ, Wilkinson JL. Surgical anatomy of double-outlet right ventricle- a reappraisal. Am J Cardiol 1983; 52:555-559.

Angelini P, Leachman RD. The spectrum of double-outlet right ventricle: an embryologic interpretation. Cardiovasc Dis 1976; 3:127-149.

Arista-Salado Martinez O, Arango Casado J, De la Cruz MV, Diaz F, Cubero O. Double outlet right ventricle-an echocardiographic stydy. Cardiol Young 1993; 3: 124-131.

Arteaga M, De la Cruz MV, Sanchez C, Diaz GF. Double outlet right ventricle: experimental morphogenesis in the chick embryo heart. Pediatr Cardiol 1982; 3:219-227.

Clarkson PM, Brandt PWT, Barratt-Boyes BG, et al. Isolated atrial inversion. *Am J Cardiol* 1972;29:877–81.

De la Cruz MV, Arteaga M, Espino-Vela J, Quen-Jiménez M. Complete transposition of the great arteries: types and morphogenesis of ventriculo-arterial discordance. Am Heart J 1981; 271–281.

De la Cruz MV, Cayre R, Arista-Salado Martinez O, Sadowinski S. The infundibular interrelationships and the ventriculoarterial connection in double outlet right ventricle, Clinical and surgical implications. Int J Cardiol 1992; 35: 153-164.

Foran RB, Becourt C, Nanton MA, et al. Isolated infundibulo-arterial inversion {S,D,I}: a newly recognized form of congenital heart disease. *Am Heart J* 1988;116:1337–50.

Goor DA, Dische R, Lillehei CW. The conotruncus. Its normal inversion and conus absorption. Circulation 1972; 46: 375–385.

Goor DA, Edward JE. The spectrum of transposition of the great arteries with specific reference to developmental anatomy of the conus. Circulation 1973; 48:406-415.

Howell CE, Ho SY, Anderson RH, Elliott MJ. Fibrous skeleton and ventricular outflow tracts in double-outlet right ventricle. Ann Thorac Surg 1991; 51:394-400.

Huai-Min Chen , Chau-Chi Chiu , Jin-Ren Wu, Ying-Fu Chen*. A Simple Model for Variant Congenital Cardiac Anomalies. Thoracic CardioVasc Surgeon 2007, 55:433-7.

Huai-Min Chen, Po-Chih Chang, Meng-Shin Lee, Jin-Ren Wu, Chaw-Chi Chiu*. Easy Category for Complex Congenital Cardiac Segmental Connections. Kaohsiung J Med Sci, 2007,23(1):30-3.

Lev M, Bharati S, Meng CCL, Liberthson RR, Paul MH, Idriss F. A concept of double-outlet right ventricle. J Thorac Cardiovasc Surg 1972; 64:271-281.

Lincoln C, Anderson RH, Shinebourne EA, English TAH, Wilkinson JL. Double outlet right ventricle with l-malposition of the aorta. Br Heart J 1975; 37:453-463.

Pasquini L, Sander SP, Parness I, et al. Echocardiographic and anatomic findings in atrio-ventricular discordance with ventricular-arterial concordance. *Am J Cardiol* 1988;62:1256–61.

Piccoli G, Pacifico AD, Kirklin JW, Blackstone EH, Kirklin JK. Changing results and concepts in the surgical treatment of double-outlet right ventricle: analysis of 137 operations in 126 patients. Am J Cardiol 1983; 52:549-554.

Quero-Jiménez M, Raposo-Sonnenfeld I. Isolated ventricular inversion with situs solitus. Br Heart J 1975; 37: 293–304.

Rosenquist GC, Sweeney LJ. Anomalous semilunar valve relationships in transposition of the great arteries. Ped Cardiol 1982; 2:195–202.

Snider AR, Enderlein MA, Feitel DF, et al. Isolated ventricular inversion: two-dimensional echocardiographic findings and a review of the literature. *Pediatr Cardiol* 1984;5:27–33.

Sridaromont S, Feldt RH, Ritter DG, Davis GD, Edwards JE. Double outlet right ventricle: hemodynamic and anatomic correlations. Am J Cardiol 1976; 38:85-94.

Stellin G, Zuberbuhler JR, Anderson RH, Siewers RD. The surgical anatomy of the Taussig-Bing malformation. J Thorac Cardiovasc Surg 1987; 93:560-569.

Tynan MJ, Becker AE, Macartney FJ, Anderson RH. Nomenclature and classification of congenital heart disease. Br Heart J 1979; 41:544-553.

Van Praagh R, Van Praagh S. Isolated ventricular inversion. A consideration of the morphogensis, definition and diagnosis of nontransposed and transposed great arteries. Am J Cardiology 1966; 17: 395–406.

Van Praagh R, Perez-Trevino C, Lopez-Cuellar M, Baker FW. Transposition of the great arteries with posterior aorta, anterior pulmonary artery, subpulmonary conus and fibrous continuity between aortic and atrioventricular valves. Am J of Cardiology 1971; 28: 621–631.

Van Praagh R. The segmental approach to diagnosis in congenital heart disease. Birth Defects (Original Article Series) 1972; 4–22.

Van Praagh R. The segmental approach to diagnosis in congenital heart disease. *Birth Defects: Original Article Series* 1972;Vol III, 5:4–22.

Van Praagh R, Durnin RE, Jockin H, et al. Anatomically corrected malposition of great arteries {S,D,L}. *Circulation* 1975;51:20–31.

Van Praagh R, Durnin RE, Jockin H, Wagner HR. Anatomically corrected malposition of the great arteries (S,D,L). Circulation 1975; 51: 20–31.

Van Praagh R. Transposition of the great arteries: history, pathologic anatomy, embryology, etiology, and surgical consideration. Cardiac Surgery: State of the Art Reviews. 1991; 5: 7–83.

Wilcox BR, Ho SY, Macartney FJ, Becker AE, Gerlis LM, Anderson RH. Surgical anatomy of double-outlet right ventricle with situs solitus and atrioventricular concordance. J Thorac Cardiovasc Surg 1981; 82: 405-417.

Witham AC. Double outlet right ventricle: a partial transposition complex. Am Heart J 1957; 53: 929-939.

Print Books

Antoon F.M. Moorman. (2010). Embryology of the Heart, In: *Pediatric Cardiology,* Robert H. Anderson, Edward J. Baker, Daniel J. Penny, et al. pp. 37-56, Churchill Livingstone, 978-0-7020-3064-2, Philadelphia, New York.

Deepak Srivastava, Scott Baldwin. (2001). Molecular Determinants of Cardiac Development, In: Moss and Adams' Heart Disease in Infants, Children, and Adolescents, Hugh D. Allen, Howard P. Gutgesell, et al, pp. 3-23, Lippincott Williams & Wilkins, 0-683-30742-8, Philadelphia, PA.

Jonas RA. (2004). Tetralogy of Fallot with Pulmonary Stenosis, In: *Comprehensive Surgical Management of Congenital Heart Disease,* Richard A Jonas, James DiNardo, pp. 279-293, Arnold, 0-340-80807-1, London.

Jonas RA. (2004). Double noutlet right ventricle, In: *Comprehensive Surgical Management of Congenital Heart Disease,* Richard A Jonas, James DiNardo, pp. 413-428, Arnold, 0-340-80807-1, London.

Lee N. Benson. (2010). The Arterial Duct: Its Persistence and its Patency, In: *Pediatric Cardiology,* Robert H. Anderson, Edward J. Baker, Daniel J. Penny, et al. pp. 875-893, Churchill Livingstone, 978-0-7020-3064-2, Philadelphia, PA.

Lilliam M. Valdes-Cruz. (1999). Double-outlet ventricle, In: *Echocardiographic Diagnosis of Congenital Heart Disease,* Lilliam M. Valdes-Cruz, Paul O. Cayre, pp. 409-422, Lippincott-Raven, 0-7817-1433-8, Philadelphia, New York.

Lilliam M. Valdes-Cruz. (1999). Embryological Development of the Heart and Great Vessels, In: *Echocardiographic Diagnosis of Congenital Heart Disease,* Lilliam M. Valdes-Cruz, Paul O. Cayre, pp. 3-18, Lippincott-Raven, 0-7817-1433-8, Philadelphia, New York.

Van Praagh R, Geva T, Van Praagh S. (1990). Segmental situs in congenital heart disease: recent rare findings. In: Development Cardiology: Morphogenesis and Function. Clark EB, Takao A, Future Publishing Co, NY.

Van Praagh R. (1991). Transposition of the great arteries: history, pathologic anatomy, embryology, and surgical considerations, In: *Cardiac Surgery: State of the Art Reviews.* Pp. 7-82, Hanley & Belfus,Philadelphia.

Van Praagh R. (1998). Cardiac anatomy, In :*Pediatric Cardiac Intensive Care,* Anthony C. Chang, Frank L. Hanley, Gil Wernovsky, David L. Wessel, pp. 1-15, Williams& Wilkins, 0-683-01508-7, Baltimore, Maryland.